Psychopathology in Epilepsy: Social Dimensions

Psychopathology in Epilepsy

SOCIAL DIMENSIONS

Edited by
Steven Whitman
and
Bruce P. Hermann

New York Oxford
OXFORD UNIVERSITY PRESS
1986

Oxford University Press

Oxford New York Toronto
Delhi Bombay Calcutta Madras Karachi
Petaling Jaya Singapore Hong Kong Tokyo
Nairobi Dar es Salaam Cape Town
Melbourne Auckland

and associated companies in
Beirut Berlin Ibadan Nicosia

Published by Oxford University Press, Inc.,
200 Madison Avenue, New York, New York 10016

Library of Congress Cataloging-in-Publication Data
Main entry under title:
Psychopathology in epilepsy.
Includes bibliographies and index.
1. Epilepsy—Social aspects. 2. Epilepsy—Psychological aspects.
3. Epilepsy—Complications and sequelae.
4. Epileptics—Psychology.
I. Whitman, Steven. II. Hermann, Bruce P.
[DNLM: 1. Epilepsy—complications. 2. Epilepsy—psychology.
3. Mental Disorders—etiology. 4. Social Adjustment
5. Social Environment. WL 385 P9743]
RC372.P77 1986 616.8'5307 85-18806
ISBN 0-19-503656-5

Printing (last digit): 9 8 7 6 5 4 3 2 1

Printed in the United States of America
on acid-free paper

This book is dedicated to people with epilepsy.

Acknowledgments

We owe many debts to many people. Shelley Reinhardt, our editor, welcomed the idea for the book, helped us construct it, answered all of our questions, read and critiqued each chapter, and facilitated the entire process at every turn.

In the finest sense, this book was a collective effort by all the authors who not only wrote chapters but critiqued others, participated in long conversations with us, and showed an overwhelming willingness to respond to the comments made by readers of their chapters. As a result, chapters were improved, ideas were exchanged, and the book is better for all of this.

Barbara Stewart coordinated much of the administrative work. She typed and retyped many of the chapters, facilitated correspondence among all the authors, and kept things flowing. She was invaluable.

In addition to those of our colleagues who wrote for this book, an equal number did not write this time but have worked with us in the past and have taught us a great deal. Among them are Fred Annegers, Andrew C. Gordon, Alan Mirsky, Janice Stevens, and Quentin D. Young.

We would like to thank four other colleagues in slightly greater detail. John S. Garvin, Professor and Head of the Department of Neurology at the University of Illinois Health Sciences Center at Chicago, provided continued encouragement and support for our work. Especially invaluable has been his ability to facilitate an atmosphere in which the members of his department can pursue their scientific interests.

John R. Hughes has been a tireless source of information, encouragement, and constructive criticism. For the past eight years we have relied heavily on his expertise in both epilepsy and electroencephalography. He has helped us in innumerable ways and we value him in his roles as teacher, colleague, and friend.

Bindu T. Desai has been the neurologist for the Epilepsy in the Urban Environment Project since its inception. She has worked on many projects and coauthored many papers with us and has taught us a great deal of neurology. More important, she has always been available to answer our questions, share insights with us, and help us think critically.

John L. McKnight was one of the originators of the idea for the Epilepsy in the Urban Environment Project and has been its principal investigator. His goal has always been to maximize the good we do for people with epilepsy.

He has put an enormous amount of intellectual and spiritual energy into the project—and taken out nothing for himself. His selflessness and integrity create a model for researchers wishing to do "good work."

Finally, we are now, and have always been, surrounded by wonderful friends and loving family who support us through good times and bad times. We would be nothing without them all.

Contents

Contributors

PAUL ARNTSON, PHD
Department of Communication Studies
Northwestern University
Evanston, Illinois

CHRISTOPHER BAGLEY, PHD
Faculty of Social Welfare
University of Calgary
Calgary, Alberta

GABOR BARABAS, MD
Department of Pediatrics
University of Medicine and Dentistry of New Jersey
Rutgers Medical School
New Brunswick, New Jersey

NICKY BRITTEN, MSC
Medical Research Council National Survey of Health and Development
Department of Epidemiology and Community Medicine
University of Bristol
Bristol, England

ROBERT L. COHEN, MD
Montefiore Medical Center
Rikers Island Jail
Bronx, New York

PETER CONRAD, PHD
Department of Sociology
Brandeis University
Waltham, Massachusetts

JADE DELL, MRE
Center for Urban Affairs and Policy Research
Northwestern University
Evanston, Illinois

BRENDA MCEVOY DEVELLIS, PHD
Department of Health Education
University of North Carolina School of Public Health
Chapel Hill, North Carolina

ROBERT F. DEVELLIS, PHD
Rehabilitation Program
University of North Carolina School of Medicine
Chapel Hill, North Carolina

DAVID DROGE, PHD
Department of Communication and Theater Arts
University of Puget Sound
Tacoma, Washington

WERNER EVEN, MD
Abteilung für Neurologie
Freie Universität Berlin
West Berlin

PETER B. C. FENWICK, MRCPSYCH
The Maudsley Hospital
London, England

BRUCE P. HERMANN, PHD
Epilepsy Center
Baptist Memorial Hospital
and
Department of Psychiatry
University of Tennessee Center for the Health Sciences
Memphis, Tennessee

LAMBERT N. KING, MD, PHD
St. Vincent's Hospital and Medical Center
New York, New York

WENDY S. MATTHEWS, PHD
Multimodal Therapy Institute
Rocky Hill, New Jersey

Robert J. Mittan, PhD
Departments of Psychology and Neurology
Sepulveda Veterans Administration Medical Center
Los Angeles, California

Ellen Murray, PhD
Department of Speech Communication
University of New Mexico
Albuquerque, New Mexico

Robert Norton, PhD
Department of Communication
Purdue University
Lafayette, Indiana

Joseph W. Schneider, PhD
Department of Sociology
Drake University
Des Moines, Iowa

Rupprecht Thorbecke, MD
Abteilung für Neurologie
Freie Universität Berlin
West Berlin

Michael E. J. Wadsworth, PhD
Medical Research Council National Survey of Health and Development
Department of Epidemiology and Community Medicine
University of Bristol
Bristol, England

Patrick West, PhD
Medical Research Council
Medical Sociology Unit
Glasgow, Scotland

Steven Whitman, PhD
Center for Urban Affairs and Policy Research
Northwestern University
Evanston, Illinois

Peter Wolf, MD
Abteilung für Neurologie
Freie Universität Berlin
Berlin

Janusz Zielinski, MD, DSc
Epilepsy Center of Michigan and Wayne State University School of Medicine
Department of Neurology
Detroit, Michigan

Introduction

Epilepsy has been recognized and pondered since at least the time of Hippocrates—over 2,000 years ago. And always this malady has presented a twofold opportunity for those who wanted to contemplate it. On the one hand there was the nature of the malady itself. What caused a person to acquire epilepsy? What triggered seizures in a person who had epilepsy? How could the seizures be prevented from occurring? And much more. On the other hand, there has always been the belief that the study of epilepsy could facilitate an understanding of even more far-reaching matters like the relationship between the mind and the brain. Observers 2,000 years ago believed that epilepsy was "the sacred disease" (Temkin, 1971) and that the workings of the Deity would be revealed through a better understanding of the malady. Today, many believe that epilepsy carries with it an increased risk for psychopathology and that the workings of the brain can be revealed through a better understanding of the malady. The form has thus remained the same—although the content has changed. The specifics of this content have given rise to this book.

In 1948, Gibbs, Gibbs, and Fuster suggested that patients with epileptiform discharges emanating from the temporal lobe(s) and/or their associated limbic structures were especially likely to manifest psychopathology, thus initiating a new paradigm in this area. Since then, numerous clinical observations of such an association in humans have been reported and have been supported by studies suggesting relationships between limbic system dysfunction and behavioral disorders in lower animals. These clinical observations and animal studies have reinforced the belief that the study of epilepsy could facilitate an understanding of the cerebral determinants of psychopathology in particular, and brain–behavior correlates in general. Unfortunately, the results from systematic and methodologically rigorous research in this area have been ambiguous and controversial, and it is fair to suggest that there currently exists little consensus regarding many aspects of the relationship between psychopathology and temporal lobe epilepsy (Hermann & Whitman, 1984).

Nonetheless, research continues that attempts to untangle the relationship between behavioral disorder and temporal lobe epilepsy. Also proceeding apace is research to locate other biological factors or markers related to behavioral disorders in people with epilepsy. Among these are electroencephalographic patterns, lateralization of the epileptogenic focus, seizure frequency, and etiology of the epilepsy.

There is an important conceptual problem with such research. Epilepsy is not only a biological condition. It is a medical condition, and as such, people with epilepsy are subject to substantial amounts of medications. Epilepsy is also a social condition, and people with epilepsy are subject to the stigmatization and discrimination that society imposes on people who experience seizures.

In contrast to biological theories of epilepsy, a multidimensional approach suggests that when a person with epilepsy experiences psychological difficulties, the cause may be traced not only to biological factors but also to medication or social factors. The fact is, however, that research about psychopathology in people with epilepsy generally ignores both social and medication variables. In a recent review of the last 20 years of the adult literature (consisting of 78 studies), we found that of the 530 variables used in this literature in an effort to predict or explain psychopathology in epilepsy, only 17 (3%) involved medication variables and only 7 (1%) involved social variables (Whitman & Hermann, submitted for publication, 1985).

In defense of the focus of this research, it is often maintained that social issues are not investigated in this area because the relevant theory is weak, or because variables that measure societal phenomena like stigma and discrimination cannot be developed and used appropriately in this field. Neither of these explanations for ignoring the social dimensions of psychopathology in people with epilepsy is appropriate. Indeed, discussions we have had with various investigators over the years suggest that good empirical and theoretical research about the social dimensions of epilepsy is being implemented but has not yet been applied in investigations of psychopathology.

This book is the first to gather scientific research about the social dimensions of epilepsy and to discuss in as much detail as possible the empirical and hypothesized links between social factors and psychopathology. We have undertaken this effort because we believe that the prevailing model, which suggests that psychopathology in epilepsy is largely a function of biological factors, is incorrect and that establishing a multifactorial approach to the etiology of psychopathology in epilepsy will yield a closer approximation to the truth. There are several additional important consequences of such an approach.

First, the chapters in this book will suggest realistic implications for treatment, i.e., psychological/psychiatric intervention. Although much has been written about the personality and behavior of people with epilepsy, the literature to date has been deficient in suggesting effective treatment modalities (Tan, 1982). This is probably due in part to the emphasis on biological risk factors, factors over which we have little or no control or means of intervention. One positive by-product of expanding the serious consideration of social variables as etiology of psychopathology is that these are more "treatable" or "intervenable" factors than seizure type, laterality of lesion, and other biological variables. The information presented in this book should thus encourage and facilitate research on intervention and treatment.

Second, it is likely that social issues are involved in the etiology of psychopathology in other neurological disorders. If current research on these other disorders is similar to that on epilepsy, then emphasis on biological precursors likely exists in these fields as well. It may not be unreasonable to suggest that the approach used in this book has relevance for conceptualizing, investigating, and treating psychopathology in other neurological disorders.

Third, despite the fact that the relationship between epilepsy and psychopathology has been studied extensively, many of the findings remain unclear. We believe that one important reason for this is that this research has been conceptually inadequate. We think that if biological variables are viewed as only some of a multitude of potentially relevant variables, and that if social and medication variables are also considered, a clearer picture of the determinants of psychopathology will result. Hence, we think that this book offers the potential to contribute to the structure of research about epilepsy/psychopathology relationships and thus about human psychopathology in general and related, but broader, themes like brain–behavior relationships and kindling theories of psychopathology.

Finally, the manner in which the potential etiologic force of biological and social factors is studied in the epilepsy/psychopathology field has an intimate connection to the age-old nature–nurture controversy. As in all such connections, the specific instance (the epilepsy/psychopathology study) both informs the general (the nature–nurture controversy) and is informed by it. In such a case only an empirical investigation of both potential biological and social etiologic factors can bring us toward a full understanding of the matter at hand. This point has been demonstrated in recent books about genetics (Lewontin, 1983), biological determinism (Lewontin, Rose, & Kamin, 1984), and neurophysiology (Rose, 1976). In these studies the authors emphasize that it is both biology *and* society that shape us and that the two are entwined in such a manner that makes it impossible to understand reality without understanding their relationship to one another. Such a formulation suggests the benefits that may accrue from the multietiologic model being pursued in this book.

One last, central point needs to be made. There is a tendency in this area to dismiss concern for the social dimensions of epilepsy as good and kind but not as important or scientific as neurophysiological variables. There is no evidence to suggest that such a perspective is correct and every reason to believe that it is just this perspective that turns discussions of psychopathology in epilepsy into neurobiology seminars—with people and their relationships to society nowhere present. As we point out in chapter 1, there is absolutely no tenable evidence that biological factors predict psychopathology in people with epilepsy better than do social factors.

We expect that social scientists, sociologists, and psychologists will find the perspective advocated in this book a convivial one. But we also invite neurologists, psychiatrists, and neuropsychologists to consider seriously the potential relevance of the many social factors discussed throughout this volume. We hope that many of our readers will select from what follows those considerations that might help them with their patients and research.

This book contains 13 chapters. The authors of these chapters comprise a diverse collection of researchers. They are sociologists, psychologists, epidemiologists, and physicians; they hail from Canada, England, Germany, Poland, Scotland, and the United States; their methodologies are theoretical and empirical, quantitative and qualitative; some are established members in this field and others are just starting out. What unites these authors is the belief that the social dimensions of epilepsy are inadequately understood and that more and better research in this area can and must be done. It was to this theme that the authors responded when we sent out our initial letters of inquiry.

Considerable effort went into finalizing each chapter prior to its publication here. Each was read and critiqued by at least two other contributors to the book and by us. We then summarized all comments, much as it is done for journal refereeing, and returned the chapter to the author(s) for appropriate revisions. Critiques were long and thorough and, as a result, summary letters were often three or four single-spaced pages long. Occasionally there were disagreements among reviewers as well as among reviewers and authors. Always the final decision was left to the authors. Thus, although the book is a collective effort, every chapter is shaped by the perspective of its author(s). As one would expect from such an approach, the authors do not share a uniform vision. We view this as a positive aspect of the book.

Finding the optimal structure for a volume of individually authored chapters is always challenging. We have chosen to group the 13 chapters into four parts, each of which pursues the explication of the social dimensions of psychopathology in epilepsy in a different manner.

Part I is meant to provide a perspective for the remainder of the book. In chapter 1, we produce a concrete, testable multietiologic model for psychopathology in people with epilepsy and indicate which parts of the model have been investigated and which have not, and we suggest potentially fruitful areas for future research. In chapter 2, Janusz Zielinski uses an epidemiologic perspective to explain what is known and, more relevantly, what is not known, about epilepsy, psychopathology, and their interaction.

Part II consists of five chapters, each of which considers social dimensions of epilepsy as potential high-risk variables for psychopathology. Included here is an investigation by Joseph Schneider and Peter Conrad concerning the extent and organization of information about epilepsy (chapter 3), an analysis of fear of seizures by Robert Mittan (chapter 4), of learned helplessness by Robert DeVellis and Brenda McEvoy DeVellis (chapter 5), of locus of control in adults by Paul Arntson, David Droge, Robert Norton, and Ellen Murray (chapter 6), and of locus of control in children by Wendy Matthews and Gabor Barabas (chapter 7).

Part III pursues the notion of stigma in epilepsy. Jade Dell, in chapter 8, critically reviews the extensive history of this pervasive problem. Then Christopher Bagley (chapter 9), Nicky Britten, Michael Wadsworth, and Peter Fenwick (chapter 10), and Patrick West (chapter 11) all examine new data in an effort to delineate empirically how and when stigma operates on people with epilepsy.

In Part IV two specific behavioral disorders alleged to be common in people with epilepsy are examined. In chapter 12, Peter Wolf, Rupprecht Thorbecke, and Werner Even examine the social determinants of psychosis in people with epilepsy. In chapter 13, Steven Whitman, Lambert King, and Robert Cohen offer a social and political analysis of the alleged link between epilepsy and violence. This relationship is the most controversial issue in the literature, and it is our hope that examining it in this unique way will shed light on analyses of epilepsy/psychopathology relationships in general and thus serve as a suitable conclusion to the book.

The area of investigation that sees some social factors as potential causes of psychopathology in people with epilepsy is a new one. It is our hope that the data, methodology, and concepts described in these 13 chapters will serve as a foundation that will facilitate future research and, eventually, improve care for people with epilepsy.

REFERENCES

Gibbs, F. A., E. L. Gibbs, & B. Fuster. (1948). Psychomotor epilepsy. *Archives of Neurology and Psychiatry* 60, 331–39.

Hermann, B. P., & S. Whitman. (1984). Behavioral and personality correlates of epilepsy: A review, methodological critique, and conceptual model. *Psychological Bulletin* 95, 451–97.

Lewontin, R. C. (1983). *Human diversity.* New York: Freeman.

Lewontin, R. C., S. Rose, & L. J. Kamin. (1984). *Not in our genes.* New York: Pantheon Books.

Rose, S. (1976). *The conscious brain.* New York: Vintage Books.

Tan, S. Y. (1982, August). Psychosocial functioning of epileptic patients referred for psychological intervention. Paper presented at the 14th Epilepsy International Symposium. London, England.

Temkin, O. (1971). *The falling sickness: A history of epilepsy from the Greeks to the beginnings of modern neurology* (2nd ed.). Baltimore, MD: Johns Hopkins University Press.

Whitman, S., & B. P. Hermann. (Submitted for publication, 1985). The structure of research in the epilepsy/psychopathology debate and its relationship to sociopolitical themes.

Psychopathology in Epilepsy: Social Dimensions

I / *Setting a Perspective*

In a recent plea to bring order (and, we would add, the scientific method) to neurological investigations, Schoenberg (1982; see References section of Chapter 1) suggests that research based on clinical exeriences is "analogous to blindfolded men examining different parts of an elephant, with each coming to an entirely different conclusion as to the characteristic of the beast" (p. 3). He goes on to quote philosopher George Boas as stating that "some scientists will study two or three dozen pigeons in a laboratory and then write a book entitled *Pigeons*. They should call it *Some Pigeons I Have Known*" (p. 3).

The study of the relationship between epilepsy and psychopathology has been suggested by some to be a good example of the use of selected perceptions generated by selected samples. The first two chapters of this book may be seen as providing alternative perspectives for those who wish to view epilesy/psychopathology relationships from a more broad-based and epidemiologic orientation. If you will, chapter 1 is about seeing the whole elephant and chapter 2 is about understanding the characteristics of all pigeons.

Chapter 1 reviews the acrimonious debate about the causes (etiology) of psychopathology in people with epilepsy. We review the arguments of those who contend that the etiology is due to neuroepilepsy factors, those who believe it is due to social factors, and those who believe it is due to factors related to antiepilepsy medications. We note that this acrimony is not unusual in scientific debates but suggest that the fact that no one has tried to evaluate this debate empirically is indeed surprising. We present evidence that suggests that such an evaluation is both necessary and possible.

In 1974 Janusz Zielinski published a report on epilepsy in Warsaw, Poland. He first gathered data about people with epilepsy that were available from all medical sources in Warsaw and then performed an unprecedented random door-to-door survey of the city. The discrepancies between the epilepsy known to medical sources and that which existed in the community were enormous in terms of prevalence and clinical characteristics. The insights gained from this study are still essential to the understanding of the nature of epilepsy, and Zielinski's work is regarded as among the most influential in this area. From his epidemiologic perspective Zielinski explains why many aspects of the research that pursues the epilepsy/psychopathology link are both conceptually and scientifically problematic. Zielinski does not simply assert this: He repeatedly demonstrates the methodological errors being made in this field—and the resulting, equally serious, erroneous conclusions that can be reached as a result of these errors.

It is our hope that these two chapters will provide useful ideas and suggestions for future research and that they will, at the same time, set a perspective for the chapters that follow.

1 / Psychopathology in Epilepsy: A Multietiologic Model

BRUCE P. HERMANN and
STEVEN WHITMAN

During the past decade a large number of review articles, symposia, edited books, and position papers have been devoted to the relationship between epilepsy and interictal psychopathology. Despite this plethora of publications, an impartial observer could derive only one accurate conclusion—that consensus on many fundamental issues has yet to be reached among investigators in this field. In fact, disagreements abound on such a wide variety of issues that one eventually begins to wonder if it is not possible that matters are involved that are deeper and larger than research technology. This chapter will focus on the central and most troublesome controversy, the nature of the determinants of psychopathology in epilepsy.

Although few researchers in this field contest the observation that rates of psychopathology in epilepsy appear significantly elevated relative to the general population, discussions of the determinants of this elevated psychopathology elicit spirited discussions as well as temporary lapses of the usual and appropriate social graces. Much of this controversy centers around the role of specific variables (e.g., seizure type, laterality of lesion, stigma, folic acid levels). However, we think that disagreements regarding the etiology of psychopathology in epilepsy can be placed in a broader perspective that would help clarify the larger issues and problems involved, and lend suggestions for future research and progress.

To that end this chapter argues that the controversies regarding the etiology of psychopathology in adults with epilepsy become more understandable if one posits that broad hypotheses of thought exist. We identify three major hypotheses and document how they compete with each other, both explicitly and implicitly, and guide research and thinking in this area. We next briefly examine the evidence supporting their claims and investigate the problems within each of them. Finally, we offer a preliminary model that we believe can be used to advance knowledge in this area.

THREE ETIOLOGIC HYPOTHESES

We suggest that virtually all the known or suspected etiologic variables in epilepsy/psychopathology research can be subsumed under one of three hypotheses. Generalities concerning the thrust and orientation of these hypotheses are well known and have been discussed extensively by previous investigators. However, we believe that they are rarely conceptualized and promoted as an organizing force in this literature. A major benefit of a perspective such as the one we propose is that it will help present the many known or suspected etiologic variables in a manner that encourages new empirical and conceptual issues to become manifest. We will now briefly overview these three hypotheses.

THE NEUROEPILEPSY HYPOTHESIS

The most prominent hypothesis reflects the belief that behavior disorder in epilepsy is largely a function of central nervous system dysfunction that is either the cause of, associated with, or a result of the patient's epilepsy. For the past 30 years most interest has centered on the relationship between psychopathology and a specific seizure type (i.e., psychomotor, temporal lobe, or complex partial epilepsy), an interest first stimulated by Frederic Gibbs and his colleagues in 1948. Many other biological and seizure-related risk variables have been implicated as being among the primary precursors of psychopathology in epilepsy. These include the etiology of the epilepsy, laterality of lesion, duration of disorder, presence of multiple seizure types, and seizure control, as well as many others that will be discussed later.

Interest in these brain-related determinants is substantial. In a recent review of the adult epilepsy/psychopathology literature from the past 20 years, we found that 79% of the nondemographic variables that had been investigated empirically as potential risk factors would be subsumed under the neuroepilepsy hypothesis (Whitman & Hermann, submitted for publication, 1985). With so much empirical investigation devoted to these variables, one might reasonably expect them to be relatively powerful, i.e., to explain a significant amount of variance in the dependent measures. However, we are aware of only three studies that have inquired into their explanatory power and the results have been surprising. Specifically, we have found that several traditionally discussed high-risk factors accounted for a modest combined total of about 25% of the variance in measures of aggression and psychosis in adults, and aggression, social competence, and general behavioral dysfunction in children with epilepsy (Hermann, Schwartz, Whitman, & Karnes, 1980b, 1981b; Whitman, Hermann, Black, and Chhabria, 1982). Although our findings are limited by the selected nature of the populations under investigation (i.e., they all consist of patients attending large medical centers) as well as the dependent measures utilized, they are consistent in their estimate of the power of neuroepilepsy factors. Thus, the current structure of the field devotes a notable majority of its effort to variables that appear to have modest explanatory power.

The Psychosocial Hypothesis

The second hypothesis derives from the general observation that epilepsy exposes those who have it to many unique social and interpersonal stresses—stresses hypothesized to cause psychopathology. Specific risk factors include stigma, discrimination, social exclusion, sense of alienation and lack of social support, fear of seizures, and feelings of helplessness, hopelessness, and loss of control (Betts, 1981, 1982; Fenton, 1981a,b). Many other psychosocial risk factors have been proposed and are discussed later in this chapter.

Although there has been considerable documentation of the social consequences of epilepsy (National Commission for the Control of Epilepsy and Its Consequences, 1978), and widespread speculation as to the role of these variables in the epilepsy/psychopathology literature, we were unable to locate any *empirical* evaluations of the relationship between social–epilepsy variables and psychopathology in our review of the adult literature (Whitman & Hermann, submitted for publication, 1985).

The Medication Hypothesis

The importance of medication variables (number, type, dosage, blood levels, etc.) as risk factors for psychopathology in epilepsy is controversial but of increasing recent interest. These medications have a therapeutic effect on seizure frequency, but several investigators contend that a potential side effect of some of these drugs is their tendency to cause behavior and/or cognitive problems (e.g., Reynolds, 1981, 1983). Certainly sufficient evidence exists to warrant further empirical attention (del Ser Quijano, Pareja, Munoz-Garcia, & Sanchez, 1983; Edeh & Toone, 1983; Reynolds, 1983; Robertson & Trimble, 1983; Rodin & Schmaltz, 1983). We will say more about these variables later in this chapter.

How do these three hypotheses interact and compete with each other in the epilepsy/psychopathology literature? Before we attempt to answer this question, three issues need clarification. First, we have used the term *psychopathology* repeatedly up to this point. This is, however, a nonspecific term. In the epilepsy literature there are actually six major areas of behavioral investigation: psychosis, aggression, sexual dysfunction, affective disorder, personality and behavioral *change,* and a large and heterogeneous category—general psychopathology—characterized by the use of standardized measures of personality and other indicators of psychopathology (e.g., rates of psychiatric hospitalization). Thus, it is important to keep in mind that whereas many investigators speak of "psychopathology in epilepsy," at least six specific areas are separate foci of investigation.

Second, briefly consider Table 1-1, to which we will devote considerable discussion later in this chapter. This table provides the reader with a more detailed overview of some of the known or suspected individual etiologic variables that can be subsumed under each hypothesis. This list is meant to be illustrative and not definitive. Other researchers will surely want to add or delete specific variables. However, we hope that Table 1-1 will provide a better sense of how we are conceptually organizing and arranging the relevant etiologic variables.

Finally, for the sake of the discussion that follows, we describe certain rsearchers as advocates of one or another of the three preceding hypotheses. It is relevant to note that if a researcher is, or has been, a strong advocate of a particular variable (e.g., seizure type), we will for the sake of argument consider him or her to be a representative of the general hypothesis (e.g., neuroepilepsy). In other words, one need not espouse all the variables within a given category to be considered a proponent of that hypothesis. Furthermore, there are of course researchers who are interested in more than one of these hypotheses. We think that such examples are generally useful as they allow us to delineate the overriding tensions in this field.

We now turn to a discussion of how the hypotheses interact and compete in this literature.

COMPETITION AMONG THE HYPOTHESES

The epilepsy/psychopathology field is similar to other areas of scientific inquiry where different schools of thought exist; that is, there is competition among the schools for primacy of their perspective. Although this competition can and often does become acrimonious, such tension is positive because it ultimately should result in the generation of empirical data that permit more informed selection among the competing hypotheses. This in turn would advance the state of the field and facilitate future investigation.

How do the specifics of the epilepsy/psychopathology field fit into this context? On the one hand, the three hypotheses actually have existed for quite some time and the expected controversy and conflict have occurrred and continue to occur. Yet, unlike controversies in other fields, *no direct empirical comparisons between the hypotheses have yet been effected.* Nonetheless, as we

TABLE 1-1. High-Risk Variables for Psychopathology in Epilepsy, Grouped According to Hypothesis

Neuroepilepsy	*Psychosocial*	*Medication*
Age at onset	Fear of seizures	Number of medications
Seizure control	Perceived stigma	Serum level
Duration of disorder	Perceived discrimination	Medication type
Seizure type	Adjustment to epilepsy	Folic acid level
Multiple seizure types	Locus of control	
Etiology	Life event changes	
Type of aura	Social support	
Neuropsychological status	Socioeconomic status	
	Childhood home environment	

will demonstrate, proponents exist for each of the hypotheses and in many cases these proponents have argued for the primacy of their orientation, always in the face of an absence of adequate data that might allow for evaluation of such an argument. We hope the following examples will demonstrate our contentions.

Gibbs and his colleagues were among major early proponents of the neuroepilepsy hypothesis. Indeed, as early as 1958 the battle lines between neuroepilepsy and psychosocial camps were drawn when Gibbs and Stamps wrote:

> The patient's emotional reactions to his seizures, to his family and to his social situation are less important determinants of psychiatric disorder than the site and type of the epileptic discharge. (p. 78)

Twenty-four years later Sherwin (1982) similarly has argued for the relevance of neuroepilepsy factors such as seizure type and laterality of lesion. He contends that psychosocial and medication factors are unlikely to be the primary etiologic factors because they cannot account for the entire spectrum of reported behavior problems:

> Social factors may aggravate the problems of psychological adjustment faced by epilepsy patients. However, in themselves they cannot account for certain characteristic psychopathological entities (for example, the schizophrenic-like psychoses) reportedly noted in epileptics. (p. 80)

Similarly, he questions the importance of anticonvulsant medications:

> Although it is well established that both acute and chronic psychiatric syndromes may occur as toxic manifestations, it appears most unlikely that this can account for the bulk of the psychiatric features occuring in epilepsy patients. (p. 80)

On the other hand, proponents of the psychosocial school assert that the psychosocial variables associated with epilepsy are dominant in this controversy. For example, the Professional Advisory Board of the Epilepsy Foundation of America (EFA) states:

> Since personality is regarded as a socially-acquired characteristic, *there is no convincing evidence suggesting any particular set of behavioral attitudes or disorder resulting directly from seizures.* However, the fact of epilepsy may have considerable impact on the individual's social experiences. Persons with epilepsy may encounter very similar social situations—overprotectiveness or a wide swing in emotional reactions on the part of parents, ostracism or taunting from peers—which have damaging effects on personality whether epilepsy is present or not. The child who faces these social and family problems compensates by fighting back. Thus, while some persons with epilepsy may display behavioral problems, *it should be remembered that these may be normal reactions to abnormal situations* [our emphasis]. (EFA, 1975, p. 61)

Serious consideration of another important social variable, socioeconomic status (SES), has been slow to develop since Stevens's (1966, 1975) suggestion that this variable may play an important role in this field. We recently have become increasingly interested in the relevance of this matter:

> Within the last few years, however, it has become clear that there is a significantly increased prevalence of epilepsy in lower SES groups. It is well known that lower SES groups also manifest a higher rate of various psychiatric disorders relative to higher SES groups. As much of the epilepsy/psychopathology literature has been derived from individuals attending epilepsy clinics at large university medical centers which serve a high proportion of unemployed, public-aid and other disadvantaged populations in the United States, the reported rates of psychopathology may be seriously confounded by SES effects. (Hermann and Whitman, 1984, p. 485)

This general concern is given specific content by Zielinski in chapter 2.

In an interesting clash between the neuroepilepsy and psychosocial paradigms it has been posited that some of the psychosocial problems widely postulated to be associated with epilepsy (e.g., social ostracism) are not only *not* the cause of psychopathology, but may actually be the end result of unattractive personality traits that are caused by neuroepilepsy factors (i.e., seizure types). For instance, Blumer (1982) hypothesizes that a personality trait indigenous to temporal lobe epilepsy (TLE) is a tendency toward "circumstantiality," i.e., excessive speech that is often quite tangential. He has stated in this regard:

> Their talk may seem incoherent, branching out from the direct line of thought—yet they will stubbornly get back to and complete the original thought if permitted to do so. They tend to be verbose and have a marked difficulty in terminating a conversation. *As a result they may be shunned* [our emphasis]. (p. 100)

Similarly, when discussing sexual dysfunction and mental state in epilepsy, Blumer minimizes the contributing effect of the anticonvulsant medications:

> It is incorrect to blame anticonvulsant medication for the hyposexuality. Rather, with sufficient control of the seizure activity by medication, a revival of sexual interest and genital arousal may occur. (p. 103)

And

> Of greater practical and theoretical significance than the direct effect of the anticonvulsant drugs on the mental state is their indirect effect via modification of the seizure disorder. (p. 99)

Reynolds (1983) has been a primary proponent of the medication hypothesis, which has met with considerable resistance:

> Considering the long-term nature of antiepileptic therapy and the widespread practice of polytherapy, it hardly seems surprising that such therapy should have subtle effects on mental functon. It has always seemed more surprising that so many doubted or overlooked this possibility. (p. S86)

As a possible explanation for this neglect Reynolds suggests:

> Physicians are usually reluctant to blame their own well-intentioned treatments for their patients' symptoms, especially when other alternative explanations appear readily available. This may partly explain the extraordinary neglect of the possible influence of antiepileptic therapy on cognitive function, mood, and behavior in the literature in the last century. (p. S85)

These quotations demonstrate that proponents of each of the hypotheses are aware of the competing hypotheses, often tend to argue for the preeminence of the etiologic effect of variables within their domain, and sometimes directly or indirectly minimize the importance of the other hypotheses. The opinions are frequently strong, often dogmatic, and not uncommonly stated with an air of authority and finality. In essence we have the expected tension between various viewpoints regarding the determinants of some phenomenon—a usual stepping-stone in the process of scientific progress. Most interestingly, for some reason the scientific development of the epilepsy/psychopathology field has been arrested in this state for over 25 years. That is, the typical next step of direct empirical contrast of alternative hypotheses has never occurred in any meaningful manner. We leave it to philosophers and sociologists of science to determine why.

We wish to make it very clear at this point that some researchers have indeed speculated that some combination of specific neuroepilepsy, psychosocial, and medication variables is involved in the genesis of disordered behavior in epilepsy (Betts, 1981; Fenton, 1981a,b; Reynolds, 1981; Serafetinides, 1965; Stevens, 1975; Taylor, 1969a,b). Hence we are discussing an old problem, albeit in a new way.

As severe and limiting as these hypothesis arguments have been, there is futher confusion in two related areas that demand at least brief review: the potential intercorrelation among risk factors, and the presumed effects of the hypothesis of interest across most or all of the specific behavior problem categories. We turn to this latter issue first.

HYPOTHESIS EFFECTS ACROSS BEHAVIORAL CATEGORIES

An interesting tendency in this literature is for proponents of a given hypothesis to posit that variables exert similarly powerful effects across the majority or all of the six major behavioral categories of interest in this field. That is, it is often implicitly assumed that individual risk factors for one specific behavior disorder will be the risk factors for other specific behavior disorders. Thus, for example, neuroepilepsy factors such as seizure type are considered by some to be just as potent for understanding aggressive behavior in epilepsy as they may be for sexual dysfunction, personality change, or psychosis (e.g., Bear, 1979; Blumer, 1982; Geschwind, 1983; Sherwin, 1982). Similarly, psychosocial factors such as stress, stigma, and discrimination have been posited to be responsible for affective disorders, aggression, sexual dysfunction, and even psychosis (EFA, 1975; Williams, 1981). Medication factors have been cited as risk factors for psychosis (Reynolds, 1971), affective disorder (Rodin, 1982), conduct disorder (Trimble, Thompson, & Corbett, 1982), and sexual dysfunction (Toone, Wheeler, Nanjee, Fenwick, & Grant, 1983), but proponents of this hypothesis have much less often espoused a dominant role for their etiologic factor.

Despite the arguments and rhetoric, there exist no relevant data. Furthermore, a close reading of the literature suggests that the relative etiologic importance of the hypotheses may vary as a function of the specific behavioral abnormality under consideration. For instance, Lishman (1978) and Standage (1981) suggest that psychosocial factors may be the primary determinants of affective disorders and Toone (1981), Trimble (1977), and Stevens and Hermann (1981) hypothesize that neuroepilepsy factors are the primary precursors of schizophrenialike psychoses in epilepsy. We are aware of no published empirical data or even serious theoretical consideration that the relative explanatory power of neuroepilepsy, psychosocial, and medication risk factors may vary as a function of the specific behavior disorder.

INTERCORRELATIONS AND REDUNDANCY AMONG RISK FACTORS

It is generally unappreciated that many of the identified or postulated risk factors within each of the hypotheses may be highly intercorrelated and may not in reality be *independent* risk factors. This can be seen most clearly in the neuroepilepsy hypothesis as most empirical investigation has occurred in this area. Several different investigative teams have identified a myriad of potential etiologic variables, e.g., presence of multiple seizure types, early age at onset, poor seizure control, and symptomatic etiology. What usually occurs in the studies themselves or in reviews of the literature is that these variables are implicitly considered to be *independent* risk factors. This generates the perception that the more factors any one patient possesses, the greater the probability of psychopathology. Rarely considered, however, is that these variables may not be independent of one another at all, but may instead be highly intercorrelated and reflect a more general factor, for example, severity of epilepsy (see Fenwick, Master, & Brown [1981], Tables 7 and 8, for examples of such intercorrelation). The same consideration would most likely apply to the psychosocial and medication hypotheses as well. In short, generation of empirically derived independent risk factors has yet to be seriously attempted in this field.

COMPONENTS OF THE THREE HYPOTHESES

In the next section we present analytic techniques for evaluating the relationships that exist among the three hypotheses. However, before we attempt that, it would be helpful to look at the literature concerning some of the variables that comprise these hypotheses. These variables are presented in Table 1-1. As noted earlier, this list is not meant to be exhaustive, but it does include a substantial number of the variables hypothesized to be high-risk factors for psychopathology in epilepsy.

Neuroepilepsy Variables

Neuroepilepsy variables have been the major factors of interest in attempts to understand the determinants of psychopathology in epilepsy. Despite the considerable theoretical and empirical attention paid to these factors, the evidence remains contradictory and confusing for reasons to be discussed shortly. Further, our analyses of certain subsets of these variables suggest that they are relatively modest in terms of their overall explanatory power. Nonetheless, these variables constitute a very important set of potential risk factors for psychopathology in epilepsy and a subset of eight of these variables is reviewed here.

It will be somewhat difficult to provide the reader with a sense of the absolute explanatory power of these variables for several reasons. First, different neuroepilepsy variables or sets of neuroepilepsy variables typically have been evaluated in limited behavioral areas using heterogeneous groups of epilepsy patients obtained from different clinical settings using a variety of selection criteria and sampling procedures. Hence, it is often difficult to untangle the reasons for the existing contradictory findings that concern a given neuroepilepsy variable. Second, the effects of some neuroepilepsy variables have been investigated in only some seizure types (or only one seizure type), and their effects for epilepsy patients in general therefore may remain unknown. Finally, there is a considerable degree of intercorrelation among several of the neuroepilepsy variables, and the degree to which this intercorrelation contributes to the contradictory findings is generally unappreciated or unknown.

We offer the preceding comments because we suspect that readers unfamiliar with the epilepsy/psychopathology literature may come away confused and uncertain as to the importance of some of the neuroepilepsy variables. These perceptions are justified and we think that such a state of affairs suggests the need for, and importance of, simultaneously evaluating the *same* set of neuroepilepsy factors in the *same* well-defined population of consecutively selected epilepsy patients across *each* of the major behavioral problem areas of interest to investigators in this field.

The eight variables we will review are age at onset, seizure control, duration of disorder, seizure type, multiple seizure types, etiology, type of aura, and neuropsychological status.

Age at Onset

The age at onset of the patient's epilepsy has long been thought to be a significant predictor of psychopathology (Notkin, 1928), and it continues to be a variable of considerable interest (Betts, 1982; Fenton, 1981b). Many contemporary investigators have reported an association between various indexes of psychopathology and the age at onset of the patient's epilepsy although considerable conflicting evidence exists.

Early age at onset of epilepsy has been reported to be associated with a generally increased risk of psychopathology (Gudmundsson, 1966) and in the area of sexual dysfunction, specifically hyposexuality, onset of TLE prior to puberty has been found to be associated with global hyposexuality. Later onset has been reported to be associated with impotence but with intact libido (Blumer, 1970; Saunders & Rawson, 1970; Shukla, Srivastava, & Katiyar, 1979; Taylor, 1969b). Serafetinides (1965) found onset of TLE prior to age 10 to be associated with increased aggression. Onset of TLE around puberty has been reported to be associated with an increased risk of psychosis (Taylor, 1965) and an adolescent onset with elevated MMPI scale scores, particularly on the psychotic tetrad (Hermann, Schwartz, Karnes, & Vahdat, 1980a). Late-onset epilepsy has been reported to be associated with significant depression (Dominian, Serafetinides, & Dewhurst, 1963).

Other investigators have failed to find an association between the age of onset of the patient's epilepsy and general indexes of psychopathology (Kogeorgos, Fonagy, & Scott, 1982), psychosis (Jensen & Larsen, 1979; Kristensen & Sindrup, 1978), and aggression (Hermann et al., 1980b). We are not aware of a failure to find an age-at-onset effect in association with sexual dysfunction in TLE nor are we aware of other attempts to examine its relationship with affective disorders.

Seizure Control

It is logical to expect poor seizure control to be associated with poor behavioral adjustment, and clinical observations have tended to support this expectation (Betts, 1982; Fenton, 1981a,b). Surprisingly, relatively little direct empirical consideration has been devoted to this relationship (e.g., Brady, 1964), but there is some indirect evidence to suggest that its effect is not trivial. Kogeorgos et al. (1982) found a relationship between *seizure severity* (of which seizure control was a composite variable) and significantly increased scores on the General Health Questionnaire (which indicated the presence of psychopathology). Jensen and Larsen (1979) noted a relationship between psychosis and seizure severity in patients with TLE. Several other lines of evidence also point to the role of seizure control or seizure severity in this literature. Patients with TLE who undergo temporal lobectomy (and who must have intractable seizures to be selected for this operation) manifest higher rates of aggression, sexual dysfunction, and general psychopathology relative to patients with TLE who are treated as outpatients (Hermann & Whitman, 1984). Further, patients treated by primary care physicians, and hence suspected to have relatively mild seizure disorders, manifest less psychopathology than patients with epilepsy treated in outpatient neurological clinics (Edeh & Toone, 1983).

Substantially more interest has centered on the observation, reported by some, of an inverse relationship between seizures, particularly complex partial or temporal lobe, and psychosis (Flor-Henry, 1969; Kristensen & Sindrup, 1978) and depression (Betts, 1974; Flor-Henry, 1969). The possible theoretical ramifications of this relationship have generated considerable interest (Flor-Henry, 1969, 1983; Trimble, 1977) even though it has not been noted consistently (e.g., Ramani & Gumnit, 1982).

Duration of Disorder

The duration of the patient's epilepsy has often been postulated to be associated with both psychopathology and intellectual functioning and has been an important variable in attempts to determine whether intellectual deterioration occurs in epilepsy. More specifically, the type and estimated total lifetime number of seizures have been found to be related to cognitive function (Dean, 1981; Dodrill, 1982; Lennox & Lennox, 1960). The duration of TLE has been reported by some to be associated with psychosis (e.g., Jensen & Larsen, 1979; Slater, Beard, & Glithero, 1963), but others have not found this relationship (Flor-Henry, 1969; Kristensen & Sindrup, 1978). With the relatively recent application of kindling theory to clinical psychiatry and psychology, there has been speculation that prolonged interictal kindling of limbic structures (and not necessarily the ictal seizures themselves) eventually might result in personality and behavioral change (Bear, 1979), although the evidence to support such a contention is equivocal (Reynolds, 1981).

Seizure Type

The relationship between seizure type—particularly complex partial seizures (CPS) or TLE—and psychopathology has been the variable of most theoretical and empirical interest since the report of Gibbs and his colleagues in 1948 (Gibbs et al., 1948). Numerous reviews of this literature are available (e.g., Bear, 1979; Betts, 1982; Blumer, 1975, 1982; Flor-Henry, 1972; Hermann & Whitman, 1984; Lishman, 1978; Reynolds, 1981; Scott, 1978; Sherwin, 1982; Stevens, 1975; Trimble, 1983). In general, consensus has yet to be reached regarding the role that an epileptiform spike focus in the temporal lobe plays in predisposing these patients to psychopathology relative to patients with, for example, corticoreticular epilepsies. It should be pointed out, however, that the least controversy surrounds the relationship between TLE and hyposexuality, yet even here recent reports have not found the hypothesized increased rate of hyposexuality in TLE (Toone, 1983).

The few comparisons of patients with TLE to patients with focal but nontemporal lobe epilepsies generally have indicated increased psychopathology in TLE (Gunn, 1977; Hermann, Black, & Chhabria, 1981a; Sherwin, Peron-Magnan, Bancaud, Bonis, & Talairach 1982; Stevens, 1966) although there are exceptions (e.g., Glass & Mattson, 1973).

A relevant consideration concerns the laterality of the temporal lobe epileptiform focus. Some researchers have contended that failure to consider the laterality of the focus has contributed in large part to the many nonsignificant TLE/non-TLE comparisons (Flor-Henry, 1982). A brief review of the relevant literature will help shed some light on the rationale for such a contention.

The laterality of the temporal lobe epileptiform activity has been of much interest since Flor-Henry's (1969) report of an association between left hemisphere TLE and schizophrenia, and right hemisphere TLE and affective psychoses. Since Flor-Henry's original study there have been several reports indicating an association between schizophrenialike psychoses and left TLE (Flor-Henry, 1972; Lindsay, Ounsted, & Richards, 1979; Sherwin, 1981; Sherwin et al., 1982) as well as an association between left TLE and aggression (Serafetinides, 1965; Sherwin, 1977), fear (Strauss, Risser, & Jones, 1982), and ideational personality and behavioral change (Bear & Fedio, 1977).

Additionally, right TLE has been reported to be associated with depression (Shukla et al., 1979), reflective conceptual tempo (McIntyre, Pritchard, & Lombroso, 1976), and Flor-Henry (1983) has posited right TLE to be associated with sexual dysfunction. Bitemporal lobe EEG foci, particularly independent bitemporal spike foci, have been found to be associated with hypergraphia (Sachdev & Waxman, 1981), MMPI-defined psychopathology (Meier & French, 1965), and personality and behavioral change (Bear, Levin, Blumer, Chetham, & Ryder, 1982) relative to patients with a unilateral focus.

Again, considerable contradictory evidence exists. Laterality of lesion has been found not to be associated with aggression (Hermann et al., 1980b; Whitman et al., 1982), psychosis (Hermann et al., 1981b; Kristensen & Sindrup, 1979), personality and behavioral change (Nielsen & Kristensen, 1981), and measures of general psychopathology such as the MMPI (Mignone, Donnelly, & Sadowsky, 1970) or the General Health Questionnaire (Kogeorgos et al., 1982).

There are many methodological difficulties that may in part account for these contradictory findings (e.g., see Sherwin [1982] for a discussion of the possible methodological problems).

Multiple Seizure Types

One consistently reported finding involves the relationship between the presence of multiple seizure types and psychopathology. Although multiple seizure types has been defined in various ways by different investigative groups (e.g., CPS only vs. CPS and secondarily generalized seizures or CPS plus *any* other seizure type; one type of any seizure vs. two or more types of any seizures), this variable has been found to be significantly associated with increased scores on several different measures of psychopathology (e.g., depression, aggression, psychosis, MMPI scale scores, Washington Psychosocial Seizure Inventory [WPSI] scores) (Dikmen, Hermann, Wilensky, & Rainwater, 1983; Dodrill, 1983; Hermann, Dikmen, & Wilensky 1982b; Ounsted, 1969; Rodin, Katz, & Lennox 1976). We are not aware of any investigation of the relationship between multiple seizure types and sexual function.

Etiology

Patients with epilepsy of symptomatic etiology are generally posited or found to be at increased psychiatric risk relative to patients with idiopathic epilepsy (Betts, 1982; Fenton, 1981a,b; Gudmundson, 1966; Lishman, 1978; Reynolds, 1981; Rutter, Graham, & Yule, 1970). Abnormalities on the neurological exam have been found to be associated with a greater risk of psychosis in patients with TLE (Kristensen & Sindrup, 1978) and aggression in patients with epilepsy in general (Rodin, 1973). Further, in patients with TLE an increased risk of psychosis has been found to be associated with a history of prenatal complications (Jensen & Larsen, 1979), a medical history suggesting an epileptogenic lesion, and a less frequent family history of epilepsy (Kristensen & Sindrup, 1978). Taylor (1975) has delineated risk factors for psychosis in TLE based on neuropathological findings in the resected temporal lobes.

Thus, etiology of the seizure disorder cannot be ignored although knowledge of its relevance is largely confined to psychosis and patients with TLE.

Type of Aura

In 1957 Pond proposed that repeated intrusions into consciousness of bizarre and alien experiences were associated with an increased risk of emotional/behavioral dysfunction. This relationship has proven difficult to verify although there is evidence of its existence. For instance, Standage and Fenton (1975) reported that patients with TLE with complex auras manifested more psychopathology on the Present State Exam relative to patients with simple auras. Jensen and Larsen (1979) reported that psychosis in patients with TLE was associated with auras consisting of illusions and hallucinations. Hermann and his colleagues (Herman & Chhabria, 1981; Hermann et al., 1982a) found an aura of fear to be associated with increased psychopathology as indicated by psychiatric history and by MMPI scale scores.

On the other hand, Kristensen and Sindrup (1979) failed to find a relationship between the nature of the patient's aura and psychosis in TLE although a higher incidence of automatisms was associated with psychosis.

Neuropsychological Status

In 1969 Ferguson and her colleagues reported five cases of psychosis in TLE and proposed that severe psychopathology in epilepsy, particularly TLE, was associated with deficits in higher cortical functioning. Subsequent direct (Stevens, Milstein, & Goldstein, 1972) and indirect (Matthews, Dikmen, & Harley, 1977; Matthews & Klove, 1968) tests of this hypothesis were not supportive. However, it recently has been argued that these negative results were obtained because of the manner in which the measures of psychopathology—the MMPI—were analyzed. The MMPI data from two recent neuropsychological investigations of epilepsy (Batzel, Dodrill, & Fraser, 1980; Dikmen & Morgan, 1980) were reanalyzed using a technique derived from Goldberg (1972), which has been found to be quite sensitive to various psychopathological categories. Comparison of patients with epilepsy varying in their degree of neuropsychological impairment revealed an increased risk to psychosis of the groups with more widespread cognitive deficits, thereby supporting the general hypothesis of Ferguson et al. (Hermann, 1981). Further, Dodrill (1980), Camfield et al. (1984), and Hermann (1982) have all additionally reported relationships between the adequacy of neuropsychological status and psychopathology.

Again, there is contradictory evidence. Moehle, Bolter, & Long (1984) failed to find a relationship between neuropsychological status and psychopathology in 34 patients with TLE. The reasons for their findings are unclear at present but they do seem contrary to the bulk of the recently reported evidence.

Summary

Neuroepilepsy variables are important considerations in the attempt to understand the determinants of psychopathology in epilepsy. With the current growth and explosion of interest in biological psychiatry, interest in these neuroepilepsy variables will probably grow. We hope this review has indicated some of the difficulties inherent in the search for biological precursors of psychopathology in epilepsy.

Psychosocial Variables

Several discussions have highlighted ways in which the unique social and interpersonal stresses associated with having epilepsy may contribute to a predisposition to psychopathology (Fenton, 1981b; Laidlaw & Laidlaw, 1982; Lennox & Lennox, 1960; Linnett, 1982; Williams, 1981). Despite this longstanding awareness of the psychosocial consequences of epilepsy and their potential relevance to the epilepsy/psychopathology literature, there has been virtually no empirical research of this issue.

In what follows we will review several specific psychosocial variables, discuss their contentions, and cite any relevant published or pilot data.

Fear of Seizures

Mittan and his colleagues (Mittan, 1983; Mittan & Locke, 1982a,b; Mittan, Wasterlain, & Locke, 1981) have noted that discussions of the precursors of psychopathology in epilepsy have rarely considered the stresses that arise as a result of the patient's fears and misperceptions about his or her seizures. In an investigation of 378 patients with epilepsy, Mittan found pervasive fears of seizures and their consequences: for example, approximately 70% of the sample reported that they were afraid that they might die during their next seizure; about 45% reported that they lived in continual dread of seizures; and approximately 35% believed that death from seizures occurred frequently. Two thirds of Mittan's sample was clinically depressed, and he postulated that the fear of seizures and their possible consequences was a major contributor to the anxiety, depression, and other psychopathologies that were so prevalent. This hypothesis, however, remained untested until recently.

In this volume, Mittan (chap. 4) directly evaluates the relationship between depression and aggression and patients' fear of seizures. As he demonstrates, there is a strong relationship.

Perceived Stigma

Much of the literature on the social consequences of epilepsy states that the disorder bears a substantial stigma (Arangio, 1980; Betts, 1982; Fenton, 1981b; Laidlaw & Laidlaw, 1982; Ryan, Kempner, & Emlen, 1980), and patients' self-reports lend strong credence to these contentions (Mittan, 1983; Mittan & Locke, 1982b). This stigma has long been thought to be a variable that could predispose the individual to various forms of psychopathology (Bagley, 1972). However, we are not aware of any published empirical evaluations of the nature and degree of the relationship between measures of actual or perceived stigma and psychopathology.

Arntson and his colleagues (chap. 6) have recently inquired into the relationship between perceived stigma and affective disorder (anxiety and depression) and have located significant relationships.

Perceived Discrimination

One way in which the stigma associated with epilepsy is hypothesized to manifest itself is via discrimination against the person with epilepsy. This discrimination is thought to be seen in several important aspects of the patient's life, particularly in the area of employment. The problems associated with the experiences of exposure to, and coping with, such discrimination are then logically thought to underlie adjustment problems that may become evident in some individuals with epilepsy (Arangio, 1980; Betts, 1982; Laidlaw & Laidlaw, 1982). Again, although this theory is widely circulated, we are aware of no empirical evaluations of the nature and degree of the discrimination/psychopathology link.

Adjustment to Epilepsy

As is well known, many individuals with epilepsy resent their condition, are embarrassed when seizures occur, find themselves ill at ease because of possible sudden attacks, or feel they are less worthy because of their epilepsy (Dodrill, Batzel, Queisser, & Temkin, 1980). Patients with epilepsy vary widely in the degree of acceptance of the disorder, and this in turn has been thought to be linked to a variety of behavioral problems such as depression and hostility (Betts, 1982; Williams, 1981). Again, we are not aware of empirical evaluations of the nature and degree of the association between psychopathology and the patient's acceptance of the disorder.

We have, however, located some circumstantial evidence to suggest that this is indeed an important predictor variable. In their article dealing with the development of the WPSI, Dodrill et al. (1980) presented an intercorrelation matrix of the individual WPSI scales. In that matrix it can be seen that the Adjustment to Epilepsy scale correlated quite highly (r = .66) with the Emotional Adjustment scale. An association between adjustment to epilepsy and psychopathology thus appears to be present and of substantial magnitude.

In addition to the specific psychosocial aspects of epilepsy described earlier, the experiences of living and dealing with epilepsy and its consequences have been found or postulated to affect more global aspects of the patient's psychological state and perceptions and orientations toward life. They are also hypothesized to increase the probability of exposing the individual to other known risk factors for psychopathology. These more general psychosocial considerations are discussed next.

Locus of Control

Several researchers have postulated that individuals with epilepsy, by virtue of experiencing seizures as well as significant lack of control over important aspects of their lives, might be prone to develop a general expectation that reinforcements in their life result from luck, chance, or are under the control of powerful others. That is, they are more likely to develop a belief in an external locus of control (e.g., Matthews, Barabas, & Ferrari, 1982). Indeed, it has recently been reported that patients with epilepsy have significantly greater external locus of control relative to both healthy people (DeVellis, DeVellis, Wallston, & Wallston (1980) and diabetic patients (Matthews et al., 1982). As there exists a well-known relationship between locus of control and various measures of behavior and psychopathology in the general population (Lefcourt, 1976), it is important to consider this concept with respect to epilepsy.

In this volume Matthews and Barabas (chap. 7) and Arntson et al. (chap. 6) review data concerning the relationship between locus of control and psychopathology in children and adults with epilepsy. In these initial inquiries significant associations between an external locus of control and psychopathology are noted.

Life Event Changes

There is a growing literature concerned with the relationship between life event changes in general, undesirable life event changes in particular, and psychopathology and physical disease (Dohrenwend & Dohrenwend, 1981). Individuals with epilepsy clearly have a higher probability of experiencing an increased number of undesirable life changes (National Commission for the Control of Epilepsy and Its Consequences, 1978). Interestingly, although some investigators are beginning to study the relationship between life changes and seizure frequency (Temkin & Davis, 1984), no one has inquired into the relationship between life events and psychopathology in patients with epilepsy.

Social Support

The amount, degree, and quality of social support available to an individual have been postulated to be important direct or moderating variables in many areas of psychopathology research (Sarason, Levine, Basham, & Sarason, 1983). The role that social support plays in the relationship between epilepsy and psychopathology remains largely unexplored. However, that it is a potentially relevant and important consideration is suggested by the observation that one major way in which the stigma and discrimination associated with epilepsy are evidenced is through relative social isolation, disturbed interpersonal relations, or loss of social support (Betts, 1981, 1982; Fenton, 1981b). In a study of intellectually intact children with epilepsy, we have found that they have significantly fewer friends, fewer contacts with available friends, and fewer social activities and outlets relative to healthy children (Hermann, 1982). The generally accepted importance of social support, the implication in data and theory that it is decreased in epilepsy, and the fact that no one has inquired into its relevance in the epilepsy/psychopathology literature all make the investigation of social support relevant for this field.

Socioeconomic Status

Stevens, following up her earlier, unheeded plea (1966) for the consideration of SES as a confounder in epilepsy/psychopathology debate, implemented a study herself (1975). Comparison of patients with epilepsy seen by private neurologists with those attending a university-based clinic revealed a significantly lower rate of psychopathology in the former. A similar observation emerges from a comparison of the studies of MMPI-defined psychosis by Hermann et al. (1981b) and Lachar, Lewis, and Kupke (1979). Utilizing identical MMPI criteria the rate of psychosis in a predominantly white, employed, middle-class sample of patients with epilepsy derived from the Mayo Clinic (Hermann et al., 1981b) was one third that found in a sample of patients from an inner-city setting who were mostly poor and composed of minority groups (Lachar et al., 1979). Despite the obvious importance of SES in the epilepsy/psychopathology debate, our recent review (Hermann & Whitman, 1984) revealed that only 5 of the 64 studies we analyzed considered SES—and none considered it in a substantive manner. This issue becomes more urgent as it becomes clearer that poor people are more likely to have epilepsy (Whitman, Coleman, Berg, King, & Desai, 1980; Zielinski, chap. 2, this volume).

Furthermore, although unemployment and underemployment are known to be pervasive among individuals with epilepsy (Fraser, 1980), the empirical relationship of employment status to psychopathology has been virtually ignored in this area. Some investigators have suggested that unemployment contributes to emotional and behavioral adjustment problems (e.g., Taylor, 1969a), but few have inquired empirically into its effect. Rodin (1973) found that aggression in epilepsy was correlated with "less time employed." That employment status should be considered as a predictor of psychopathology in people with epilepsy is clear. In his seminal work in this area, Brenner (1973, 1976, 1984) found unemployment status in the general population to be significantly correlated with every index of psychopathology he considered (e.g., admissions to mental health facilities, psychiatric diagnosis).

Childhood Home Environment

It is important to know details about the presence or absence of psychopathology in the parents of the patients as well as details concerning other relevant aspects of their home environment. These variables are known risk factors for psychopathology in the general population and have been found to be risk factors for psychopathology in patients with epilepsy in particular (e.g., Bagley, 1971; Jensen and Larsen, 1979; Pond & Bidwell, 1960; Rutter et al., 1970).

Further, the impact of the diagnosis of epilepsy on the child's parents and their subsequent expectations and management of the child are important topics in a better understanding of epilepsy/psychopathology relationships. West (chap. 11) reviews evidence from several of his studies that document the impact of epilepsy on the family unit and the relevance of this impact for better understanding epilepsy/psychopathology relationships.

Summary

A variety of psychosocial variables have been widely hypothesized to play important roles in the genesis of psychopathology in adults with epilepsy, but empirical investigation has been lacking. As noted, several chapters in this volume will, for the first time, provide empirical data supporting the role these variables play in predisposing a person with epilepsy to psychopathology. In other instances we have been able to provide some indicators that suggest that significant relationships exist; in still others, data await collection. However, in *every* instance in which direct or indirect data are available, the findings support a relationship between psychosocial variables and psychopathology. We are therefore confident that greater consideration of these psychosocial variables will enhance considerably our understanding of psychopathology in epilepsy.

Further work will also be needed to tackle difficult conceptual issues. For instance, although an association between psychosocial variables (e.g., adjustment to epilepsy) and psychopathology may exist, the direction of causality is a priori unclear and such issues will require rigorous investigation (e.g., longitudinal studies). We should also emphasize that some of these variables are indigenous only to epilepsy (e.g., fear of seizures, adjustment to epilepsy), whereas others are not (e.g., childhood home environment, level of social support). This implies that the determinants responsible for a relationship between independent and dependent variables may reflect epilepsy per se (e.g., fear of seizures), the mediating effects of epilepsy (e.g., epilepsy might further lower the level of social support in a person who had relatively low social support to begin with), or may in fact have little or nothing to do with epilepsy per se (e.g., a person with epilepsy may come from a disordered home for reasons unrelated to his or her epilepsy).

Therefore, the demonstration of significant relationships between psychosocial variables and psychopathology is but the first step in a difficult process of understanding the nature and direction of causative factors.

Medication Variables

Collectively, individuals with epilepsy ingest a great amount and diversity of antiepilepsy drugs (AEDs). One might thus expect interest in the biobehavioral effects of AEDs to be great, but surprisingly this is not the case. Comparatively few data on this topic exist, and the first review of behavioral problems associated with anticonvulsants did not appear until 1976 (Trimble & Reynolds). In our review of the adult epilepsy/psychopathology literature, only 3% of the variables empirically evaluated as risk factors for interictal psychopathology were medication-related (Whitman & Hermann, submitted for publication 1985).

AEDs have been posited by many to play a significant role in the etiology of psychopathology in epilepsy (e.g., Betts, 1982; Fenton, 1981b; Laidlaw & Laidlaw, 1982; Reynolds, 1981; Williams, 1981). Unfortunately, in many instances the nature and magnitude of the behavioral effects of AEDs have not been specified (e.g., Betts, 1982; Fenton, 1981b) although a few investigators, particularly Reynolds and his colleagues, have suggested specific mechanisms of effect (Reynolds, 1981). A particularly troublesome problem in the task of evaluating the behavioral effect of the AED concerns the confounding influence of the patient's neurological condition.

Here we will simply note a few possible medication-related variables. For a more detailed discussion of medication-related variables, see Reynolds (1983).

Polypharmacy

It is becoming increasingly clear that polypharmacy for epilepsy may adversely affect not only seizure control, but also cognitive function, mood, and psychological state (Shorvon & Reynolds, 1979; Thompson & Trimble,

1982). Some investigators have found that the number of AEDs taken by a patient is associated with measures of psychopathology (e.g., del Ser Quijano et al., 1983).

Serum Levels of AEDs

Toxic blood serum levels of AEDs would be expected to affect behavioral and cognitive functioning adversely, and such effects have been reported (see Reynolds, 1981, for a review). Recently, however, it has become clear that adverse biobehavioral effects might be assoicated even with serum levels of some AEDs within the therapeutic range (Thompson, Huppert, & Trimble, 1981). Reynolds and Travers (1974) found that after exclusion of patients with signs of drug toxicity, mental symptoms preceding epilepsy, and/or evidence of gross cerebral lesions, those patients manifesting clinical evidence of psychomotor slowing, intellectual deterioration, psychiatric illness, or personality change had significantly higher serum phenytoin and phenobarbital levels than those without such changes. Similar differences were found when those patients whose seizures were relatively well controlled (less than one per month) were analyzed. Of importance is that none of the AED serum levels were in the toxic range.

Hence, even appropriate therapeutic use of the medications may, in some individuals, play a role in the development of psychopathology. A related variable concerns the specific type of AED.

Medication Type

Over 20 AEDs currently are approved for the treatment of epilepsy. Because some commonly used medications exert therapeutic effects for specific seizure types (e.g., carbamazepine for TLE, succinimides for absence attacks), a considerable amount of error variance in an etiologic model might be explained by understanding whether AEDs varied in the degree to which they contributed to cognitive/behavioral/mood alterations. Recent findings suggest this may be the case (e.g., Dalby, 1975; Thompson et al., 1981; Thompson & Trimble, 1981, 1982). For instance, carbamazepine has been argued to have psychotropic effects (Dalby, 1975), and phenobarbital is widely held to be associated with irritability and, particularly in children, hyperkinetic side effects (Reynolds, 1981).

Folic Acid Levels

Several investigations have noted an association between mental and/or neurological changes and folate depletion in cerebrospinal and serum fluid (e.g., Grant, Hoffbrand, & Well, 1965; Howard, 1975). Depletion of folate can have several causes, including the use of certain AEDs (Reynolds, 1976, 1981). The relation between low serum folate levels and psychiatric states includes depression (Reynolds, 1967), dementia (Melamed, Reches, & Hereshko, 1975), and fatigue, irritability, and apathy (Botez, Fontaine, Botez, & Bachevalier, 1977).

Among patients with epilepsy, low folate levels have been found to be associated with increased psychiatric risk in general, and increased risk for specific behavior disorders in particular (Callaghan, Mitchell, & Cotter, 1969; del Ser Quijano et al., 1983; Edeh & Toone, 1983; Reynolds, 1971, 1976; Robertson, 1983; Robertson & Trimble, 1983; Robin & Schmaltz, 1983; Snaith, Mehta, & Raby, 1970; Trimble, Corbett, & Donaldson, 1980, Trimble, Thompson, & Corbett, 1982), although some investigators have failed to find such a relationship (e.g., Bruens, 1971; Ramani & Gumnit, 1981). The weight of the evidence thus suggests that folate levels should be further investigated as etiologic agents for psychopathology in people with epilepsy (Reynolds, 1983).

Summary

An extended discussion of the mechanisms whereby AEDs affect behavior is beyond the scope of this chapter. However, it should be noted that Reynolds (1967, 1968, 1971, 1981, 1982) and his colleagues have suggested that AEDs could adversely affect mental functioning by (a) causing neuropathological changes in the central nervous system, (b) inducing folate deficiency, (c) altering monoamine metabolism, and/or (d) affecting hormonal or endocrine functioning.

It is apparent from this very brief and selected review that medication variables should not be ignored in the search for a better understanding of the precursors of psychopathology in epilepsy.

IMPLEMENTING THE MODEL

Thus far we have described our model in general and have selected and defined the independent variables. How might we go about empirically establishing the model in a manner consistent with the methodological and conceptual prbolems we discussed at the beginning of this chapter? The purpose of this section is to suggest an analytic procedure to accomplish this task. It is not our belief that this procedure is the only one available. Certainly there are others. However, it is our hope that explaining how such an empirical evaluation might proceed will increase understanding of the general process we have been pursuing in this chapter and following in our research.

Three steps are necessary to establish empirically the shape of our model.

STEP 1

The first step in the data analysis would involve locating nonredundant high-risk variables within each hypothesis for each of the six behavior problems (i.e., aggression, sexual dysfunction, psychosis, affective disorder, behavioral change, general psychopathology). To accomplish this, one would randomly select half of the subjects from whom the necessary information has been gathered. For these subjects one initially would regress the first dependent variable (for example, a measure of general psychopathology) on the eight predictor variables from the neuroepilepsy category (Table 1-1). Basic demographic variables (e.g., age, race, sex) would be treated as covariates. The use of "standard" regression analysis would guarantee that variables indentified as statistically significant would be so identified only if they make a significant contribution *after* the effects of all other variables have been accounted for.

After the identification of those variables from the neuroepilepsy category that are significant predictors of general psychopathology, the significant psychosocial variables and then the significant medication variables would be similarly identified. We emphasize that although the identified risk variables within any given category may be intercorrelated to some degree, the analytic procedures we suggest guarantee that they *each* will have a statistically significant relationship with the dependent measure (general psychopathology). Thus, the end product of Step 1 of the data analysis will be the identification of a subset of nonredundant, significant predictor variables from *within* each of the three categories of independent variables (neuroepilepsy, psychosocial, and medication).

STEP 2

The subjects who were not used in Step 1 of the data anlaysis would be used in Step 2. Now, all of the variables identified as being significant predictors of, e.g., general psychopathology in Step 1 would be placed in the *same* regression analysis. Thus, neuroepilepsy, psychosocial, and medication variables would now "compete" to determine which variables remain significant when the variance attributable to significant risk factors from the other categories is controlled. This will tell us, for example, if a relationship between polypharmacy and depression remains after stigma and the severity of the patient's epilepsy are taken into account. This will also tell us if there exist interactions between significant risk factors across hypotheses.

It should be pointed out that a by-product of Step 2 would be a replication of Step 1. This second analysis (effected on a completely independent sample in our split sample design) affords a rare opportunity for within-experiment verification. Thus, any variable that emerges from Steps 1 and 2 as being significantly correlated with the dependent measure under investigation would certainly demand attention as it would have "survived" two different sets of competing variables and two independent samples.

After Steps 1 and 2 are completed for the measure of general psychopathology, the same analyses will be repeated for measures of depression, aggression, psychosis, sexual dysfunction, and behavioral change.

The primary clinical implications that would result from Step 1 and Step 2 analyses are as follows. For each type of psychopathology, a regression formula would be produced that would specify the independent multietiologic risk factors for that psychopathology as well as the relative importance of each risk factor. For example, suppose the significant independent risk factors for depression (and the proportion of variance they were found to account for) were as follows:

Depression = symptomatic epilepsy (20%) + AED polypharmacy (18%)
+ fear of seizures (15%) + external locus of control (11%)
+ unemployment (9%) + low folic acid level (8%) + male sex (6%)

Such an equation would have interesting clinical implications: (1) Those variables predictive of depression and their relative importance are specified; (2) this list of risk factors indicates where intervention can and should take place in order to ameliorate depression among patients with epilepsy (polypharmacy, fear of seizures, external locus of control, unemployment, folic acid level), thereby also suggesting the nature of the multidisciplinary team needed to help such patients. Further, it is clear where no intervention can occur even though the factor is a significant predictor of depression (symptomatic epilepsy, sex); (3) Also suggested is how to *prevent* depression in patients with epilepsy, for example, among those patients with newly diagnosed epilepsy.

Although this is a hypothetical example, we hope it makes clear to the reader that the results would have the potential to make practical clinical and preventative contributions. Further, the findings would have significant theoretical and conceptual merit by answering the following questions: What proportion of the variance in the dependent measures have we accounted for via this multietiologic approach? Does the overall explanatory power of the neuroepilepsy, psychosocial, and medication categories vary as a function of the specific behavior disorder under investigation? If so, do they vary in the direction we have previously hypothesized (Hermann & Whitman, 1984)?

Step 3

The final step would involve exploration of the regression model in order to initiate and facilitate discussion of this and related models derived from similar efforts. In our example of depression, various numeric values of the variables would be inserted into the resulting regression equation to provide the clinician with a feeling for what depression levels might be expected when these terms are at their maxima, minima, and various combinations in between. Clearly there are many such combinations and we would be able to evaluate only a few. However, by providing the regression equations and the methodology, readers would be allowed to explore any such combinations that may be of specific interest to them and that would help them predict the degrees of behavioral change expected via modification of particular risk factors.

We emphasize that the analytic technique we have used to illustrate how we would establish our model is not the only one available. Furthermore, any number of absolutely essential statistical issues would have to be taken into consideration. Among these would be the number of degrees of freedom available, the power of the tests, mathematical assumptions of the model, validity and reliability of the measures employed, and so on.

CONCLUSION

This chapter has two main goals: to point out the need for a multietiologic model for psychopathology in epilepsy and to show how such a model could be empirically established. We hope we have succeeded in the pursuit of these goals and that the reader is convinced that such a model is both needed and possible.

We assert once more that neither the analytic technique we suggest nor the specific variables we have discussed need to be central to the *process* we have proposed. What we have described in this chapter is only the first phase in what must become a sustained effort to refine continuously the specifics, the methodology, and the concepts of this model.

REFERENCES

Arangio, A. (1980). The social worker and epilepsy: A description of assessment and treatment variables. In B. P. Hermann (Ed.), *A multidisciplinary handbook of epilepsy.* Springfield, IL: Thomas.

Bagley, C. (1971). *The social psychology of the epileptic child.* Coral Gables: University of Miami Press.

Bagley, C. (1972). Social prejudice and the adjustment of people with epilepsy. *Epilepsia* 13, 33–45.

Batzel, L. W., C. B. Dodrill, & R. T. Fraser. (1980). Further validation of the WPSI Vocational Scale: Comparisons with other correlates of employment in epilepsy. *Epilepsia* 21, 235–42.

Bear, D. (1979). Temporal lobe epilepsy: A syndrome of sensory-limbic hyperconnection. *Cortex* 15, 357–84.

Bear, D., & P. Fedio. (1977). Quantitative analysis of interictal behavior in temporal lobe epilepsy. *Archives of Neurology* 34, 454–67.

Bear, D., K. Levin, D. Blumer, D. Chetham, & J. Ryder. (1982). Interictal behavior in hospitalized temporal lobe epileptics: Relationship to idiopathic psychiatric syndromes. *Journal of Neurology, Neurosurgery, and Psychiatry* 45, 481–88.

Betts, T. A. (1974). A follow-up study of a cohort of patients with epilepsy admitted to psychiatric care in an English city. In P. Harris & C. Maudsley (Eds.), *Epilepsy—proceedings of the Hans Berger Centenary Symposium.* Edinburgh: Churchill-Livingstone.

Betts, T. A. (1981). Epilepsy and the mental hospital. In E. H. Reynolds & M. R. Trimble (Eds.), *Epilepsy and psychiatry.* Edinburgh: Churchill-Livingstone.

Betts, T. A. (1982). Psychiatry and epilepsy. In J. Laidlaw & A. Richens (Eds.), *A textbook of epilepsy* (2nd ed.). Edinburgh: Churchill-Livingstone.

Blumer, D. (1970). Hypersexual episodes in temporal lobe epilesy. *American Journal of Psychiatry* 126, 1099–1106.

Blumer, D. (1975). Temporal lobe epilepsy and its psychiatric significance. In D. F. Benson & D. Blumer (Eds.), *Psychiatric aspects of neurologic disease.* New York: Grune & Stratton.

Blumer, D. (1982). Specific psychiatric complication in certain forms of epilepsy and their treatment. In H. Sands (Ed.), *Epilepsy: A handbook for the mental health professional.* New York: Bruner/Mazel.

Botez, M. I., T. Botez, J. Léveillé, P. Bielmann, & M. Cadotte. (1979). Neuropsychological correlates of folic acid deficiency: Fact and hypotheses. In M. I. Botez & E. G. Reynolds (Eds.), *Folic acid in neurology, psychiatry and internal medicine.* New York: Raven Press.

Botez, M. I., F. Fontaine, T. Botez, & J. Bachevalier. (1977). Folate responsive neurological and mental disorders: Report of 16 cases. *European Neurology* 16, 230–36

Brady, J. P. (1964). Epilepsy and disturbed behavior. *Journal of Nervous and Mental Disease* 138, 468.

Brenner, M. H. (1973). *Mental illness and the economy.* Cambridge, MA: Harvard University Press.

Brenner, M. H. (1976). *Estimating the social costs of national economic policy: Implications for mental and physical health and criminal aggression.* Washington, DC: U.S. Government Printing Office.

Brenner, M. H. (1984). *Estimating the effects of economic change on national health and social well-being.* (Joint Economic Committee, Congress of the United States). Washington, DC: U.S. Government Printing Office.

Bruens, J. H. (1971). Psychoses in epilepsy. *Psychiatria, Neurologia, Neurochirurgia* 74, 175–92.

Bruens, J. H. (1974). Psychoses in epilepsy. In. P. L. Vinken & L. W. Bruyn (Eds.), *Handbook of clinical neurology* (Vol. 15). Amsterdam: North Holland.

Callaghan, N., R. Mitchell, & P. Cotter. (1969). The relationship of serum folic acid and vitamin B_{12} levels to psychosis in epilepsy. *Irish Journal of Medical Science* 2, 497–505.

Camfield, P. R., R. Gates, G. Ronen, C. Camfield, A. Ferguson, & G. W. McDonald. (1984). Comparison of cognitive ability, personality profile, and school success in epileptic children with pure right versus pure left temporal EEG foci. *Annals of Neurology* 15, 122–26.

Dalby, M. A. (1975). Behavioral effects of carbamazepine. In J. K. Penry & D. D. Daly (Eds.), *Advances in neurology* (Vol. 11). New York: Raven Press.

Dean. R. S. (1981). Neuropsychological correlates of total seizures with major motor epileptic children. *Clinical Neuropsychology* 5, 1–3.

del Ser Quijano, T., F. B. Pareja, D. Munoz-Garcia, & A. P. Sanchez. (1983). Psychological disturbances and folic acid in chronic epileptic outpatients. *Epilepsia* 24, 588–96.

DeVellis, R. G., B. M. DeVellis, B. S. Wallston, & K. A. Wallston. (1980). Epilepsy and learned helplessness. *Basic and Applied Social Psychology* 1, 241–53.

Dikmen, S., B. P. Hermann, A. Wilensky, & G. Rainwater. (1983). The validity of the MMPI to psychopathology in epilepsy. *Journal of Nervous and Mental Disease* 171, 114–22.

Dikmen, S., & S. F. Morgan. (1980). Neuropsychological factors related to employability and occupational status in persons with epilepsy. *Journal of Nervous and Mental Disease* 168, 236–40.

Dodrill, C. B. (1980). Interrelationships between neuropsychological data and social problems in epilepsy. In R. Canger, F. Angeleri, & J. K. Penry (Eds.), *Advances in epileptology: XIth Epilepsy International Symposium*. New York: Raven Press.

Dodrill, C. B. (1982). Neuropsychology. In J. Laidlaw & A. Richens (Eds.), *A textbook of epilepsy*. Edinburgh: Churchill-Livingstone.

Dodrill, C. B. (1983). Development of intelligence and neuropsychological impairment scales for the Washington Psychosocial Seizure Inventory. *Epilepsia* 24, 1–10.

Dodrill, C. B., L. W. Batzel, H. R. Queisser, & N. R. Temkin. (1980). An objective method for the assessment of psychological and social difficulties among epileptics. *Epilepsia* 21, 123–35.

Dohrenwend, B. S., & B. P. Dohrenwend. (1981). *Stressful life events and their contexts*. New York: Neale Watson Academic Publications.

Dominian, J., E. A. Serafetinides, & M. Dewhurst. (1963). A long-term follow-up of late onset epilepsy. II. Psychiatric and social. *British Medical Journal* 1, 431–35.

Edeh, J., & B. Toone. (1983). *A general practice study of the prevalence of psychiatric morbidity and social handicap in epilepsy and related clinical, neurophysiological, biochemical and therapeutic aspects*. Presented at the XVth Epilepsy International Symposium, Washington, DC.

Epilepsy Foundation of America (EFA). (1975). *Basic statistics on the epilepsies*. Philadelphia: F. A. Davis.

Fenton, G. W. (1981a). Psychiatric disorders of epilepsy: Classification of phenomenology. In E. H. Reynolds & M. R. Trimble (Eds.), *Epilepsy and psychiatry*. Edinburgh: Churchill-Livingstone.

Fenton, G. W. (1981b). Personality and behavioral disorders in adults with epilepsy. In E. H. Reynolds & M. R. Trimble (Eds.), *Epilepsy and psychiatry*. Edinburgh: Churchill-Livingstone.

Fenwick, P. B., D. Master, & D. Brown. (1981). Relationship between ventricular volume, cortical atrophy, and epilepsy. In M. Dam, L. Gram, & J. K. Penry, (Eds.), *Advances in epileptology: XIIth Epilepsy International Symposium*. New York: Raven Press.

Ferguson, S. M., M. Rayport, R. Gardner, W. Kass, H. Weiner, & M. F. Reiser. (1969). Similarities in mental content of psychotic states, spontaneous seizures, dreams, and responses to electrical brain stimulation in patients with temporal lobe epilepsy. *Psychosomatic Medicine* 31, 479–97.

Flor-Henry, P. (1969). Psychosis and temporal lobe epilepsy: A controlled investigation. *Epilepsia* 10, 363–95.

Flor-Henry, P. (1972). Ictal and interictal psychiatric manifestations in epilepsy: Specific or non-specific? *Epilepsia* 13, 773–83.

Flor-Henry, P. (1982). Hemisyndromes of temporal lobe epilepsy: Review of evidence relating psychopathological manifestations in epilepsy to right and left-sided epilepsy. In M. Myslobodsky (Ed.), *Hemisyndromes: Psychobiology, neurology, and psychiatry*. New York: Academic Press.

Flor-Henry, P. (1983). Determinants of psychosis in epilepsy: Laterality and forced normalization. *Biological Psychiatry* 18, 1045–57.

Fraser, R. T. (1980). Vocational aspects of epilepsy. In B. P. Hermann (Ed.), *A multidisciplinary handbook of epilepsy*. Springfield, IL: Thomas.

Geschwind, N. (1983) Interictal behavioral changes in epilepsy. *Epilepsia* 24 (Supp. 1), 523–30.

Gibbs, F. A., E. L. Gibbs, & B. Fuster. (1948). Psychomotor epilepsy. *Archives of Neurology and Psychiatry* 60, 331–39.

Gibbs, F. A., & F. W. Stamps. (1958). *Epilepsy handbook*. Springfield, IL: Thomas.

Glass, D. H., & R. J. Mattson. (1973). Psychopathology and emotional precipitation of seizures in temporal lobe and nontemporal lobe epileptics. *Proceedings of the 81st Annual Convention of the American Psychological Association* 8, 425–26.

Goldberg, L. R. (1972). Man versus mean: The exploitation of group profiles for the construction of diagnostic classification systems. *Journal of Abnormal Psychology* 79, 121–31.

Grant, H. C., A. V. Hoffbrand, & D. G. Well. (1965). Folate deficiency and neurological disease. *Lancet* 2, 763–67.

Gudmundsson, G. (1966). Epilepsy in Iceland. *Acta Neurologica Scandinavica* (Supp. 25), 43.

Gunn, J. (1977). *Epileptics in prison*. New York: Academic Press.

Hermann, B. P. (1981). Deficits in neuropsychological functioning and psychopathology in epilepsy: A rejected hypothesis revisited. *Epilepsia* 22, 161 67.

Hermann, B. P. (1982). Neuropsychological functioning and psychopathology in children with epilepsy. *Epilepsia* 23, 545–54.

Hermann, B. P., R. B. Black, & S. Chhabria. (1981a). Behavioral problems and social competence in children with epilepsy. *Epilepsia* 22, 703–10.

Hermann, B. P., & S. Chhabria. (1981). Interictal psychopathology in patients with ictal fear: Examples of sensory-limbic hyperconnection? *Archives of Neurology* 37, 667–68.

Hermann, B. P., S. Dikmen, M. S. Schwartz, & W. E. Karnes. (1982a). Psychopathology in TLE patients with ictal fear: A quantitative investigation. *Neurology* 32, 7–11.

Hermann, B. P., S. Dikmen, & A. Wilensky. (1982b). Increased psychopathology associated with multiple seizure types: Fact or artifact? *Epilepsia* 23, 587–96.

Hermann, B. P., M. S. Schwartz, W. E. Karnes, & P. Vahdat. (1980a). Psychopathology in epilepsy: Relationship of seizure type to age at onset. *Epilepsia* 21, 15–23.

Hermann, B. P., M. S. Schwartz, S. Whitman, & W. E. Karnes. (1980b). Aggression and epilepsy: Seizure type comparisons and high risk variables. *Epilepsia* 22, 691–98.

Hermann, B. P., M. S. Schwartz, S. Whitman, & W. E. Karnes. (1981b). Psychosis and epilepsy: Seizure type comparisons and high risk variables. *Journal of Clinical Psychology* 37, 714–21.

Hermann, B. P., & S. Whitman. (1984). Behavioral and personality correlates of epilepsy: A review, methodological critique and conceptual model. *Psychological Bulletin* 95, 451–97.

Howard, J. S. (1975). Folate deficiency in psychiatric practice. *Psychosomatics* 16, 112–15.

Jensen, I., & J. K. Larsen. (1979). Psychoses in drug resistant temporal lobe epilepsy. *Journal of Neurology, Neurosurgery and Psychiatry* 42, 948–54.

Kogeorgos, J., P. Fonagy, & D. F. Scott, (1982). Psychiatric symptom profiles of chronic epileptics attending a neurologic clinic: A controlled investigation. *British Journal of Psychiatry* 140, 236–43.

Kristensen, O., & E. H. Sindrup. (1978). Psychomotor epilepsy and psychosis. I. Physical aspects. *Acta Neurologica Scandinavica* 57, 361–69.

Kristensen, O., & E. H. Sindrup. (1979). Psychomotor epilepsy and psychosis. III. Social and psychological correlates. *Acta Neurologica Scandinavica* 59, 1–9.

Lacher, D., R. Lewis, & T. Kupke. (1979). MMPI in differentiation of temporal lobe and non-temporal lobe epilepsy: Investigation of three levels of test performance. *Journal of Consulting and Clinical Psychology* 47, 186–88.

Laidlaw, J., & M. V. Laidlaw. (1982). People with epilepsy—living with epilepsy. In J. Laidlaw & A. Richens (Eds.), *A textbook of epilepsy.* Edinburgh: Churchill-Livingstone.

Lefcourt, H. M. (1976). *Locus of control: Current trends in theory and research.* New York: Erlbaum.

Lennox, W. G., & M. A. Lennox. (1960). *Epilepsy and related disorders* (2 vols.). Boston: Little, Brown.

Lindsay, J., C. Ounsted, & P. Richards. (1979). Long term outcome in children with temporal lobe epilepsy. III. Psychiatric manifestations in adult life. *Developmental Medicine and Child Neurology* 21, 630–36.

Linnett, M. F. (1982). People with epilepsy—the burden of epilepsy. In. J. Laidlaw & A. Richens (Eds.), *A textbook of epilepsy* (2nd ed.). Edinburgh: Churchill-Livingstone.

Lishman, W. A. (1978). *Organic psychiatry: The psychological consequences of cerebral disorder.* Oxford: Blackwell Scientific Publications.

Matthews, C. G., S. Dikmen, & J. P. Harley. (1977). Age at onset and psychometric correlates of MMPI profiles in major motor epilepsy. *Diseases of the Nervous System* 38, 173–76.

Matthews, C. G., & H. Klove. (1968). MMPI performance in major motor, psychomotor and mixed seizure classifications of known and unknown etiology. *Epilepsia* 9, 43–53.

Matthews, W. S., G. Barabas, & M. Ferrari. (1982). Emotional concomitants of childhood epilepsy. *Epilepsia* 23, 671–81.

McIntyre, M., P. B. Pritchard, & C. Lombroso. (1976). Left and right temporal lobe epileptics: A controlled investigation of some psychological differences. *Epilepsia* 17, 377–86.

Meier, M. J., & L. A. French, (1965). Some personality correlates of unilateral and bilateral EEG abnormalities in psychomotor epileptics. *Journal of Clinical Psychology* 21, 3–9.

Melamed, E., A. Reches, & C. Hereshko. (1975). Reversible central nervous system dysfunction in folate deficiency. *Journal of Neurological Science* 25, 93–98.

Mignone, R. J., E. F. Donnelly, & D. Sadowsky. (1970). Psychological and neurological comparisons of psychomotor and non-psychomotor epileptic patients. *Epilepsia* 11, 345–59.

Mittan, R. (1983). *Patients fears about seizures: A greater psychosocial stressor?* Presented at the XVth Epilepsy International Symposium, Washington, DC.

Mittan, R., & G. E. Locke. (1982a). The other half of epilepsy: Psychosocial problems. *Urban Health,* January/February, 38–39.

Mittan, R., & G. E. Locke. (1982b). Fear of seizures: Epilepsy's forgotten problem. *Urban Health,* January/February, 40–41.

Mittan, R., C. Wasterlain, & G. E. Locke. (1981). *Medical misinformation, fears about seizures, and their potential contribution to epileptics' poor psychosocial adjustment.* Presented at the Annual Meeting of the American Epilepsy Society, New York.

Moehle, K. A., J. F. Bolter, & C. J. Long. (1984). The relationship between neuropsychological functioning and psychopathology in temporal lobe epileptic patients. *Epilepsia* 25, 418–22.

National Commission for the Control of Epilepsy and Its Consequences. (1978). *Plan for nationwide action on epilepsy.* (DHEW Publication No. NIH 78-276). Washington, DC: U.S. Government Printing Office.

Nielsen, H., & O. Kristensen. (1981). Personality correlates of sphenoidal EEG foci in temporal lobe epilepsy. *Acta Neurologica Scandinavica* 64, 289–300.

Notkin. J. (1928). Is there an epileptic personality make-up? *Archives of Neurology and Psychiatry* 20, 799–803.

Ounsted, C. (1969). Agression and epilepsy: Rage in children with temporal lobe epilepsy. *Journal of Psychosomatic Research* 13, 237–42.

Pond, D. A. (1957). Psychiatric aspects of epilepsy. *Journal of the Indian Medical Profession* 3, 1441–51.

Pond, D. A., & B. H. Bidwell. (1960). A survey of epilepsy in fourteen general practices. II. Social and psychological aspects. *Epilepsia* 1, 285–99.

Ramani, V., & R. J. Gumnit. (1981). Intensive monitoring of epileptic patients with a history of episodic aggression. *Archives of Neurology* 38, 570–71.

Ramani, V., & R. J. Gumnit. (1982). Intensive monitoring of interictal psychosis in epilepsy. *Annals of Neurology* 11, 613–22.

Ray, J. J. (1982). Toward a definitive alienation scale. *Journal of Psychology* 112, 67–70.

Reynolds, E. H. (1967). Schizophrenia-like psychosis of epilepsy and disturbances of folate and B_{12} metabolism induced by anticonvulsant drugs. *British Journal of Psychiatry* 113, 911–19.

Reynolds, E. H. (1968). Epilepsy and schizophrenia: Relationship and biochemistry. *Lancet* 1, 398–401.

Reynolds, E. H. (1971). Anticonvulsant drugs, folic acid metabolism, fit frequency and psychiatric illness. *Psychiatria, Neurologia, Neurochirurgia* 74, 167–74.

Reynolds, E. H. (1976). Neurological aspects of folate and B_{12} metabolism. In A. V. Hoffbrand (Ed.), *Clinics in haematology* (Vol. 5). London: Saunders.

Reynolds, E. H. (1981). Biological factors in psychological disorders associated with epilepsy. In E. H. Reynolds and M. R. Trimble (Eds.), *Psychiatry and epilepsy.* Edinburgh: Churchill-Livingstone.

Reynolds, E. H. (1982). Anticonvulsants and mental symptoms. In M. Sandler (Ed.), *Psychopharmacology of anticonvulsants.* New York: Oxford University Press.

Reynolds, E. H. (1983). Mental effects of antiepileptic medication: A review. *Epilepsia* 24 (Supp. 2), S85–S96.

Reynolds, E. H., & R. D. Travers. (1974). Serum anticonvulsant concentrations in epileptic patients with mental symptoms. *British Journal of Psychiatry* 124, 440–45.

Robertson, M. (1983). *Depression and epilepsy.* Presented at the XVth Epilepsy International Symposium, Washington, DC.

Robertson, M., & M. R. Trimble. (1983). Depressive illness in patients with epilepsy: A review. *Epilepsia* 24 (Supp. 2), S109–S116.

Rodin, E. (1973). Psychomotor epilepsy and aggressive behavior. *Archives of General Psychiatry* 28, 210–13.

Rodin, E. A. (1982). Aggression and epilepsy. In T. L. Riley & A. Roy (Eds.), *Pseudoseizures.* Baltimore, MD: Williams & Wilkins.

Rodin, E., M. Katz, & D. Lennox. (1976). Differences between patients with temporal lobe seizures and those with other forms of epileptic attacks. *Epilepsia* 17, 313–20.

Rodin, E., & S. Schmaltz. (1983). The Bear-Fedio personality inventory and temporal lobe epilepsy. *Epilepsia* 24, 260.

Rutter, M., P. Graham, & W. Yule. (1970). *A neuropsychiatric study in childhood.* Philadelphia: Lippincott.

Ryan, R., K. Kempner, & A. C. Emlen. (1980). The stigma of epilepsy as a self-concept. *Epilepsia* 21, 433–44.

Sachdev, H. S., & S. G. Waxman. (1981). Frequency of hypergraphia in temporal lobe epilepsy: An index of interictal behavior syndrome. *Journal of Neurology, Neurosurgery and Psychiatry* 44, 358–60.

Sarason, I. G., H. M. Levine, R. B. Basham, & B. R. Sarason. (1983). Assessing social support: The Social Support Questionnaire. *Journal of Personality and Social Psychology* 44, 127–39.

Saunders, M., & M. R. Rawson. (1970). Sexuality in male epileptics. *Journal of the Neurological Sciences* 10, 577–83.

Schoenberg, B. (1982). The scope of neuroepidemiology from Stone Age to Stockholm. *Neuroepidemiology* 1, 1–16.

Scott, D. F. (1978). Psychiatric aspects of epilepsy. *British Journal of Psychiatry* 132, 417–30.

Serafetinides, E. A. (1965). Aggressiveness in temporal lobe epileptics and its relation to cerebral dysfunction and environmental factors. *Epilepsia* 6, 33–42.

Sherwin, I. (1977). Clinical and EEG aspects of temporal lobe epilepsy with behavior disorder: The role of cerebral dominance [Special issue]. *McLean Hospital Journal,* 40–50.

Sherwin, I. (1981). Psychosis associated with epilepsy: Significance of the laterality of the epileptogenic lesion. *Journal of Neurology, Neurosurgery and Psychiatry* 44, 83–85.

Sherwin I. (1982). Neurobiological basis of psychopathology associated with epilepsy. In H. Sands (Ed.), *Epilepsy: A handbook for the mental health professional.* New York: Brunner/Mazel.

Sherwin, I., P. Peron-Magnan, J. Bancaud, A. Bonis, & J. Talairach. (1982). Prevalence of psychosis in epilepsy as a function of the laterality of the epileptogenic lesion. *Archives of Neurology* 39, 621–25.

Shorvon, S. D., & E. H. Reynolds. (1979). Reduction of polypharmacy for epilepsy. *British Medical Journal* 2, 1023–25.

Shukla, G. D., O. N. Srivastava, & B. C. Katiyar. (1979). Sexual disturbances in temporal lobe epilepsy: A controlled study. *British Journal of Psychiatry* 134, 288–92.

Slater, E., A. W. Beard, & E. Glithero. (1963). The schizophrenia-like psychoses of epilepsy. *British Journal of Psychiatry* 109, 95–150.

Snaith, R. P., S. Mehta, & A. H. Raby. (1970). Serum folate and vitamin B_{12} in epileptics with and without mental illness. *British Journal of Psychiatry* 116, 179–83.

Standage, K. F. (1981). Psychopathology in epilepsy. *Journal of the Irish Medical Association* 74, 271–82.

Standage, K. F., & G. W. Fenton. (1975). Psychiatric symptom profiles of patients with epilepsy: A controlled investigation. *Psychological Medicine* 5, 152–60.

Stevens, J. R. (1966). Psychiatric implications of psychomotor epilepsy. *Archives of General Psychiatry* 14, 461–71.

Stevens, J. R. (1975). Interictal clinical manifestation of complex partial seizures. In J. K. Penry & D. D. Daly (Eds.), *Advances in neurology* (Vol. 11). New York: Raven Press.

Stevens, J. R. & B. P. Hermann. (1981). Temporal lobe epilepsy, psychopathology, and violence: The state of the evidence. *Neurology* 31, 1127–32.

Stevens, J. R., V. Milstein, & S. Goldstein. (1972). Psychometric test performance in relation to the psychopathology of epilepsy. *Archives of General Psychiatry* 26, 532–38.

Strauss, E., A. Risser, & M. W. Jones. (1982). Fear response in patients with epilepsy. *Archives of Neurology* 39, 626–30.

Taylor, D. B. (1969a). Sexual behavior and temporal lobe epilepsy. *Archives of Neurology* 21, 510–16.

Taylor, D. C. (1969b). Aggression and epilepsy. *Journal of Psychosomatic Research* 13, 229–36.

Taylor, D. C. (1975). Factors influencing the occurrence of schizophrenia-like psychoses in patients with temporal lobe epilepsy. *Psychological Medicine* 5, 249–54.

Temkin, N. R., & G. R. Davis. (1984). Stress as a risk factor for seizures among adults with epilepsy. *Epilepsia* 25, 450–56.

Thompson, P., F. A. Huppert, & M. R. Trimble. (1981). Phenytoin and cognitive function: Effects on normal volunteers and implications for epilepsy. *British Journal of Clinical Psychology* 20, 155–62.

Thompson, P. J., & M. R. Trimble. (1981). Further studies on anticonvulsant drugs and seizures. *Acta Neurologica Scandinavica* 64 (Supp. 89), 51–58.

Thompson, P. J., & M. R. Trimble. (1982). Anticonvulsant drugs and cognitive functions. *Epilepsia* 23, 531–44.

Toone, B. (1981). Psychoses of epilepsy. In E. H. Reynolds & M. R. Trimble (Eds.), *Epilepsy and psychiatry.* Edinburgh: Churchill-Livingstone.

Toone, B. (1983). *Sexual function and sex hormone patterns in male epileptics on anticonvulsants.* Presented at the XVth Epilepsy International Symposium, Washington, DC.

Toone, B. K., M. Wheeler, M. Nanjee, P. Fenwick, & R. Grant. (1983). Sex hormones, sexual drive and plasma anticonvulsant levels in male epileptics. *Journal of Neurology, Neurosurgery and Psychiatry* 46, 824–26.

Trimble, M. R. (1977). The relationship between epilepsy and schizophrenia: A biochemical hypothesis. *Biological Psychiatry* 12, 299–304.

Trimble, M. R. (1983). Personality disturbances in epilepsy. *Neurology* 33, 1332–34.

Trimble, M. R., J. A. Corbett, & D. Donaldson. (1980). Folic acid and mental symptoms in children with epilepsy. *Journal of Neurology, Neurosurgery, and Psychiatry* 43, 1030–34.

Trimble, M. R., & E. H. Reynolds. (1976). Anticonvulsant drugs and mental symptoms: A review. *Psychological Medicine* 6, 169–78.

Trimble, M. R., P. J. Thompson, & J. A. Corbett. (1982). Anticonvulsant drugs, cognitive function, and behavior. In M. Sandler (Ed.), *Psychopharmacology of anticonvulsants*. Oxford: Oxford University Press.

Whitman, S., T. Coleman, B. Berg, L. King, & B. Desai. (1980). Epidemiological insights into the socioeconomic correlates of epilepsy. In B. P. Hermann (Ed.), *A multidisciplinary handbook of epilepsy*. Springfield, IL: Thomas.

Whitman, S., & B. P. Hermann. (Submitted for publication, 1985). The structure of research in the epilepsy/psychopathology debate and its relationship to sociopolitical themes.

Whitman, S., B. P. Hermann, R. B. Black, & S. Chhabria. (1982). Psychopathology and seizure type in children with epilepsy. *Psychological Medicine* 12, 843–53.

Williams, D. (1981). The emotions and epilepsy. In E. H. Reynolds & M. R Trimble (Eds.), *Epilepsy and psychiatry*. London: Churchill-Livingstone.

2 / Selected Psychiatric and Psychosocial Aspects of Epilepsy as Seen by an Epidemiologist

JANUSZ J. ZIELINSKI

Epilepsy is one of the most common of all chronic conditions and *the* most common among chronic neurological disorders. Its multiple, varying psychiatric and psychosocial implications have been studied for decades and reviewed in numerous papers, but there remains a great deal of controversy among various authors. Although for centuries a seizure has been considered the basic manifestation of epilepsy, the contemporary criteria for the diagnosis and classification of seizures were established only recently. Still less is known about the more permanent psychic phenomena that occur interictally in some individuals with epilepsy. No satisfactory answers to the many questions pertaining to the psychosocial implications of epilepsy can, however, be fully provided by studying small case series distorted by sampling bias. Psychiatric and psychosocial implications of epilepsy preferably should be studied in the general population or its random samples—in other words, in an epidemiologist's laboratory.

Epidemiology is concerned not only with the frequency and distribution of various disorders, disabilities, and deaths in the human population, but also with identifying biological, clinical, physical, and social factors related to the occurrence, course, and outcome of a disease. The epidemiologic methods, terms, rates, and indexes must always be defined as clearly and unequivocally as possible. There is no doubt that the very basic condition of any evaluative research is to define clearly the subjects studied, along with the methodological approached used. Unfortunately, both epidemiology and epidemiologic terms are occasionally misused in the epilepsy/psychopathology literature.

The purpose of the present chapter is to discuss some of the more crucial findings in the field of research concerned with the psychiatric, psychosocial, and socioeconomic implications of epilepsy. As the controversy between the findings and conclusions of various authors frequently may result from different methodological approaches, special attention will be paid to these approaches. As will be seen, many of these are severe enough to influence the reliability of the investigators' results and conclusions.

The first topic discussed involves shortcomings that stem from unrecognized mechanisms underlying the formation of case series (sampling bias), absence of clear definitions of epilepsy and psychopathology, improperly chosen or missing control groups, negligence of methodological differences in comparing results from various studies, and finally, tendencies toward generalization of findings from small case series.

Next to be discussed will be the frequency of epilepsy as based on the results of variously designed studies. Included in this discussion will be a review of the methodological problems involved in the epidemiology of epilepsy. Next, the psychiatric manifestations of epilepsy as reflected in case series studies will be reviewed followed by a discussion of the same topic as reflected in epidemiologic studies. Finally, the importance of socioeconomic variables will be reviewed.

EPILEPSY: CASE SERIES STUDIES VERSUS EPIDEMIOLOGIC RESEARCH

Epidemiologic research has to be carried on in a strictly defined population (at least in terms of numbers, time, geographic area, and basic demographic variables) or in a random sample from such a population. Contrary to this, case series usually stem from undefined populations and the authors are often not aware of the actual mechanisms responsible for the formation of their sample. As a rule, such case series are liable to be severely biased. However, if an attempt is made to ascertain all the patients diagnosed in a defined population, such an "extended case series," especially if collected over a period of time, might then become "a register" that in turn can be used for an epidemiologic survey.

Definitions, Selection of Patients, and Mechanisms of Case Series Formation

As mentioned earlier, the definition of "a case" is a crucial factor when considering the reliability of the results obtained and the conclusions derived from a study. Epilepsy is primarily a clinical diagnosis based on the presence of recurring seizures. Most physicians, however, rarely have an opportunity to observe a seizure personally, and they therefore have to rely on the reports of witnesses. This can seriously influence the accuracy of the physician's diagnosis and classification of the patient's seizures. Similarly, the patient's ability to report experiences occurring before or during the seizure is very important for proper diagnosis and classification, especially in cases of temporal lobe epilepsy. Moreover, diagnosis and classification of some seizures may remain questionable even if they are recorded and observed by the expert. Obtaining such information can be even more difficult, if not impossible, among patients with concomitant mental retardation.

Problems of definition and classification are not limited to neurological concepts. Definitions of *psychosis*, *schizophrenia*, *schizophrenialike syndrome*, or *depression* may also be difficult, and comparisons of results obtained by various authors may be invalid because of different or nonspecified diagnostic criteria. Diagnoses made by means of questionnaires or scales may allow for better comparability of results obtained from various samples, assuming that the same questionnaire is used. Thus, comparisons of the results obtained by means of different tools may be difficult and/or unreliable.

The mechanisms underlying the formation of a case series are important, as little-appreciated sources of bias may generate incorrect conclusions. An "unselected case series" or a series of "consecutive admissions" is frequently considered sufficient proof of the "representativeness" of an analyzed sample of patients. In fact, the precise mechanisms underlying the formation of a case series may be largely unknown to investigators. Generally speaking, case series can be derived from the following sources:

- Primary health-care services (primary care physicians, pediatric clinics, etc.)
- Neurological facilities
- Psychiatric facilities
- Neurosurgical facilities
- Special centers (e.g., for epilepsy)
- Death certificates
- Postmortem series.

The more benign the case of epilepsy, the lower the probability that the patient will appear beyond the level of primary care. Even at the primary health-care level many benign cases of epilepsy will be unknown and the only way of finding such cases is through a population-based epidemiologic survey. This can be demonstrated from the results of an epidemiologic survey of epilepsy in Warsaw, Poland, conducted in 1969.

In the Warsaw population study, only 35% of the people identified as having epilspsy were being treated at the time of the survey, and 26% had never been previously diagnosed; that is, they were discovered to have epilepsy during the course of the survey (Zielinski, 1974, 1976). Of the latter, a majority had brief partial seizures, mostly of temporal lobe origin, which the patients considered unworthy of treatment even if they had suffered from sporadic major motor seizures in the past. Another 10% had been seen previously by doctors and diagnosed as having epilepsy but refused to start taking anticonvulsants. Again, most of these people suffered from partial seizures only or infrequent major motor attacks (or both). These patients were either unconcerned about their seizures, afraid of hospitalization (e.g., for diagnostic tests; at the time of this survey CAT scan techniques were not available), or did not believe the treatment was effective. Finally, 29% were diagnosed and treated in the past; half of them (or 15% of the total group) had discontinued anticonvulsant medications on their own for various reasons, such as disappearance of seizures, side effects of medications, or the high cost of the drugs.

Thus, in neurological and especially in neurosurgical facilities, more severe and complicated cases of epilepsy prevail. Contrary to that, there is little chance of someone being admitted to a *psychiatric* department only because of epileptic seizures, with the exception of prolonged confusional states or temporal lobe status epilepticus, both of which are rare. Thus, the mechanisms responsible for the formation of a case series selected from a psychiatric or neurosurgical facility might actually be attributable to the previous level of care (i.e., general or neurological facilities) and ultimately be a function of the severity of the patient's epilepsy.

Factors other than medical may also play a role in the formation of a case series: Patients seeking medical care in specialty centers or university hospitals may do so because of severe epilepsy, multiple health problems, or low socioeconomic position (Hauser, 1972; Rodin, 1968; Rodin, Shapiro, & Lennox, 1977; Stevens, 1975; Zielinski, 1972). Additionally, a significant percentage of patients with poorly controlled epilepsy will be mentally handicapped. This observation is not novel. In 1907 Turner wrote: "There is a direct association between frequency of seizures and the mental state, for the more frequent the attacks, the greater degree of mental impairment and vice versa." (p. 153).

It should also be mentioned that admission rates to psychiatric hospitals yield a misleading estimate of the number of patients actually admitted, unless only first admissions are considered, since the more severe the course of epilepsy or psychiatric disorder, the higher the chance of readmission. Socioeconomic features might also play a role in hospital admissions processes (see Socioeconomic Variables). Admissions with a diagnosis of epilepsy constitute from 3% to 19% of all admissions to mental hospitals (Slater & Roth, 1969), but this finding has little epidemiologic value. Thus, case series of patients with epilepsy selected from such settings are very likely to be biased.

The preceding considerations similarly apply to the pediatric population. Recently Ellenberg and Nelson (1980), on the basis of an extensive review of the literature concerning febrile seizures, concluded that the prognosis of developing epilepsy was much worse in selected case series of children than in population-oriented studies.

Overdiagnosis of Epilepsy

Not only are real cases of epilepsy missed at some levels of care, but individuals commonly are mistakenly diagnosed as having epilepsy. Overdiagnosis of epilepsy is especially frequent among case series derived from primary health-care facilities, although this also occasionally occurs in psychiatric facilities. For example, a diagnosis of epilepsy could not be confirmed during reexamination in approximately 15% of patients previously diagnosed as "epileptic" in the Warsaw study. The highest percentage of overdiagnosis was found in pediatric and psychiatric facilities, especially child psychiatry facilities (Zielinski, 1974). Similar problems of overdiagnosis were recently encountered in the National Child Developmental Study in Great Britain: Of 103 children reported by their general practitioners or consultants as having epilepsy, the diagnosis could not be substantiated in 39 (Ross & Peckham, 1983).

Control Groups

Even when cases of epilepsy are appropriately identified, comparisons to control groups are needed to inform us of relevant risk factors. Numerous studies based on selected case series make no attempt whatsoever to compare their findings to a control group. For example, a recent review of the literature revealed that only 8 of 64 studies (12%) had used nonepilepsy control groups (Hermann & Whitman, 1984). The distribution of clinical findings and other features nevertheless is reported and/or compared between variously selected subgroups. Despite the use of sophisticated statistical methods, such conclusions must be limited to the case series under investigation or, at best, may be extended only to other similarly selected case series. Results derived from such studies are frequently unrepresentative of all people with a history of seizures in a general population.

However, finding a satisfactory control group is not always easy. In 1946 Joseph Berkson, a physician at the Mayo Clinic, noted that the relative frequency of a disease among hospitalized patients may be different when compared to that of a population in a hospital catchment area. Because the risk of hospitalization is higher for those suffering from more than one disease, epidemiologic studies based on hospitalized populations will likely be biased. The same consideration pertains to hospitalized patients entered as controls in any clinical studies. Berkson's hypothesis (or "paradox") has recently been confirmed by Roberts, Spitzer, Delmore, and Sackett (1978) for some internal diseases. There are no known psychiatric or neurological studies on similar topics, but in a random sample of general practices in England a positive relationship was found between the occurrence of physical and psychiatric disorders (Eastwood & Trevelyan, 1972).

An extensive discussion of appropriate methods for the selection of control groups is beyond the scope of this chapter. Recently, Leviton and Cowan (1981) have reviewed these problems as they pertain to childhood epilepsy. The preceding remarks, however, may illustrate the various methodological difficulties often seen in studies of selected groups of patients with epilepsy or psychosis or both.

Epidemiologic Studies of Epilepsy

Before one can meaningfully discuss the prevalence of psychosocial and emotional disorders in epilepsy, one first must have a clear understanding of the prevalence of epilepsy. This is, however, a very formidable task. A brief discussion of the literature pertaining to the epidemiology of epilepsy will be presented that will include some of the more pertinent methodological and conceptual problems. This discussion will then lead us into evaluation of the psychiatric risk associated with epilepsy.

Early studies on epilepsy usually were based on reviews of records from various medical facilities or other institutions. One of the very first epidemiologic surveys of epilepsy was carried out in Michigan (Anderson, 1936). Anderson studied nine counties in Michigan's lower peninsula, an area with a population of 73,056. He found a total of 154 cases, including 46 in various state institutions and 108 in the population at large. Among the latter, only 62% "were or had been under medical care" (a strikingly similar ratio to that of the Warsaw study some 40 years later). Anderson estimated the total prevalence rate of epilepsy to be 2.1 per 1,000. More recent studies based on known epilepsy cases, as well as data from medical facilities, yielded very similar prevalence rates: 1.5/1,000 in Niigata City, Japan (Sato, 1964), 3.5/1,000 in Northern Norway (De Graaf, 1974), and 2.8/1,000 in sampled areas of Poland (Zielinski, 1974).

Incidence and Lifetime ("Total") Prevalence

It may be helpful to briefly review the definitions of the basic epidemiologic indexes that illustrate the frequency of a disorder in a community. *Incidence rate* is calculated according to the number of new cases of a disorder in a defined population. For neurological and psychiatric disorders an interval of 1 year is usually considered. If the incidence is calculated on the basis of new cases diagnosed in medical facilities, the term *first attendance rate* might be preferred.

Prevalence rate refers to the proportion of people afflicted with a disorder in a defined population. In most chronic disorders with low mortality, incidence rates may be relatively small whereas prevalence rates may be high. This is true for epilepsy and many psychiatric disorders, especially for schizophrenia. Point prevalence rates (rates computed for a specific moment in time rather than an interval of time) are frequently underestimated: Persons who died or, more often, have dropped out from medical care might not be counted in the survey.

Another effective measurement is the *accumulated incidence,* or the sum of the age-specific incidence rates. If the mortality rate is low and case ascertainment methods effective, the accumulated incidence rate at each specific age interval will be close to the point-prevalence rate for that age. In epilepsy, however, with the exception of severe cases, the case ascertainment procedure is usually incomplete. Therefore, the accumulated incidence gives a better estimation of the number of people with epilepsy (or history of epilepsy) in the population. Calculation of the accumulated incidence is possible only if a defined population is carefully observed for the occurrence of new cases of epilepsy over a longer period of time (decades).

Average annual incidence rates for epilepsy that have been estimated by various authors vary between 11 and 54 per 100,000, but most often fall between 20 and 50 per 100,000 (Hauser, 1978; Zielinski, 1982). Incidence and prevalence rates for epilepsy are usually at least twice as high among younger poeple than among adults. Such trends in prevalence rates could be explained in two ways: Either a great number of children with epilepsy die before reaching adulthood, or in a considerable percentage of these children the seizures cease for an indefinite period of time if not forever. The former hypothesis has been supported in studies of highly selected series of individuals with severe epilepsy (e.g., Lindsay, Ounsted, & Richards, 1979), and the latter hypothesis has been found to be consistent with the results derived from many population-oriented, longitudinal studies. These latter studies provide a definitely more optimistic outlook for epilepsy. Twenty years after diagnosis, 70% of the Rochester, Minnesota, patients were found to be seizure free for at least 5 years, and 50% of those were no longer on anticonvulsants (Annegers, Hauser, & Elveback, 1979). A follow-up of the Warsaw patients determined that 37% had been seizure free for over 5 years and over 60% for 2 years. This latter estimate is reliable because the patient's seizure-free status was confirmed not only by the patients themselves, but also by their family members, doctors, and other knowledgeable informants. Those individuals who were seizure free for long periods of time, however, were most reluctant to provide information during the follow-up interview as they considered themselves "cured" and unwilling to discuss their "past disorder" (Zielinski, Kuran, & Witowska-Olearska, 1978).

Seizure Type

The distribution of seizure types is often analyzed in case series derived from various outpatient and inpatient departments, epilepsy centers, or electroencephalographic (EEG) laboratories. Unfortunately, only a few epidemiologic or population-oriented studies have inquired into seizure type distributions.

The percentage of individuals with "primary generalized" seizures is similar in series derived from Rochester, Warsaw, and France, ranging from 34% to 38%. (See Table 2-1.) Individuals with temporal lobe seizures constituted the highest percentage among population samples from Warsaw, France, and Denmark, whereas in India and Rochester they comprised the lowest percentage. In view of population-based studies, the percentage of temporal lobe epilepsy can be considered to constitute about 40% of all epilepsies and even this figure may be an underestimation. Complex partial seizures, if not secondarily generalized, might be very difficult to identify even during a population survey (Zielinski, 1976).

Undiagnosed Epilepsy

As in many other chronic disorders (including psychiatric ones) it seems virtually impossible to ascertain all cases of epilepsy in a surveyed population. A previous investigation by this author can be used to illustrate the difficulties that may arise during a population field survey. Two groups of persons with epilepsy were compared: patients from various medical facilities in Warsaw with diagnosed epilepsy ("known epilepsy"—Group K) and persons with epilepsy selected from a sample of the Warsaw population irrespective of their medical attendance ("field study"—Group F). Prevalence rates per 1,000 by various clinical variables in these groups were as follows:

	Group K	*Group F*
Overall	4.3	9.2
In remission for over 5 years	0.5	1.4
On antiepileptic drugs when examined	3.3	3.2
On antiepileptic drugs at any time	3.9	5.2
Seizures or on drugs during last 5 years ("active cases")	4.2	7.8
Number of subjects	312	98

Moreover, among the subjects in Group F, 26% had never been previously diagnosed. In summary, of those with epilepsy living in a given area at a given time, only 30%–40% consulted a physician, 25% were treated sometime in the past, and over 35% were never treated, including the 25% never previously diagnosed (Zielinski, 1974).

In conclusion, epidemiologic studies can provide data whose value extends far beyond the evaluation of the actual frequency of seizure disorders in a given population. From the results of these studies we can learn more about the actual distribution of various clinical and social features of the people with

TABLE 2–1. Relative Frequency of Generalized and Partial Seizures in Case Series of Patients with Epilepsy and Individuals with Epilepsy Found During Selected Studies (in %)

	Epidemiological Surveys				Case Series		
	Rochester[a]	Warsaw[b]		Bogotá[c]			
Type of Seizure		Known Cases	Field Survey		4,590 Private Patients with Epilepsy, France[d]	265 Outpatients Epilepsy Clinic, India[e]	1508 "Consecutive" Patients, Age 15+ Epilepsy Clinic University Hospital, Denmark[f]
Generalized	34	48	35	73	38	18	24
Partial	66	52	65	27	62	82	76
Temporal lobe (psychomotor, complex partial)	27	34	43		40	13	40

[a]Hauser & Kurland (1975).
[b]Zielinski (1974).
[c]Gomez et al. (1978).
[d]Gastaut et al. (1975).
[e]Joshi et al. (1977).
[f]Alving (1978).

epilepsy in a community. That epileptic seizures may disappear without medications seems to have been known for centuries but has been proven recently only by means of population-oriented studies. Thus, medical prognosis for the "total" population of persons with epilepsy appears to be far better than has been generally thought.

PSYCHIATRIC MANIFESTATIONS IN EPILEPSY

Studies of Case Series and Methodological Shortcomings

The more frequent a disorder, the higher the chance of its coinciding with other frequent disorders. Both epilepsy and mental and psychiatric disorders are common. Many papers have focused on the frequency of various psychiatric disorders in case series of patients with epilepsy derived from outpatient and inpatient specialty facilities, and this topic has been recently reviewed by numerous authors (Betts, 1981; Fenton, 1981; Hermann & Stevens, 1980; Leviton & Cowan, 1981; Parnas & Korsgaard, 1982; Robertson & Trimble, 1983, Stevens, 1982; Trimble, 1982). Much less frequent, however, are attempts to analyze and discuss not only the results of the studies reviewed, but also the adequacy of the methodological approaches employed. The most extensive and analytic reviews covering the methodological shortcomings of the literature were recently published by Stevens (1982), Leviton and Cowan (1981), and Parnas and Korsgaard (1982).

As mentioned, the mechanisms underlying the formation of case series obtained from various facilities are frequently unappreciated. These mechanisms, however, may influence to a significant degree the distribution of clinical and social features subsequently noted by the investigators. Consequently, the results from such studies are liable to be biased. A good example of the difficulties inherent in the interpretation of findings derived from select groups can be illustrated in the widely cited study of Flor-Henry (1969). He investigated 50 patients admitted to a psychiatric hospital *because of psychosis* who also appeared to have a history of epileptic seizures (i.e., in retrospective review). The control group was selected from among patients admitted to the neurosurgical ward and psychiatric hospital for investigation and treatment of temporal lobe epilepsy. In other words, the basic reason for admission of the former group was psychosis, whereas for the latter it was poorly controlled, mostly psychomotor seizures. Due to the mechanisms underlying the formation of these groups one might naturally expect that the frequency of psychomotor seizures would be higher in the "control group" when compared with the "psychotic group." This difference was in fact statistically significant ($p < .001$). Further, of the 50 psychotic patients, 10% showed an EEG focus in the right hemisphere, whereas among the "controls" 50% showed such a focus. It may be reasonable to suggest that many of the "controls" with psychomotor seizures were referred to the neurosurgical ward because of their better suitability for surgical treatment (right temporal focus). Therefore, a preponderance of dominant hemisphere foci in the psychotic group may not necessarily be "very significantly correlated with psychosis and . . . lowered fit frequency" (Flor-Henry, 1969, p. 389), but rather associated with the mechanisms responsible for the formation of the psychotic and control groups. If one is to take seriously the extremely small number of psychotic cases among people with epilepsy and the predominant frequency of left-sided foci among these cases, one might also note that the left hemisphere has been known for years to be more susceptible to variously defined abnormalities (e.g., Hughes, 1960; Sommer, 1880).

Two other papers worth discussing came from the London Hospital and, surprisingly, produced strikingly different results. The first, by Currie, Heathfield, Henson, and Scott (1971), reported findings on 666 patients with epilepsy from an undefined population (partly from London) cited only as "attending a general hospital . . . and not deliberately selected." Of this group, 62 underwent lobectomy (9.3%) and brain tumors were diagnosed in another 9.5%. The study was retrospective and only 56% of the patients were seen by the authors personally; another 10% remained untraced. In all, 40 patients had a "florid psychiatric disorder," including 17 with "gross hysteria" and 12 with "schizophrenic illness"; another 127 were found to be "depressed." The authors concluded that among their patients with epilepsy, "severe psychiatric disorders are uncommon." They also "did not find that a psychiatric disorder or an aggressive affect was more common in those with psychomotor attacks" (p. 187).

In contrast, some 10 years later, Kogeorgos, Fonagy, and Scott (1982) performed a study *at the same hospital* and stated that nearly "half of the epileptics were classified as probable psychiatric cases." This time a small case series of 66 patients with epilepsy (half of them males) was carefully selected. A diagnosis of epilepsy "had been corroborated by one or more definitely abnormal EEGs." The psychosocial features of this small group of patients, stemming from an undefined population, were then compared to a community sample (derived from the Manual for the General Health Questionnaire [Goldberg, 1972]). After recomputation of data from one of their tables, entitled "proportion of probable psychiatric cases," it appears that among males with epilepsy, 70% were classified as "probable" psychiatric cases," whereas only 21% of females were so classified. In the neurological control group these percentages were 19% and 39%, respectively, and in the (not at all comparable) "community sample" they were 16% and 26%, respectively. Such a distribution of "probable psychiatric cases" in sex groups, along with employed methods of case selection, clearly show that the discussed group of patients cannot be considered as a "representation" either for people with epilepsy in a community or even for patients with epilepsy seen in a hospital. Nevertheless, Kogeorgos et al. concluded that the "high proportion of probable psychiatric cases among epileptics living in the community is impressive" as they felt their "group is likely to represent a substantial proportion of epileptics living in the community." (p. 242).

This may serve as a good example of an unjustified attempt to overgeneralize findings from a small and severely biased series of epileptic patients to all the people with epilepsy in a community. The most discouraging fact, however, is that some very experienced authors have cited the preceding findings with no attempt to critically analyze their value.

Other examples of attempts to generalize results obtained from studies on specifically selected case series can be found in papers of Sherwin, Peron-Magnan, Bancaud, Bonis, and Talairach (1982) as well as of Lindsay et al. (1979). Both groups of patients under study consisted of very severe (if not most severe) epilepsy cases, selected purposely (Lindsay et al.), or in terms of referral to a neurosurgical ward (Sherwin et al.). Results of both studies were quite pessimistic, as one could expect due to the selection process operating in both studies.

All the foregoing examples of methodological shortcomings illustrate the need for carefully designed, prospective studies in truly unselected or more representative and larger samples of individuals with epilepsy. The most promising approach would be a longitudinal follow-up of all cases of epilepsy diagnosed in a defined population. Risk factors purported to be responsible for later development of psychosis, aggressiveness, and other behavioral problems should be identified and analyzed from the beginning. A good example of such a methodological approach may be the Framingham study on myocardial infarction and stroke (Kannel, Rawber, Cohen, & McNamara, 1965). Until the results of such studies on epilepsy are available, conclusions based on selected case series must be considered cautiously.

Schizophrenialike Syndromes in Other CNS Disorders

Although much has been made of a possible relationship between epilepsy and schizophrenia, it should be noted that the occurrence of schizophrenia or schizophrenialike psychosis seems to exceed "chance expectations" in case series of other types of patients as well. In their extensive review of the literature, Davison and Bagley (1969) have shown that "schizophrenia" has been diagnosed more often than expected in a number of "organic CNS disorders." For instance, in people with traumatic brain injury followed for 10–20 years, schizophrenia occurs two to three times more often than expected. An increased risk of schizophrenia was found in cases of brain tumor (in all types and various cerebral localizations, but particularly in tumors of the pituitary or the temporal lobe), Sydenham's chorea and acute rheumatism, cerebral syphilis (8%–20% of cases with general paresis), Wilson's disease, Huntington's chorea, and narcolepsy but not in multiple sclerosis. Paranoid hallucinatory psychoses are reported in association with subarachnoid hemorrhage, fat cerebral embolism, or bilateral carotid artery occlusion. Schizophrenialike psychoses frequently can be seen in various cerebral intoxications (carbon monoxide, cerebral anoxia, hypoglycemia, hepatic encephalopathy, etc.). It should be clear that most, if not all, of these CNS disorders also may be associated with the occurrence of epileptic seizures. Finally, schizophrenialike psychosis also has been attributed to anticonvulsant toxicity (Franks & Richter, 1979).

Thus, underlying brain damage, and not necessarily epileptic seizures or "epilepsy," may play a causative role in the occurrence of schizophrenialike psychoses. Furthermore, persons with frequent tonic–clonic seizures, especially if severe or involving major motor status epilepticus, are more exposed to the risk of brain trauma or recurrent episodes of anoxia that might be associated with "schizophrenialike syndromes" or other mental or personality disorders. Finally, people with multiple cerebral disorders, i.e., epilepsy plus psychosis plus other CNS manifestations, have a significantly increased risk of hospitalization, or appearance in files of the highly specialized centers (see the earlier discussion of Berkson's paradox). This again shows how cautious the attempts should be to generalize results of studies on patients derived from such facilities.

Coexistence of Psychosis and Epilepsy in Studies Based on Case Series Analysis

If a person suffers from more than one disorder, possible causative relationships between them should be considered. If such a relationship exists, one may speak about "complications" of a disorder. Examples may be arterial hypertension and cerebral hemorrhage or diabetes mellitus and peripheral neuropathy. The term *coexistence* is used if an individual suffers from two or more etiologically independent disorders, e.g., arterial hypertension and compulsive neurosis or schizophrenia and epilepsy. In fact, coexistence may occur by chance and its frequency may be roughly estimated from incidence and prevalence rates of each of the coexisting disorders.

The formula for calculating the coexistence of epilepsy and schizophrenia in the general population, as proposed in the very influential paper of Slater and Beard (1963), i.e., $5/1{,}000 \times 8/1{,}000 = 40/1{,}000{,}000$, will not be applicable for patients referred to hospitals, especially psychiatric ones (Parnas & Korsgaard, 1982; Stevens, 1982). If one assumes that epilepsy does not prevent development of schizophrenia (and vice versa), then among every 100 newly diagnosed cases of schizophrenia a history of a seizure can be expected in about five cases along with one in whom the seizures were recurrent, i.e., with epilepsy. Davison and Bagley (1969) in their extensive review have shown that in various case series of schizophrenic patients, epilepsy may be diagnosed in a wide range from 0.06% to 19.5%. Interestingly enough, the larger the schizophrenic case series (6,000–50,000) the lower the percentage of those with coexistent epilepsy—0.3%.

The frequency of schizophrenialike syndrome in patients with epilepsy has been calculated in fewer, usually highly selected case series. Currie et al. (1971) estimated the frequency of schizophrenialike syndromes at 1.8%, and Sherwin, et al. (1982) and Lindsay et al. (1979) estimated it at about 10%–15%. Ferguson and Rayport (1984), after reviewing available data on the frequency of psychoses in various groups of patients with epilepsy, concluded that the "estimation of the prevalence of psychosis in epilepsy faces substantial problems" (p. 234). Thus, the available data on the coexistence of epilepsy and psychosis based on analyses of case series are inconsistent and vary widely. The need for further prospective studies on more representative patient populations is again indisputable.

Epilepsy and Depression: Studies Based on Case Series

The frequency of depression and anxiety in patients with a seizure disorder has been reviewed recently by Robertson and Trimble (1983). Unfortunately, the authors did not attempt to discuss any of the methodological approaches employed in the reviewed papers. Furthermore, no attention was given to the definitions of depression or anxiety that were used by the various authors, some of whom derived their conclusions from studies based on specifically selected case series (i.e., Betts, 1981; Currie et al., 1971; Kogeorgos et al., 1982). Similarly, no attention was given to the effects of socioeconomic factors. Robertson and Trimble's final conclusion was that depression is a common problem in patients with epilepsy, although "not directly interlinked with epileptic variables per se." An extremely high frequency of "depression" also has been recently reported by the Epilepsy Center at UCLA (Mittan & Locke, 1982a,b). Among 147 patients with epilepsy (59% of whom were white) examined by means of numerous psychological tests, including the MMPI, 80% complained of being "often depressed" and 23% admitted that they either are or were suicidal because of their epilepsy. Half of the patients considered their seizures to be worse than social stigma, and 78% were afraid they might die with the next seizure.

Opposite conclusions can be found in DeAngelis and Vizioli (1983). The authors compared their 50 neurological inpatients with epilepsy and patients with other chronic diseases. Both groups were thought to be socioeconomically homogeneous. Patients with epilepsy appeared to score much lower on the depression scale of the Middlesex Hospital Questionnaire than the controls.

Not much is known about the individuals' self-evaluation of various social and emotional needs. The level of satisfaction of basic needs was studied in Warsaw among 188 patients with "uncomplicated epilepsy" (Bejnarowicz & Zielinski, 1979). In the area of social needs (including employment) low need satisfaction occurred in 72%, whereas emotional needs were not satisfied in 47% and family needs in 27%. The patients' level of education and IQ positively and significantly correlated with poor satisfaction of basic needs as well as with anxiety levels. These findings may illustrate the extent to which people with "uncomplicated epilepsy" may suffer from social and emotional difficulties. Unfortunately, lack of a control group and the fact that the study was performed in a group of patients under a comprehensive treatment program restrict the appropriateness of generalizing these findings to all people with epilepsy in a community.

All in all, a review of studies based on various epilepsy case series has shown that the results almost invariably cannot be directly compared. This is due to significant variability in methodological approaches, particularly because of the different means of patient selection. Multiple factors have been shown to be involved in the process of forming the various samples of patients with epilepsy (e.g., variability in health service systems, health insurance and various disability benefit policies, hospital admission threshold, medical attitudes in a community). These selection factors may significantly influence the results of studies performed in various countries and geographic areas. Studies based on selected groups of patients with epilepsy, e.g., from mental hospitals or special centers in contrast to population-oriented surveys, usually provide pessimistic results regarding the frequency of mental handicap and the general prognosis in epilepsy. The "epileptic label" originating from these studies might easily stick to every individual who has the misfortune of being recognized as an "epileptic" in his or her milieu. Thus, it should be kept in mind that results of studies based on selected groups of patients cannot be directly generalized to all people with epilepsy in a community.

PSYCHIATRIC MANIFESTATIONS IN EPILEPSY: EPIDEMIOLOGIC STUDIES

Frequency of Psychiatric Hospitalization

Perhaps the best way to study the nature and degree of psychiatric risk associated with epilepsy would be via epidemiologic surveys. Unfortunately, in most of the epidemiologic surveys of epilepsy, psychiatric manifestations and disorders have not been analyzed. Neither Gudmundsson in Iceland nor this author in Warsaw employed a structured type of psychiatric examination. Both relied on clinical interviews. In Gudmundsson's (1966) national sample of 916 people with epilepsy, 71 were diagnosed as psychotic (7.7%), and more females received such a diagnosis. In two thirds of the patients with psychosis, "ixoid" or "iothymic" personality (equivalents to a "viscous" or "epileptoid" personality trait) were diagnosed. However, wide discrepancies were noted between various psychiatric diagnoses made by the author and by the other examining physicians. The differences were most substantial in the class of "normal personality" (46% vs. 70%) and "neurotic personality" (19% vs. 5%).

Of people with known epilepsy in Warsaw (Group K), 3% were diagnosed as "psychotic" as were only 2% in the field survey (Group F). Features of the so-called epileptic characteropathy or epileptic dementia could be traced in 11% and 6% of cases, respectively. Among those with "behavioral problems" hysterical traits or emotional immaturity were frequently diagnosed. The tendency toward alcohol abuse was noted in 14% of males in Group K and 20% in Group F, an observation similar to that of Oleanders and Steinwall (1965).

As far as psychiatric hospitalization is concerned, less than 5% of all patients with epilepsy in Iceland reported such an admission. In the Warsaw study, in the sample of known patients (Group K) a history of admission to a neurological department was noted in 41% and to a psychiatric department in 11%. In Group F (98 persons with epilepsy identified in the random population sample), these percentages were 11% and 1%, respectively (Zielinski, 1974). It should be mentioned, however, that in Group F a history of psychiatric hospitalization for reasons other than epilepsy was reported by two respondents. Thus, some 3% of those afflicted with epilepsy in a population are exposed to a risk of psychiatric hospitalization. This percentage is significantly lower when compared to known epilepsy cases. These epidemiologic data demonstrate that rates of psychopathology derived from medical facilities are significant overestimates of the true prevalence of psychopathology in epilepsy that is obtained when all individuals with the disorder are considered.

Psychiatric Disorders in Children with Epilepsy

Rutter, Graham and Yule (1970) examined a general population of 2,288 school children on the Isle of Wight. Using a "clinical diagnostic approach," they classfied 6.8% of all children as having a "psychiatric disorder." Children with nonneurological chronic disorders had nearly double the percentage of psychiatric disorders. Among children with epilepsy, however, this percentage was much higher (34%), and if epilepsy was associated with "lesion above brain stem," 58% had a psychiatric disorder. Among the 63 children with "uncomplicated epilepsy" a neurotic disorder was diagnosed in 8 (12.9%) compared with only 1.9% of all the children. Antisocial or conduct disorder was diagnosed in 9.5% vs. 1.2%, respectively. Possible epilepsy cases not diagnosed by doctors and not reported by parents or teachers were not identified, and accordingly the proportion of children with both psychiatric and seizure disorders might have been somewhat overestimated.

Epidemiology of Psychiatric Disorders: A Chance of Coexistence with Seizures

A number of psychiatric-epidemiologic studies conducted in the general population reviewed by this author (Zielinski, 1984) have shown quite a wide range of prevalence rates for psychoses and psychiatric disorders. Rates for all psychoses appear to vary depending on the diagnostic method employed. Similar to studies on epilepsy, the cohort analysis yielded one of the highest estimates for lifetime prevalence (44 per 1,000 population in Bornholm), whereas most of the point prevalence estimated varied between 3.9 and 6.7 per 1,000. Most of the studies done in the United States yield results in that range. Prevalence rates of schizophrenia were the highest in Bornholm and northern Sweden (9 and 9.6 per 1,000), and in the United States they vary between 1.0 and 2.9 per 1,000. Babigian (1975) has given an estimate between 2.3 and 4.7 per 1,000.

Depression is not only one of the most frequent psychiatric conditions, but it also seems to be one of the most difficult to define. In the 1930s, the prevalence of depression in the U.S. population was estimated at 0.8–0.9 per 1,000 (Cohen & Fairbank, 1938; Lemkau, Tietze, & Cooper, 1941). In 1943 Roth and Luton found psychotic depression alone in 0.7 per 1,000 and depressive neurotic reaction in an additional 1.4 for a total of 2.1 per 1,000. More recently, Leighton, Harding, Macklin, Hughes, and Leighton (1963) in Canada estimated the prevalence of depression at 3.0 per 1,000. A longitudinal survey of a U.S. urban community yielded much higher rates (Weisman, Myers, & Harding, 1978). "Major depression" was diagnosed in 3.7%, "minor" in 2.0%, and "depressive personality" in another 4.5% of the inhabitants.

Review of the studies on psychiatric morbidity in general medical practice suggests that the percentage of patients at risk for various psychiatric disorders (neuroses, anxiety states, and others) falls between 4% and 13% within 1 year of the survey. One study estimated a prevalence of psychiatric morbidity, according to patient consulting, to be 102 per 1,000, including 4.9 per 1,000 for psychoses, 2.3 for mental subnormality, 1.4 for dementia, 88.5 for neuroses, and 5.5 for personality disorders. Organic illnesses with psychiatric overlay account for an additional 15 per 1,000 (Shepherd, Cooper, Brown, & Kalton, 1981).

In their review of the U.S. mental health services system, Regier, Goldberg, and Taube (1978) estimated that at least 15% of the U.S. population is affected by mental disorders. Sixty per cent of them will be identified in the primary care sector while an unknown percentage will not be in treatment. This estimate is consistent with the recent findings of D'Arcy (1982) in Canada, who by means of mailed Goldberg's General Health Questionnaire found 15% of the respondents suffering from nonpsychotic psychiatric symptoms.

In summary, one may contend that the frequency of various psychiatric disorders in case series of persons with epilepsy may not be higher than prevalence rates of these disorders in the general population. This may be particularly true among children and adolescents in whom prevalence rates of epilepsy are high as well. Additionally, the question of the actual frequency of psychoses and depression among the people suffering from epileptic seizures remains open.

SOCIOECONOMIC VARIABLES

Socioeconomic factors, if discussed at all, are considered as dependent variables in almost all epidemiologic and clinical surveys. There are numerous papers on the social implications of epilepsy and the impact of this disorder on the employment, education, or economic status of the individual. Only a few authors have considered these factors as independent variables, that is, risk factors in the development of mental and/or neurological disorders (Weissman & Klerman, 1978).

In the 1930s Faris and Dunham (1965) found that the highest rates of first admissions to mental hospitals in Chicago occurs in inhabitants of areas with the highest social disorganization. Although the "drift hypothesis" of the authors can be disputed, they have demonstrated the role of social variables as risk factors with regard to one's chance of admission to a mental hospital. Later, Hollingshead and Redlich (1958), in their classic study, found that the prevalence of schizophrenia was much higher in lower socioeconomic strata and lowest among people from upper socioeconomic classes. The authors also concluded that patients from low socioeconomic strata did not receive sufficient treatment for their condition and therefore many of them became "chronic inpatients." The impact of socioeconomic changes on mental health has been carefully documented by Leighton et al. (1963).

More recently, Frerichs, Aneshensel, and Clark (1981), in a multiethnic probability sample of 1,000 adults in Los Angeles County, found an overall prevalence of depression (defined as a score above 16 on a 20-item "scale of depression") of 19%. Prevalence was greatest among Hispanics (27%), lower in blacks (22%), and lowest in whites (16%). Females were nearly twice as likely to be depressed as males (24% and 13%, respectively). The highest prevalence of depression was found in families with low-level income ($8,500 or less, 31%; $25,000 and above, 10%) and lower educational level (27% in those with below high school level and 8% in people with college or postgraduate education). Employment status was significantly associated with frequency of depression as well.

Prenatal care is essential for reducing risk of fetal infections, malnutrition, perinatal trauma, and so on, all of which are more likely to be met in children with epilepsy (Pasamanick & Lilienfeld, 1955). In a careful, nationwide study Taffel (1978b) has shown that timing of initiation of prenatal care and number of prenatal visits are directly related to the mother's educational level. Racial differences were not as noticeable for women with low education as for those with 9 years of schooling and over. The same author (1978a), accepting the mother's educational level as an index of socioeconomic status, found that congenital anomalies show an inverse correlation with level of education. This difference may be attributed to less satisfactory prenatal care, poor hygiene, a higher incidence of infections, and malnutrition among mothers of lower socioeconomic status. The latter also has been associated with an increased risk of anencephaly and spina bifida in newborns in Boston hospitals (Naggan & McMahon, 1967). Thus, socioeconomic status not only may be related to psychopathology, but also may be associated with an increased exposure of the fetus to factors known to be associated with or responsible for brain damage and/or seizure disorders.

Further effects of socioeconomic status can be seen in national statistics. The National Health Survey (1973) yielded substantial data on the frequency of various disorders. Table 2-2 presents relative frequencies of selected conditions reported by sampled inhabitants, by race and socioeconomic level. Epilepsy, diabetes, and especially anemia are reported more frequently by nonwhites, with thyroid conditions and migraine reported more frequently by whites. All conditions, however, are more frequently reported in families with the lowest income level. Thus, this survey yields further data corroborating the possibility of a higher incidence of epilepsy in lower socioeconomic strata. Moreover, 38% of those reporting seizures have not recently visited a doctor, a finding consistent with the results of Anderson (1936), Gudmundsson (1966), and Zielinski (1974). Another indirect index suggesting a higher prevalence of epilepsy among poor and nonwhite people has been derived from a study of prisoners (Whitman et al., 1984).

Low socioeconomic status can also be responsible for the more severe course of epilepsy. Among patients of the Epilepsy Center of Michigan (ECM), only 23% are considered to suffer from "uncomplicated epilepsy"

TABLE 2–2. Frequency of Reported Conditions per 1,000 Interviewed Persons and Frequency Rates by Race, Education, and Economic Level (from the U.S. National Health Survey, 1973)

Rate of Reporting the Condition per 1,000 Interviewed	*Epilepsy*	*All Thyroid Conditions*	*Goiter, All Forms*	*Diabetes Mellitus*	*Anemia (All)*	*Migraine*
Total (= 1.00)	3.1	13.9	2.0	20.4	14.5	21.8
Ratios:						
Race						
Whites	0.97	1.07	1.05	0.98	0.94	1.03
All others	1.19	0.59	1.00	1.17	1.41	0.77
Economic level						
Lower	1.84	1.19	1.85	2.21	1.90	1.34
Higher	0.68	1.11	0.80	0.63	0.70	1.05
Educational level						
Lower	1.29	1.03	1.35	1.86	1.10	0.83
Higher	0.81	1.08	0.80	0.63	0.87	1.10

(Rodin, Shapiro, & Lennox, 1977). This relatively low percentage of people whose major problem constitutes only epileptic seizures can be attributed, at least in part, to the fact that the ECM patients come "primarily from lower socioeconomic classes" (Rodin, 1972) and that a considerable proportion of them is unemployed (Zielinski & Rader, 1984). The same situation probably applies to case series seen in various university departments and clinics resulting from mechanisms of formation of these case series.

The only population-oriented study of epilepsy that considers race and socioeconomic level as independent variables has been conducted by Shamansky and Glaser (1979) in the New Haven Standard Metropolitan Statistical Area (SMSA). The authors reviewed the files of the two major EEG laboratories in the area, believing that the resulting case ascertainment bias was minimal. All basic data on children up to 14 years of age referred for routine EEG because of the occurrence of a seizure (or seizures) were derived from routine EEG requisitions and reports. The cases were classified into three categories: definite epilepsy (557 cases), probable epilepsy (123 cases), and neonatal seizures (53 cases). The last category included cases of perinatal hypoxia, infections, and transient biochemical disorders. These three categories were not analyzed separately and therefore the authors accepted "cumulative incidence rates" as a measure of prevalence. Cumulative incidence and average annual incidence rates are summarized in Table 2-3. As can be seen, both the cumulative incidence and average annual incidence rates were higher in the second period of the study in all subgroups. This was particularly true among black males (almost twofold increase) though no explanation is offered for this phenomenon. In general, rates were higher for black people than for whites. Similar to Faris and Dunham (1965), the authors found an excess of children from lower socioeconomic areas referred for an EEG because of seizures.

Although the authors were fully aware of numerous possible sources of bias, they discussed only those that might be responsible for the underestimation of their rates. Among several methodological shortcomings of this study, apart from the retrospective analysis of EEG lab files, there was no attempt to analyze the accuracy of clinical data and the methods of diagnosis. It should be pointed out that the general tendency to overdiagnose seizures and epilepsy, especially among children, is a well-known and frequent finding during epidemiologic surveys. Thus, the estimated vector of bias might well be multidirectional. The survey of Shamansky and Glaser, however, is another example that strongly points to the urgent necessity of further and more detailed studies on socioeconomic status and race as possible risk factors for epilepsy.

Socioeconomic Variables in Epilepsy: Need for Further Studies

Until recently, socioeconomic variables in epilepsy usually have been considered secondary to epilepsy, and research has been directed toward determining the extent to which the occurrence of seizures and social stigma attached to epilepsy may reduce the quality of an individual's social life, e.g., education, employment, economic level, and family life. Thus, epilepsy has been considered the independent variable, and the social implications the dependent variables. In psychiatric epidemiology and social psychiatry various socioeconomic variables have long been considered probable risk factors for psychiatric disorder. In epilepsy research, however, little or no attention has been paid to possible risk factors more or less directly related to socioeconomic level.

The few papers that have considered a direct relationship between low socioeconomic status and a higher incidence of epilepsy have provided sufficient data to allow us to strongly suspect such a relationship, but there are still no well-documented studies showing that socioeconomic status and ethnicity are the direct risk factors for epilepsy. It should be mentioned, however, that several of the preceding studies have shown a significant association between social-educational and racial variables and CNS abnormalities, birth injuries, and congenital malformations, all of which are potentially related to

TABLE 2–3. Cumulative Incidence and Average Annual Incidence Rates of Epilepsy by Sex, Race, and Survey Period in New Haven (from Shamansky & Glaser, 1979)

	CUMULATIVE INCIDENCE RATES PER 1,000					
	MALES			FEMALES		
Years Studied	White	Black	White + Spanish Speaking	White	Black	White + Spanish Speaking
1960–64	8.01	13.16	8.48	8.92	14.28	9.00
1965–70	10.91	23.59	12.00	9.29	15.28	10.08
1960–70	9.53	19.63		9.10	15.00[a]	
	AVERAGE ANNUAL INCIDENCE PER 1,000					
1960–64	0.54	0.98	0.50	0.60	0.93	0.60
1965–70	0.71	1.50	0.78	0.61	1.03	0.66
1960–70	0.63	1.36		0.60	0.99	

[a]As calculated by this author; in the original paper the rate was 19.51.

the occurrence of epileptic seizures. Moreover, these variables are also associated with less complete and effective prenatal care.

There are other fields of research on epilepsy in which the instances of socioeconomic variables have not been explored sufficiently or even considered. If one accepts that both epilepsy and mental and psychiatric disorders are more frequent in people from lower socioeconomic strata, and if the same people predominate in case series of specialty centers and university hospitals, then the introduction of socioeconomic status as a variable in surveys of the frequency of psychiatric disorders in epilepsy (and vice versa) becomes imperative.

Furthermore, the prognosis of epilepsy may depend on many factors. For thousands of years experts have agreed that there is an association between initiation of treatment and prognosis in epilepsy. According to Hippocrates, "It was . . . of great importance to treat the patient before disease [epilepsy—JJZ] has become chronic . . . Inveterate cases are incurable" (Temkin, 1971, p. 65). Most recently Shorvon and Reynolds (1982) have written: " . . . early, effective treatment may be important to prevent evolution into chronic and more intractable epilepsy . . . " (p. 1,699). Hippocrates' statement seems to be based on careful observation of the natural history of epilepsy, whereas that of the latter authors appears to be based on the effective action of modern anticonvulsants. A survey on the "natural course" of epilepsy in various socioeconomic and ethnic groups may provide important prognostic data. Even if one accepts no significant differences in the delay of initiation of treatment at various socioeconomic levels, there still may be differences regarding the drugs used and the intensity of monitoring, e.g., frequency of medical visits, laboratory tests, or anticonvulsant serum levels. Both phenobarbital and phenytoin (Dilantin) are known to suppress levels of mental functioning as well as to exacerbate behavioral problems. More modern anticonvulsants, such as carbamazepine and sodium valproate, have fewer side effects in terms of mental and behavioral deterioration, but they are more expensive. Therefore, differences in treatment patterns and difficulties in obtaining more expensive medications may substantially influence not only the prognosis in terms of the frequency of epileptic seizures, but also the occurrence of mental and psychiatric disorders. Studies on the "natural course" of epilepsy in various communities or countries defined by actual socioeconomic status, health insurance policies, and accessibility of effective, updated medical care are urgently needed.

Another problem, which may contribute to a poorer prognosis, involves medical compliance, which may be more of a problem among those with less education (Zielinsky & Nowak, 1971). Additionally, nutritional factors, especially folic acid depletion, may result in mental deterioration and the occurrence of psychiatric problems (Reynolds, 1983). It is quite probable that people from lower socioeconomic strata are more often exposed to risk of nutritional deficiency, including vitamins and mineral salts.

Finally, psychosocial factors may play a causative role in the development of psychiatric problems in epilepsy. It sounds like a truism that negative attitudes toward epilepsy in a community may result in the worsening of various psychiatric problems (neurotic reactions, personality and behavioral disorders). In the Warsaw study the lowest social acceptance of epilepsy was noted among people with elementary or lower education and among unskilled workers, and the best level of social acceptance was found among senior white-collar workers and those with unversity education (Zielinski, 1974). Similarly, an average level of knowledge of epilepsy was positively correlated with the level of education. Thus, poorly educated and vocationally poorly trained people with epilepsy will become even more socially suppressed, being exposed to insufficient knowledge of the disorder and negative attitudes in their social milieu. Furthermore, depression was diagnosed more often among the unemployed persons (Frerichs et al., 1981), and this seems quite reasonable. Thus, keeping in mind the higher than average unemployment rate among people with epilepsy, one may also expect a higher frequency of depression among them. If this is true, unemployment due to epilepsy may be considered as an independent, causative factor in development of depressive mood and possibly other psychiatric disorders.

CONCLUSION

Our knowledge of the psychiatric implications of epilepsy based on results of studies of various select case series appears very incomplete and controversial. One of the most discouraging problems is the tendency to overgeneralize results of these studies, some of which are flawed by significant methodological shortcomings. This tendency and the associated methodological problems discussed throughout this chapter indicate the urgent need for population-oriented, prospective studies on incidence of epilepsy and prognosis in terms of frequency of seizures, mental abnormalities, psychiatric disorders, and neurological handicaps. Such surveys should consider socioeconomic variables as independent risk factors, and not only as dependent outcomes of epilepsy. Along with socioeconomic variables, racial-specific differences should also be analyzed.

REFERENCES

Alving, J. (1978). Classification of the epilepsies: An investigation of 1,508 consecutive adult patients. *Acta Neurologica Scandinavica* 58, 205–12.

Anderson, C. L. (1936). Epilepsy in the state of Michigan. *Mental Hygiene* 20, 441–62.

Annegers, J. F., W. A. Hauser, & L. R. Elveback. (1979). Remission of seizures and relapse in patients with epilepsy. *Epilepsia* 20, 729–37.

Babigian, H. M. (1975). Schizophrenia: Epidemiology. In A. M. Freedman, H. I. Kaplan, & B. T. Saddock (Eds.), *Comprehensive textbook of psychiatry*. Baltimore: Williams & Wilkins.

Bejnarowicz, J. H., & J. J. Zielinski. (1979). The level of basic human need satisfaction and its variations. In J. J. Zielinski (Ed.), *Program of medical treatment and course of epilepsy and social functioning of patients* (Rehabilit. Services Administration, DHEW, report on research program 19-P-58335). Washington, DC: U.S. Government Printing Office.

Berkson, J. (1946). Limitations of the application of fourfold table analysis to hospital data. *Biometrics Bulletin* 2, 47–53.

Betts, T. A. (1981). Depression, anxiety and epilepsy. In E. H. Reynolds & M. R. Trimble (Eds.), *Epilepsy and psychiatry*. New York: Churchill-Livingstone.

Cohen, B. M., & R. E. Fairbank. (1938). Statistical contributions from the mental hygiene study of the Eastern Health District in Baltimore. II. Psychosis in the Eastern Health District. *American Journal of Psychiatry 94*, 1377–95.

Currie, S., H. G. Heathfield, R. A. Henson, & D. F. Scott. (1971). Clinical course and prognosis of temporal lobe epilepsy. A survey of 666 patients. *Brain* 94, 173-90.

D'Arcy, C. (1982). Prevalence and correlates of nonpsychotic psychiatric symptoms in the general population. *Canadian Journal of Psychiatry* 4, 316–24.

Davison, K., & C. R. Bagley. (1969). Schizophrenia-like psychoses associated with organic disorders of the central nervous system: A review of the literature. In

R. N. Herrington (Ed.), Current problems in neuropsychiatry—schizophrenia, epilepsy, and temporal lobe. *British Journal of Psychiatry: Special Publ. No. 4,* Ashford, UK: Healey Brothers.

DeAngelis, G., & R. Vizioli. (1983). Epilepsy and depression. In M. Parsonage (Ed.), *Advances in epileptology: XIVth Epilepsy International Symposium.* New York: Raven Press.

DeGraaf, A. S. (1974). Epidemiological aspects of epilepsy in Northern Norway. *Epilepsia* 15, 291–99.

Eastwood, M. R., & M. H. Trevelyan. (1972). Relationship between physical and psychiatric disorder. *Psychological Medicine* 2, 363–72.

Ellenberg, J. H., & K. B. Nelson. (1980). Sample selection and the natural history of disease. *Journal of the American Medical Association* 243, 1337–40.

Faris, R. E. & H. W. Dunham. (1965). *Mental disorders in urban areas, an ecological study of schizophrenia and other psychoses.* Chicago: University of Chicago Press.

Fenton, G. W. (1981). Personality and behavioural disorders in adults with epilepsy. In E. H. Reynolds & M. R. Trimble. (Eds.), *Epilepsy and psychiatry.* Edinburgh: Churchill-Livingstone.

Ferguson, S. M., & M. Rayport. (1984). Psychosis in epilepsy. In D. Blumer (Ed.), *Psychiatric aspects of epilepsy.* Washington, DC: American Psychological Association.

Flor-Henry, P. (1969). Psychosis and temporal lobe epilepsy. A controlled investigation. *Epilepsia,* 10, 363–95.

Franks, R. D., & A. J. Richter. (1979) Schizophrenia-like psychosis associated with anticonvulsant toxicity. *American Journal of Psychiatry 136,* 973–74.

Frerichs, R. S., C. S. Aneshensel, & V. A. Clark. (1981). Prevalence of depression in Los Angeles County. *American Journal of Epidemiology 113,* 691–99.

Gastaut, H., J. L. Gastaut, G. E. Goncalves Silva, & G. E. Fernandez-Sanchez. (1975). Relative frequency of different types of epilepsy: A study employing the classification of the International League Against Epilepsy. *Epilepsia* 16, 457–61.

Goldberg, D. (1972). *Manual of the General Health Questionnaire.* New York: Oxford University Press.

Gomez, J. G., E. Arciniegas, & J. Torres. (1978). Prevalence of epilepsy in Bogota, Colombia. *Neurology* 28, 90–94.

Gudmundsson, G. (1966). Epilepsy in Iceland: A clinical and epidemiological investigation. *Acta Neurologica Scandinavica* 25 (Supp. 43), 1–124.

Hauser, W. A. (1972). Sex and socioeconomic status. In M. Alter & W. A. Hauser (Eds.), *The epidemiology of epilepsy: A workshop* Washington, DC: U.S. Government Printing Office (DHEW Publ. No. NIH 73-390).

Hauser, W. A. (1978). Epidemiology of epilepsy. In B. S. Schoenberg, (Ed.), *Advances in neurology* (Vol. 19). New York: Raven Press.

Hauser, W. A. & L. T. Kurland. (1975). The epidemiology of epilepsy in Rochester, Minnesota, 1935 through 1967. *Epilepsia* 16, 1–66.

Hermann, B. P., & J. R. Stevens. (1980). Interictal behavioral correlates of the epilepsies. In B. P. Hermann (Ed.), *A mutidisciplinary handbook of epilepsy.* Springfield, IL: Thomas.

Hermann, B. P., & S. Whitman. (1984). Behavioral and personality correlates of epilepsy: A review, methodological critique and conceptual model. *Psychological Bulletin* 95, 451–97.

Hollingshead, A. B., & F. C. Redlich. (1958). *Social class and mental illness.* New York: Wiley.

Hughes, J. R. (1960). A statistical analysis on the location of EEG abnormalities. *EEG Journal* 12, 906–909.

Joshi, V., B. C. Katiyar, P. K. Mohan, S. Misras, & G. D. Shukla. (1977). Profile of epilepsy in a developing country: A study of 1000 patients based on international classification. *Epilepsia* 18, 549–54.

Kannel, W. B., T. R. Rawber, M. E. Cohen, & P. M. McNamara. (1965). Vascular disease of the brain—epidemiologic aspects: The Framingham study. *American Journal of Public Health* 55, 1355–66.

Kogeorgos, J., P. Fonagy, & D. F. Scott (1982). Psychiatric symptom patterns of chronic epileptics attending a neurological clinic: A controlled investigation. *British Journal of Psychiatry* 140, 236–43.

Leighton, D. C., J. S. Harding, D. B. Macklin, C. C. Hughes, & A. H. Leighton. (1963). Psychiatric findings of the Stirling County study. *American Journal of Psychiatry* 119, 1021–26.

Lemkau, P., C. Tietze, & M. Cooper. (1941). Mental hygiene problems in an urban district. *Mental Hygiene* 26, 275–88.

Leviton, A., & L. D. Cowan. (1981). Methodological issues in the epidemiology of seizure disorders in children. *Epidemiological Review* 3, 67–89.

Lindsay, J., C. Ounsted, & P. Richards. (1979). Long term outcome in children with temporal lobe seizures: Social outcome and childhood factors. *Developmental Medicine and Child Neurology 21*, 285–98.

Mittan, R. J., & G. E. Locke. (1982a). The other half of epilepsy: Psychological problems. *Urban Health*, January/February, 38–39.

Mittan, R. J., & G. E. Locke. (1982b). Fear of seizures: Epilepsy's forgotten problem. *Urban Health*, January/February 40–41.

Naggan, L., & B. McMahon. (1967). Ethnic differences in the prevalence of anencephaly and spina bifida in Boston, Massachusetts. *New England Journal of Medicine 277*, 119–23.

National Health Survey (1973). *Prevalence of chronic conditions of the genito-urinary, nervous, endocrine, metabolic and blood and blood-forming systems and of other selected conditions.* (DHEW Publ. No. HRA 77-1536). Washington, DC: U.S. Government Printing Office.

Oleanders, S., & O. Steinwall. (1965). Preliminary evaluation of early prognostication in epilepsy. *Acta Neurologica Scandinavica* 41 (Supp. 13), 509–16.

Parnas, J., & S. Korsgaard. (1982). Epilepsy and psychosis. *Acta Psychiatrica Scandinavica* 66, 89–99.

Pasamanick, B., & A. M. Lilienfeld. (1955). Maternal and fetal factors in the development of epilepsy. 2. Relation to some features of epilepsy. *Neurology* 5, 77–83.

Regier, D. A., I. D. Goldberg, & C. A. Taube. (1978). The de facto U.S. mental health services system. A public health perspective. *Archives of General Psychiatry* 35, 685–93.

Reynolds, E. H. (1983). Biological factors in psychiatric disorders associated with epilepsy. In M. Parsonage (Ed.), *Advances in epileptology: XIVth Epilepsy International Symposium* New York: Raven Press.

Roberts, R. S., W. O. Spitzer, T. Delmore, & D. Sackett. (1978). An empirical demonstration of Berkson's bias. *Journal of Chronic Disorders* 31, 119–28.

Robertson, M. M., & M. R. Trimble. (1983). Depressive illness in patients with epilepsy: A review. *Epilepsia* 24 (Supp. 2), 109–16.

Rodin, E. A. (1968). *The prognosis of patients with epilepsy.* Springfield, IL: Thomas.

Rodin, E. A. (1972). Race. In M. Alter & W. A. Hauser (Eds.), *The epidemiology of epilepsy: A Workshop.* (DHEW Publ. No. NIH 73-390). Washington, DC: U.S. Government Printing Office.

Rodin, E. A., H. Shapiro, & K. Lennox. (1977). Epilepsy and life performance. *Rehabilitation Literature* 38, 34–39.

Ross, E. M., C. S. Peckham. (1983). School children with epilepsy. In M. Parsonage (Ed.), *Advances in Epileptology: XIVth Epilepsy International Symposium.* New York: Raven Press.

Roth, W. F., F. H. Luton. (1943). Mental health program in Tennessee. *American Journal of Psychiatry* 99, 662.

Rutter, M., P. Graham, & W. Yule. (1970). *A neuropsychiatric study in childhood clinics in developmental medicine.* Philadelphia: J. P. Lippincott & Co.

Sato, S. (1964). An epidemiologic and clinicostatistical study of epilepsy in Niigata City. Epidemiologic study (in Japanese). *Clinical Neurology* 4, 461–71.

Shamansky, S. L., & G. H. Glaser. (1979). Socioeconomic characteristics of childhood seizure disorders in New Haven area: An epidemiological study. *Epilepsia* 20, 457–74.

Shepherd, M., B. Cooper, A. C. Brown, & G. Kalton. (1981). *Psychiatric illness in general practice* (2nd ed). New York: Oxford University Press.

Sherwin, I., P. Peron-Magnan, J. Bancaud, A. Bonis, & J. Talairach. (1982). Prevalence of psychosis in epilepsy as a function of the epileptogenic lesion. *Archives of Neurology* 39, 621-25.

Shorvon, S. D., & E. H. Reynolds. (1982). Early prognosis in epilepsy. *British Medical Journal* 285, 1699–1701.

Slater, E., & A. W. Beard. (1963). The schizophrenia-like psychoses of epilepsy. *British Journal of Psychiatry* 109, 95–150.

Slater, E., & Roth, M. (1969). *Clinical psychiatry* (3rd ed.). London: Bailiere, Tindall & Cassell.

Sommer, W. (1880). Disorders of the Ammon's Horn as an etiological factor in epilepsy (in German). *Archiv für Psychiatrie und Nervenkrankheiten* 10, 631-75.

Stevens, J. R. (1975). Interictal clinical manifestations of complex partial seizures. In J. K. Penry (Ed.), *Advances in neurology* (Vol. 11). New York: Raven Press.

Stevens, J. R. (1982). Risk of factors for psychopathology in individuals with epilepsy. In W. P. Koella & M. R. Trimble (Eds.), *Advances in Biological Psychiatry* 8, 56–80. Basel: Karger.

Taffel, S. (1978a). *Congenital anomalies and birth injuries among live births: United States, 1973–1974* (Vital and Health Statistics: Series 21, No. 31, DHEW Publ. No PHS 79-1909). Washington, DC: U.S. Government Printing Office.

Taffel, S. (1978b). *Prenatal care in the United States, 1969–1975* (Vital and Health Statistics: Series 21, No. 33 DHEW Publ. No. PHS-78-1911). Washington, DC: U.S. Government Printing Office.

Temkin, O. (1971). *The falling sickness. A history of epilepsy from the Greeks to the beginning of modern neurology* (2nd ed.) Baltimore: Johns Hopkins University Press.

Trimble, M. R. (1982). Phenomenology of epileptic psychosis: A historical introduction to changing concepts. In W. P. Koella & M. R. Trimble (Eds.), *Advances in Biological Psychiatry* 8, 1–11. Basel: Karger.

Turner, W. A. (1907). *Epilepsy. A study of the idiopathic disease.* London: Macmillan.

Weissman, M. M., & G. L. Klerman. (1978). Epidemiology of mental disorders. Emerging trends in the United States. *Archives of General Psychiatry* 35, 705–12.

Weissman, M. M., J. K. Myers, & P. S. Harding. (1978). Psychiatric disorders in a U.S. urban community, 1975–1976. *American Journal of Psychiatry* 135, 459–62.

Whitman, S., T. E. Coleman, C. Patmon, B. T. Desai, R. Cohen, & L. N. King. (1984). Epilepsy in prison: Elevated prevalence and no relationship to violence. *Neurology* 34, 775–82.

Zielinski, J. J. (1972). Social prognosis in epilepsy. *Epilepsia* 13, 133–40.

Zielinski, J. J. (1974). *Epidemiology and medical social problems of epilepsy in Warsaw* (Final report on research program No. 19-P-58325-F-01. DHEW, Social and Rehabilitation Services). Washington, DC: U.S. Govenment Printing Office.

Zielinski, J. J. (1975). Epidemiology of epilepsy in Poland on the basis of visits to physicians (in Polish). *Przeglad Epidemiologiczny* 29, 123–32.

Zielinski, J. J. (1976). People with epilepsy who do not attend doctors, in epileptology. In D. Janz, (Ed.), *Proceedings of the Seventh International Symposium on Epilepsy*. Stuttgart: Thiem.

Zielinski, J. J. (1982). Epidemiology. In J. Laidlaw & A. Richens (Eds.), *A textbook of epilepsy*. Edinburgh: Churchill-Livingstone.

Zielinski, J. J. (1984). Epidemiological overview of epilepsy: Morbidity, mortality, clinical implications. In D. Blumer (Ed.), *Psychiatric aspects of epilepsy*. Washington, DC: American Psychological Association.

Zielinski, J. J. & S. Nowak. (1971). A contribution to the problem of medical compliance of outpatients with epilepsy (in Polish). *Neurologia i Neurochirurgia Polska* 5, 379–82.

Zielinski, J. J., W. Kuran, & K. Witowska-Olearska, (1978). The course of epilepsy and drug taking in randomly selected groups of patients in the light of 5-year follow-up (in Polish). *Polski Tygodnik Lekarski* 33, 1927–30.

Zielinski, J. J., & B. Rader. (1984). Employability of persons with epilepsy: Difficulties of assessment. In R. J. Porter, R. H. Mattson, A. A. Ward, Jr., & M. Dam (Eds.), *Advances in epileptology: XVth Epilepsy International Symposium*. New York: Raven Press.

II / *The Social Dimensions of Epilepsy as High-Risk Variables for Psychopathology*

As we have noted in the Introduction and argued in chapter 1, the potential for social factors to cause psychopathology in people with epilepsy is substantial and heretofore empirically unexplored. The chapters in this section respond to this issue.

In chapter 3, Joseph Schneider and Peter Conrad present new data from an ethnographic investigation of 80 people with epilepsy. Both the methodology and the information growing out of that methodology are new in this field. For one of the first times, the perceptions and words of people with epilepsy are the center of research. There is much of importance in what they have to say, including a great deal about the stressful nature of the restrictive control of information about epilepsy by physicians and family. Might the resulting lack of information cause psychological distress in people with epilepsy?

Robert Mittan examines data relevant to this hypothesis in chapter 4. Testing several hundred people from three ethnic groups, Mittan establishes that fear of seizures, often stemming from patients' misunderstanding of the medical knowledge of epilepsy, is significantly related to psychopathology. Not only is Mittan's empirical investigation the first in this area, but he leaves us a well-defined "fear of seizures scale" to be continually retested and reevaluated, thus facilitating a good deal of future research into this very important matter.

In chapter 5, Robert and Brenda DeVellis review the similarity between epilepsy and experimental models of learned helplessness. They explain how learned helplessness might develop in people with epilepsy and review its potential to generate interictal psychopathology. They culminate their discussion by providing an analytic model that may be used to test their hypotheses.

In chapter 6, Paul Arntson, David Droge, Robert Norton, and Ellen Murray replicate previous findings that epilepsy is associated with a variety of interpersonal and social problems. They also replicate previous findings that psychopathology is increased in epilepsy relative to healthy controls. They then demonstrate, for the first time, the interrelationship between these areas of inquiry. That is, perceived stigma, helplessness, and external locus of control (thought to result from the psychosocial consequences of epilepsy) are found to be significantly associated with increased depression, anxiety, somatic problems, and decreased life satisfaction.

In chapter 7, Wendy Matthews and Gabor Barabas continue their series of studies of children with epilepsy, this time concentrating on the children's perceptions of cause–effect relationships (locus of control). By relating locus of control to social competence and psychopathology, and by comparing these results to those obtained from children with diabetes and from healthy children, Matthews and Barabas are able to gain important insights into these relationships.

These five chapters provide specific data that explicitly suggest a relationship between social factors and psychopathology in people with epilepsy, a hypothesis that is tested formally in chapters 4, 6, and 7. Beyond the data, the chapters provide a conceptual structure and a methodology that can facilitate much work in this area. Whether all hypotheses in this section will be borne out after further investigation, and whether all results will be replicated, is a secondary issue. The primary issue is that there is now a research agenda before us that can be responsibly and effectively pursued.

3 / Doctors, Information, and the Control of Epilepsy: A Patients' Perspective

JOSEPH W. SCHNEIDER and
PETER CONRAD

People with epilepsy, like all people with chronic illness, are confronted with many new problems and experiences to manage. Not only must they take a variety of medications, follow a variously elaborate regimen of medically prescribed "dos and don'ts," submit to the often frightening scrutiny of medical experts and technicians, they must also face a host of their own questions about ("What might happen if . . . "; "What does this feeling mean?") along with questions about their worth as friends, members of their families, and even of society. In short, having epilepsy brings many new unknowns that can cause considerable emotional strain and upheaval. In this situation, people with epilepsy are likely to see information as a valuable resource to help them maintain a sense of order and control in their lives.

Surely one of the nearest sources of information about epilepsy for most people who have it is their doctors. Patients rely on their doctors not only for medical and scientific information about epilepsy—what it is as a medical "condition" or "disorder"—but for an understanding of what *their* case is like and what having epilepsy means *for them* as well. To properly "treat" and care for themselves, they need to know about epilepsy in general and about its details in their lives. Such information, then, has both emotional and instrumental value. It reduces anxiety and unfounded fears, and provides grounds for specific directions about what to do about epilepsy-related "trouble."

It is usually assumed that the flow of information between physician and patient is relatively smooth and predictable. Doctors collect initial diagnostic information from patients and tell them what they "have" and how it should be treated. Subsequently, with the aid of patients' answers to doctors' questions, doctors monitor relevant changes and maintain appropriate medical regimens. Doctors tell patients what they need to know to comply with medical directions and thus improve their condition or retard its deterioration. Medical and even popular culture portrays patients' troubles typically as a result of a lack of compliance with medical rules and directions (for an alternative view of "compliance problems," see Schneider & Conrad, 1983, chap. 9, and Trostle, Hauser, & Susser, 1983).

In fact, however, we have few systematic data on how the patient–physician relationship looks from the inside, and particularly from the patient's viewpoint. We know little about how such assumptions about information exchange between doctors and patients fit experience. In this chapter, we attempt to shed light on this question by using depth interview data from people who have epilepsy to examine how patients see doctors as providers of information about epilepsy and its effects on their lives. We want to consider, in a preliminary way, the possibility that some of the "emotional problems" people with epilepsy may have could be a product, not of biophysiology, but rather of their relationships with doctors (and, of course, many other people as well). First, we describe the nature of our data, sample, and method. Next we present our analysis, which considers information as a scarce resource for patients. We discuss information problems for patients before they are given a diagnosis, how diagnosis is an important form of information, what information is gained from routine visits to the doctor, and how patients use sources of information other than their doctors in an attempt to cope. Finally, we examine the connections between shared information and the control of epilepsy by both physician and patient.

DATA AND METHOD

Our data come from a larger study in which we conducted depth interviews with people who had epilepsy about their lives and experiences, including experiences with physicians (Schneider & Conrad, 1983). Between 1976 and 1979 we interviewed 80 people with epilepsy. We each did roughly half of the interviews and we interviewed each person just once. The interviews lasted from 1 to 3 hours, were guided by roughly 50 open-ended questions, were tape-recorded, and yielded over 2,000 single-spaced verbatim transcribed pages. We asked no fixed-response or "forced-choice" format questions, and although we asked each person most of the relevant standard questions, each interview contains lines of questions, answers, and commentary peculiar to the person's experience.

Our sample was chosen on the basis of the availability and cooperation of volunteers. Because epilepsy is a stigmatized illness, many hesitate or refuse to disclose their diagnosis. No complete list of the population of people with epilepsy exists, and we believed that physicians, quite properly, would protect the identities of their patients. It is surely possible that this self-selection produced a sample made up of people predisposed to tell their stories, and even predisposed to tell negative stories or make complaints about doctors. Our respondents, however, had both positive and negative things to say about their experiences with physicians. Fully three fourths made clearly positive remarks about some experiences with some doctors. In fact, 40% had *both* positive and negative things to report.

We knew from the outset that our sample would not be in any sense statistically representative, measured either in terms of the personal or social characteristics of all people with epilepsy or in terms of the "population" (that is, all the kinds) of experiences these people have that involve epilepsy. Indeed, it seems clear that no one knows what this latter population of experiences looks like. This makes talk about "representativeness" (or its absence) even more problematic. It also seemed clearly preferable to discover as much as we could about *some* of these experiences from *some* people than to abandon the project because our sample would be statistically flawed. Generalizations from our data in terms of these criteria are thus hypothetical, akin to what might be called "informed speculation."

We drew on our personal contacts with a local epilepsy self-help group to obtain our first six respondents. Then we placed classified advertisements in local newspapers, including a statewide, mass-circulation paper, a university weekly, and several suburban "shoppers." The advertisement read, "Drake University sociologists studying people's experiences with epilepsy. Need volunteers to interview. Confidentiality assured. Call . . . " We did not pay the people we interviewed or otherwise materially reward them. We did not record systematically the effectiveness of our various strategies to get respondents, but our sense is that these newspaper advertisements yielded the largest number of people.

Each person interviewed was asked if he or she knew anyone who had epilepsy. If they did, we asked them to pass on a letter from us describing our research and asking the person to call us or return an enclosed postcard to find out more about the project. This is called a "snowball" sampling strategy. As the sample grew, it gained more volunteers through these personal referrals. This is an often-used sampling technique in nonquantitative social science research. It is particularly useful in the absence of available population lists. None of our respondents provided more than two others by this procedure. Most denied they knew anyone else with epilepsy. We also posted similarly worded announcements about our research in a variety of public places. Finally, roughly 10 people from a local vocational rehabilitation program volunteered and were interviewed, after the program director told them about our project.

Given these sampling constraints, we tried to select volunteers so as to maximize variation in age, sex, and social and economic background, although we were only moderately successful. Our respondents ranged in age from 14 to 54 years (average age 28; median age, 27); the sex distribution is 44 women and 36 men. Of our respondents, 25% said they were diagnosed prior to adolescence, 44% during adolescence, and 7% as young adults. Sixty-eight interviews came from a metropolitan area in the Midwest, twelve from a major city on the East Coast. These latter respondents were interviewed by one of the authors after a move. We were curious to see if stories from another part of the country would vary substantially from what we had been hearing. They did not, at least not in any ways we could determine as significant. These people were of similar age and social and economic backgrounds to those from the Midwest.

Table 3-1 contains descriptive data on the demographic characteristics of the sample. The table should be approached with some caution, however, in that many cells represent very small frequencies. Over half of our respondents were single; 65% had some college work or beyond, yet roughly the same percent said their total family incomes were less than $16,000. Thirty-two percent said they were employed in white collar jobs, but fully one fourth of the sample was made up of students, many of whom said they were on their way to professional and managerial occupations. Fifteen percent said they were unemployed and looking for work at the time of the interview.

None of our respondents had been institutionalized in any long-term care facility because of epilepsy; none was interviewed in a hopsital, clinic, or physician's office. In fact, our sample and study were independent of medical and institutional settings. This is unusual for research on epilepsy and illness in general. Most studies have been done with people in the hospital or patients obtained from clinics' or physicians' rosters (exceptions include Trostle et al, 1983; West, 1979a, and Whitman et al., 1984; and a small number of epidemiologic studies.)

In this research we wanted to give prime attention to the particular and detailed life experiences of people with epilepsy. Our data consist of their *perceptions* of this experience. We do not claim that these perceptions are shared by others, and we were not interested in validating them by reference to external criteria, such as official records or corroborating views from others. Since these perceptions apparently are "true" for our respondents, they provide the frames through which they define themselves, epilepsy, doctors, and medical care. As such, they become plausible as grounds on which these people think and act, quite aside from how others in the situations described, including doctors, see things. It is the *viability* and the everyday utility of these definitions *for patients,* rather than their validity in terms of some "objective" criterion, that make them fitting objects for study (cf. Spector & Kitsuse, 1977).

TABLE 3–1. Demographic Characteristics, by Gender and for Total Sample

	Men (N = 36)	*Women (N = 44)*	*Total (N = 80)*
AVERAGE AGE	27	29	28
MARITAL STATUS			
Married	25%	34%	30%
Single	58	50	54
Divorced/sep.	17	9	12
Spouse deceased	0	7	4
	100%	100%	100%
EDUCATION (level completed)			
Junior high	3%	7%	5%
High school	39	23	30
Some college	28	36	32
College	22	27	25
Grad/prof.	8	7	8
	100%	100%	100%
OCCUPATION			
Professional	11%	11%	11%
Managerial	14	7	10
Clerical/sales	11	11	11
Labor, skilled	14	3	8
Labor, unskilled	11	5	8
Unemployed	11	18	15
Student	25	25	25
Homemaker	0	20	11
Retired	3	0	1
	100%	100%	100%
INCOME			
Less than $5,000	14%	14%	14%
$5,000–$10,000	36	23	29
$11,000–$15,000	25	23	24
$16,000–$21,900	11	20	16
$22,000–$26,900	8	5	6
$27,000–$29,000	0	4	3
$30,000 & above	6	7	6
Don't know	0	4	2
	100%	100%	100%

This means we had to preserve as much as possible the meanings and feelings each person expressed to us in the interviews. We searched the transcripts, as a growing collection of stories, for patterns of common experience and perception. This "qualitative" approach to research (as distinct from the more "quantitative") runs immediately into one of the historic tensions that bedevil social science, namely, the desire to capture the nature of people's *particular* human experience versus a scientific mandate to create *general* knowledge.

This tension is both inevitable and insoluble in social science. To discard the unique and meaningful experience of the individual necessarily blurs the validity of the generalizations that follow and denies some of what is distinctive about the subject matter of social science. To pursue this detail alone precludes the possibility of "patterns" in the data and of generalizability at any level. The procedures of qualitative analysis in sociology attempt to manage this tension by staying as close to the meanings of respondents' words and stories as possible, while at the same time searching for what appear to be essentially similar kinds of expressed meaning and experience. In our research we have drawn on what is called the "grounded theory" approach of qualitative analysis (see Glaser, 1978; Glaser & Strauss, 1967; Lofland, 1971). This approach is inductive and involves identifying recurrent themes in early respondents' comments to guide subsequent sampling, questioning, and analysis.

We read and reread and then coded segments of our respondents' stories to preserve as much information as possible while trying to draw out important common features of the reported experience. We used codes made up of respondents' own words. For example, "doctors," "information," and "taking medicine" were important general codes that included several subcodes, such as "told me nothing," "gave good details, " "kind," and "in a hurry."

In the sections that follow, we occasionally use count and percentage figures to describe perceptions and experiences. These numbers should be taken as approximate, inasmuch as the particular issue at hand often emerged spontaneously in our conversations rather than as answers to direct, standard questions. Moreover, in considering these numbers it is important to remember that our sample is not statistically representative.

ANALYSIS

Information as a Scarce Resource

Starting with their initial contact and diagnosis, patients look to doctors not only for specific medical treatments, but also for correct and relevant information about epilepsy and themselves as people who have it. At the same time, doctors need information about their patients' lives and physical troubles. Doctors evaluate and process this and other information to make a diagnosis and plan treatment. Then they advise patients, prescribe treatment regimens, and suggest prognoses. This and other information can alleviate patients' fears, dispel misconceptions, and help patients better understand present troubles and plan courses of future action. An important product of this understanding can be a greater sense of control over their lives and themselves. The majority of our respondents believed that their doctors were, in general, rich in this resource but quite miserly in how they distributed it.

Patients' perceptions of the amount and kind of information doctors shared with them seemed to affect how they judged their doctors. A number of studies show that problems of "inadequate" information are perhaps the single greatest source of patient dissatisfaction with medical care received (Boreham & Gibson, 1978; Matthews, 1983; Waitzkin & Stoeckle, 1976). Twenty-two (28%) of our respondents even believed their doctors' hesitancy to share information about epilepsy with them meant the doctors neither knew nor wanted to know much about it. One woman said, "I think doctors are rather uninformed, just like the rest of us are . . . or if they were informed, they didn't let me know." This perceived reticence surely contributed to seeing doctors as aloof, distant, "too busy," or as not really caring about the patient's problems. Thirty-seven respondents (46%) expressed some variant of this view. These and similar perceptions easily became "good reasons" for not contacting doctors at all (Locker, 1981).

Doctors do limit or control the amount and kind of information they share with patients. Sociological research suggests that information about prognosis is shared most selectively with patients (Davis, 1963; Glaser & Strauss, 1965; Roth, 1963), especially with the chronically ill. But doctors control information in many if not most encounters with patients (Boreham & Gibson, 1978; Danziger, 1978; Quint, 1965). Physicians seem to allocate relatively little time for providing medical information and answering questions, at least to their patients' satisfaction (Speedling, 1982; West, 1983). Waitzkin and Stoeckle (1976) found that doctors they studied spent only about 1 minute of a 20-minute appointment giving patients information.

Researchers have offered several explanations for why physicians control information. One sociologist suggests that physicians limit information about prognosis because they are unsure what the patient's emotional reaction will be, are not sure patients will understand the information, do not want to remove hope, and want patients to make the best of the situation (Davis, 1963). Discussing certain problems may make health professionals themselves anxious, so they avoid these topics (Quint, 1965). There is some evidence that doctors may underestimate patients' abilities to comprehend medical information (McKinlay, 1972) and, as a result, do not offer very much. Medical education gives little emphasis to the importance of information for patients, compared, for instance, to the importance of "taking a history." Medical schools ill prepare doctors to handle the social and emotional apsects of being a person with illness and receiving medical care (Coombs, 1978). Finally, since much of the physician's authority in the patient–physician encounter rests on the possession of expert information, doctors may control information to maintain their authority (Waitzkin & Stoeckle, 1976).

Before Diagnosis and Discovery

Many respondents said information problems with physicians began early, before diagnosis. Although a significant minority (35%) told of "emergency" first seizures followed soon by diagnosis, most spoke of a longer process that involved several physicians, during which they received little clear information about what was happening to them and why.

Twenty-nine people (35%) saw at least three different doctors before anyone told them they had epilepsy. There is, of course, some diagnostic uncertainty about epilepsy, but it is not surprising that patients might have felt increasingly anxious as they went from one doctor and one explanation to another, with little idea of what was happening. One young man described his first seizure in high school: "The next thing I remember was waking up in an ambulance. . . . I stayed in the hospital a couple of days. . . . They sent me home and they said it was stress." We asked if anyone at the hospital told him he might have epilepsy. He said no, but remembered his school nurse at the time saying to someone that he had had a convulsion. He recalled no tests being done at the hospital. "They just said, 'You're rested up now. Go home. It was propably stress.'" We asked when he remembered first hearing the word *epilepsy* used to describe his experiences. He said: "Well, after the first [seizure] the word epilepsy never came up. I never even heard it, so I just went on, you know, normal, and three weeks later, bam, the same thing." He and his parents were perplexed and concerned by this second episode and called their family doctor, who referred them first to one neurologist and then to another at a major medical center. There, after more tests, he was told he was "very prone to convulsions" that could be controlled by medication. Dilantin was prescribed. He noted in passing, "Come to think of it, they never actually used the word epilepsy."

A 27-year-old woman spoke about regularly "passing out" as a child. It was always attributed to her being "overly heated" and "excited." Finally, at age 24 a doctor examined her and said she had epilepsy. "They figured out that I was an epileptic from birth," she said. She had seen "literally twenty-seven doctors" before being diagnosed: "Every time I would pass out they would make me go get another physical and they just kept sayin', 'Oh, she was just overheated.'"

Some (34%) said they first received diagnoses other than epilepsy. The most common alternate diagnosis was some kind of vague "emotional," "psychological," or "psychiatric" problem that was supposed to explain the person's strange feelings and conduct. All stories reporting such alternate "psychological" diagnoses came from women (who were, overall, about twice as likely as men to have received an initial diagnosis other then epilepsy). Some research shows women to be more "at risk" for such affective disorder diagnoses than men (Dohrenwend & Dohrenwend, 1974, 1976; Riessman, 1983). One study found that when patient complaints persisted in the absence of physical evidence, some physicians concluded, based on no other evidence, that the patient suffered from a psychiatric problem (Millman, 1976).

A 21-year-old woman said she had "fainting spells" from the time she was a college freshman but was not diagnosed as having epilepsy until 3 years later. During this time her doctors insisted her problem was "psychosomatic." Another woman received therapy at a mental health unit for a year after a series of "blackouts":

> I really didn't think of me having epilepsy for a long time. It was never talked about as epilepsy. They [her GP] first thought I had a psychological problem because of the death of my husband and I was blacking out. They sent me to a psychiatrist, a psychologist, for over a year. It was never regarded as epilepsy . . . it was just an emotional thing. It wasn't until [later] when I went to [a major medical center] that they used the word epilepsy.

In these and similar cases respondents presented complaints that were defined as "normal" under the circumstances, were neutralized as something unknown yet nevertheless of little lasting significance, or taken as grounds for various diagnoses other than epilepsy—most commonly some vague kind of "psychological problem." Even when these people went to a doctor, it took quite some time to get a diagnosis of epilepsy.

Nineteen respondents (24%) told us that in the face of these uncertainties about what was wrong with them, coupled with hypotheses they overheard or that medical people mentioned directly to them (e.g., "brain tumor" and "blood clot"), they thought the worst—they became pessimistic. One man's comments suggest how ambiguity, medical uncertainty, and a sense of gravity about one's condition can contribute to the problems of having epilepsy:

> Nobody would tell you things and you'd look up things on your own. You'd hear doctors talking about things, you'd pick out certain words and, you know, you're a little paranoid if you have something and you don't know what it is. And I'd been hearing things and so like I didn't know what a brain tumor was. It didn't mean anything to me, so I went and looked it up on my own and I got a lot of misinformation on my own. I got a lot of strange ideas on my own. I figured the reason they wouldn't tell me was because I was going to die and they didn't have the nerve to tell me that. And, you know, that sounds strange to me even, but at that time it was serious.

He told us later in the interview that he had tried to kill himself in reaction to his despair and anxiety. One woman said that after a protracted time with no firm answers she concluded the worst and was about to take drastic steps:

> I had built up in my mind by the time I went to the doctor [a neurologist, the last physician of several she had consulted] that I probably had a brain tumor or I was . . . there for a while I thought maybe I was . . . going crazy, you know, just to myself. Like I said, it had been going on for five years, and I just was to the point if I hadn't gone to [that] doctor when I did, I'da probably done something that I would have regretted. I was just so terribly frustrated by all of this goin' on . . . and mostly [with] doctors that I have had confidence in sayin', "Oh, I don't know what it is," and, y'know, nobody suggestin' that maybe I go see a neurologist.

That patients come to such conclusions about their condition and prognosis and consider such allegedly "pathological" acts is a product more of the *situation* than of a "suggestible" personality. It is ironic that such experiences, rather than reducing, can actually produce emotional distress.

The great expectations we have for the efficacy of medical care set the stage for seeing medical ambiguity and delay as particularly ominous. Those who found themselves in such situations reasoned that after "all these tests, if they don't know or aren't telling, it must be very bad." When fear, ambiguity, great expectations in experts, and dire possibilities come together, pessimistic conclusions and courses of action based on them are one way people attempt to cope. These resultant strategies, destructive though they may be, are understandable and not surprising.

Diagnosis as Information

Given continuing ambiguity and the search for information, it is not surprising to find a few people (9%) who said they diagnosed themselves. Sometimes this was a result of systematic study, stimulated in part by overhearing physicians' or nurses' conversations about them. One 49-year-old woman had had seizures since age 15 but said she discovered her epilepsy at 35, after reading an article in *Reader's Digest*. She had seen many physicians, taken Dilantin for years, but had never been told she had epilepsy. In fact, she said her doctors did not name her condition until about 5 years after she diagnosed it herself, when a neurologist wrote "classical epilepsy" on a consultation report to her family doctor.

Fourteen (18%) of our respondents said they were "shocked" by their diagnosis. Virtually all who had seen several doctors over a protracted period with no "answers" forthcoming, however, said they were *relieved* to "know what it is." This was particularly true for those who had become pessimistic.

Beyond telling a patient what "it" is not, a diagnosis "organizes" previously disparate events, feelings, and experiences (Balint, 1972). One woman, after years of "fainting spells," described her diagnosis as

> something I could get a handle on . . . what was happening to me and why. I got some medication, which started to control it, and I had a label on what was hap-

> pening and that was very important to me, because to be having these things happen that nobody knew anything about. It wasn't so much that it was epilepsy but it was something that people knew about at least and could be controlled and I could stop these interminable visits to doctors.

It was important to this woman and to others to be "able to get a handle on it," to have a name and an "explanation" for what was happening to them (cf. Hilbert, 1984). Given such comments, a diagnosis of "seizure disorder" or "convulsive disorder" instead of "epilepsy" may be problematic. In wanting to avoid the stigma of "epilepsy," physicians may unwittingly create new anxieties. The diagnosis "a seizure disorder" (which leads in turn to, "Which one?") may not end the anxieties and search for answers our respondents described.

One woman spoke directly to this point. She had what she later learned was a grand mal seizure while at work and was taken to the hospital. She said of her doctors:

> They never used the word [epilepsy]. They say I have a "seizure disorder." They don't like using the word epilepsy to anybody. I realized I had epilepsy 'cause the doctors kept saying, "You've got a seizure disorder and you've gotta take Dilantin," and then [when I would tell others] people would say, "Isn't that like epilepsy?" And I looked up epilepsy in the dictionary and I saw it was defined as a "seizure disorder." I went back to my doctor and said, "Do I have epilepsy?" and he said, "Well, we don't want to use that word." But for me, using the word . . . literally calmed me down, made me less anxious. Knowing I have something I could call something. I had a disorder I could give a name. *Literally* made me more relaxed. But initially I was terrified. Nobody *told* me anything except to take my medicine.

Such comments reinforce the importance of doctors' naming their patients' illness in clear language patients can understand. Such knowledge can be an important turning point in the experience and control of illness. Information can of course bring new unknowns. A diagnosis does have an ordering effect, but new questions can come quickly. One woman said, for instance, she was glad to have a medical label for her troubles, but began to ask herself a new set of "What ifs?": "What if my gums rot [from medication side effects] and all my teeth fall out? What if the driver's license people find out? What if they screw me over at work or school or at a new job? What if I can't handle the stupid things my mother or other people will say?" There is risk, then, in having as well as lacking information.

Routine Visits

After diagnosis, visits to the doctor typically become routine. Our respondents said that unless they raised a specific problem, interactions seemed cursory; doctors asked questions such as, "How are you doing—any seizures?", gave a brief physical examination, and prescribed a refill of medication. If patients did not present specific troubles (e.g., an increase in seizures, bad headaches, new medication side effects), the doctor–patient encounter tended to be brief and standardized, making exchange of new information difficult.

Half of our respondents said that both the quality and quantity of information they received were less than they expected. This is a recurrent and major complaint about medical care more generally (Mathews, 1983). One 40-year-old man recalled an early encounter that was to typify subsequent interactions with his doctor:

> You'd sit down and talk with him and he'd take notes and ask you how you were feeling and I guess he was trying to explain to me what it was, but he never did explain what it was, he explained how to live with it and asked how are you living with it? But I didn't know—I know how I was living, but I didn't know what I was living with because no one ever explained that. To this day I couldn't tell you what type of epilepsy I have.

Although this doctor *did* provide information about epilepsy, it did not, at least in this man's eyes, answer the most important question: "What *is* epilepsy?"

Doctors were perceived by our respondents as very busy and in a hurry. They only rarely asked patients if *they* had any questions or inquired about the effects of epilepsy on their everyday lives. Patients (particularly those with fewer educational and verbal resources) seemed reluctant to infringe on the doctor's time with "personal" questions.

The routine doctor-patient encounter easily becomes a technical checkup focusing on the body as machine, bypassing the person with the disorder. Patients can interrupt this routine, but only by persisting. Research suggests, moreover, that patients typically do *not* persist—they do *not* ask their doctors questions. Less than 20% of our respondents told of pursuing detailed questions about their epilepsy with their doctors. Some research suggests that patients think such questioning is a challenge to their doctors' judgment and therefore avoid it (see Boreham & Gibson, 1978). Other research suggests it is not only the doctor who tends to see the "ideal patient" as passive and compliant—attentive to the authority and judgment of the doctor, but patients as well see this as proper patient behavior (Boreham & Gibson, 1978; Lorber, 1979; Tagliacozzo & Mauksch, 1979). So, *doctors* decide what patients are interested in knowing; patients have *other* questions they usually do not ask. When they do ask, they find it difficult. One articulate professional woman described how hard it was to assert herself and ask questions:

> It's just very professional and businesslike. They often take another EEG to see what's going on and ask me, "Well, when was the last time you had a convulsion

> and are you having any problems with your medication? Do you feel like you're overmedicated? Can you still concentrate and function normally? Oh, fine. See you in six months." And so it's been real hard for me to be assertive and say, "Well, I need more than that. You know, can I ask you some questions?" And I did get to the point where I would write down questions and take them with me 'cause I'd just get so flustered. I really get intimidated by them you know, walking in, walking out. . . . That did help.

Some patients (14%) said they asked doctors specific questions about the origins and consequences of epilepsy. But with little understanding of epilepsy to begin with, it is difficult to formulate pertinent questions. As a part-time college instructor said, "I didn't know enough even to know what questions to ask. You can't ask a doctor, 'Well, if A, should I B?' unless you know B exists" (cf. Mathews, 1983). A certain level thus is required to obtain more information.

Children experience particular information problems. According to medical convention, doctors talk to the parents privately about the child's problem. It may be that doctors believe children incapable of understanding what is said or that children should be protected from knowing the details of their disorder or that parents are the most appropriate conveyors of information to minors. Whatever the reasons, this effectively limits the child's access to information.

One woman diagnosed at age 13 said no one even mentioned the word *epilepsy* to her until she was 16. One young man's doctor refused to see him without his parents until he was 21 years old. He said the information he received was very limited:

> [The doctor] never related any real information. He was [a] . . . very conservative gentleman. And when I turned eighteen, he said, "You have to listen to the four Ds: no drinking, no driving, no drugs, and no draft."

Teenagers resented being treated as if they were still children who needed protection. One young man told us:

> The first neurologist I did not like because I don't think he treated me like a person. It was more like a little kid coming in. I was thirteen and able to understand and felt I had a right to know 'cause I was the one who had it.

When patients visit specialists, such as a neurologist, the already asymmetical doctor–patient relationship (Parsons, 1951) may tip even further. People sometimes expect neurologists to minister to all their medical care needs, but the province of the specialist, at least in this case, remains disproportionately medicotechnological (cf. Speedling, 1982). It is as though neurologists treat the seizure disorder, but not the person with epilepsy. There is a certain irony here. The family doctor's orientation appears to focus more on treating the patient in social context. Family doctors are often described as more concerned, supportive, and forthcoming with information than neurologists, especially about life issues involved in managing epilepsy (cf. Dowling, 1977). But family doctors typically know relatively little about the medicotechnological details of epilepsy (Beran & Read, 1983; Beran, Jennings, & Read, 1981), and respondents saw them as less competent to treat their disorder. A recent study of the experience of heart attack (Speedling, 1982) uncovered these same perceptions. Although patients had contact with family doctors after hospitalization, they concluded in the hospital that these doctors were not competent to treat them. Only cardiac specialists were allowed to treat cardiac patients in the hospital. Patients thought their family doctors had little to offer them, but once home they no longer could turn to their specialists for routine information (much to their dismay). This and our own research suggest patients may understand poorly the routine divisions of labor within medical practice. It is another example of how a lack of information hampers effective self-care as well as cooperation with those medical providers that are available, to say nothing of increasing anxiety and uncertainty. For our respondents, family doctors are willing to give information but they have little; neurologists have information but they give little. Where do patients turn?

Alternative Sources of Information

When they felt physicians did not give them enough information about epilepsy, 25 people (32%) turned to other sources (cf. Comaroff & Maguire, 1981; Locker, 1981; Stewart & Sullivan, 1982). They said they needed to know more. Their search took them to libraries, magazines, medical books, a national epilepsy society, local self-help groups, and, occasionally, to other people with epilepsy. One man said:

> [After not getting much information from my doctor] I went out and tried to find out on my own what it was. Then I was a psychiatric technician at [hospital] . . . for a little over a year. I used to take people down to get EEGs and it's kind of interesting because I looked in these books, volumes on different types of epilepsy, and I didn't realize how many different kinds of epilepsy there were. And I kept looking for my kind.

A woman said: "[My doctor] just told me that it was like . . . a short circuit in your electrical system. . . . That everything just went haywire and that's why it happened." We asked if her doctor gave her any information about managing epilepsy. She said:

> No, he just told me to take my medication and that's about it. I was talking to my mom about it and she said that the only way we were really going to find out about epilepsy is to write one of the leagues of epilepsy . . . and they sent out pamphlets and stuff. I was calling hospitals and everything and they couldn't tell me anything.

Knowing little of epilepsy, but with a growing sense it was "something serious," these respondents' research efforts sometimes heightened rather than reduced fears. A man diagnosed at 16 recalled:

> I guess I didn't know anything about epilepsy. I was sixteen and never even heard of it. And it was kind of a shock because I decided I would find out what it was and the first thing I read about was when they used to burn people that had epilepsy. I thought, "Wait a minute, I ain't gonna tell anybody about this." I guess from the very beginning I had a lot of misconceptions about what it was, a lot of misinformation, because the doctors weren't volunteering any . . . probably because they figured I wouldn't understand it anyway.

Sharing Information and Control: Doctors, Patients, and Epilepsy

Given this dissatisfaction, it is reasonable to ask what it is these patients want from their doctors. What kind of information do they want? Beyond a medical label (a diagnosis) and professional help to control seizures (prescribing medications), they wanted to know "what epilepsy is," what is happening to *them*, what might happen, and how they might better manage epilepsy and its impact on *their* lives. They wanted doctors to listen to their questions, indeed, to facilitate their asking questions; to support them in their fears, and to be listened to and aided in making better adaptations (see also Molleman et al., 1984; Segall & Burnett, 1980). They want doctors to *share* more with them. For some, this is very general: "If some one had just sat down and said *anything* [about epilepsy and what was happening] to me, I would have been so grateful at that point." For others it can be very specific, as one woman explained:

> My GP tries to be supportive, he's just real rushed. He gives hugs and stuff and that's like a real daddy kind of person. But they don't really sit down and look at you . . . and say, "Hey, you're an intelligent person and you wanna know what's going on in your head with that seizure. What it is and what it's not." They try to allay your fears without real explanations. I wanted them to tell me [the] kinds of things I've seen in the literature. What a seizure is and basically, more important, what a seizure is not. I think that's the biggest fear I have. Can I die? Can I choke? Can I . . . ? Oh, big fears. I wanted my bigger fears allayed without [him] then saying, "Well, go for another blood test."

Our respondents appreciated doctors who were straightforward and sensitive to their situations. A young factory worker remarked about his physician: "He was a pretty good doctor. He sort of tried to explain it to me. Told me to stay calm about it, what it was like." One woman said, approvingly, that her doctor "explained that I did need to have my sleep, to eat a good balanced diet, not to skip meals 'cause that has a tendency to throw you."

But even when respondents said a doctor gave such information, a few (12%) said that *this* doctor was the first, following on less satisfying medical experiences. A young woman said: "I think the fact that he sat down with me, and was the *first* doctor that ever sat down and explained to me as an adult and made me understand [was important]." A 19-year-old man recalled:

> My doctor in [my home city] that treated me first didn't tell me much at all. The one in [a big city] I went to . . . probably explained more to me. He really laid it on the line. He told me it was like a . . . disorder of the nervous system and . . . there were a lot of people who have it. . . . And he said, "You can just live a normal life, the only thing is to keep on medication.

This more satisfying relationship typically involved a give-and-take, with both patients and doctors asking and answering questions. It is almost as though the form and sensitivity of information giving by doctors are as important as the specific information given.

In a very few instances (4 of 80), patients and doctors engaged in a type of mutual participation (Danziger, 1978; Szasz & Hollender, 1956). This cooperation is likely to reduce the degree of dependence typical of the traditional doctor–patient relationship and to increase the likelihood that doctors will consider in more detail the influence of the social context on seizures and epilepsy. Doctors may see this mode as more appropriate for specific forms of epilepsy, since three of our four coparticipating respondents had psychomotor or complex partial seizures. It is reasonable to expect, as Szasz and Hollender (1956) point out, that the likelihood of this kind of coparticipation would vary according to the illness. Illnesses that are more immediately and profoundly disabling would seem not to offer the same opportunities for such relationships as epilepsy does.

One woman said she and her doctor together concluded that some of her seizures had psychological causes:

> So [the doctor] and I talked. And then I did a lot of research on epilepsy on my own. Not to sit down and memorize all, but enough to educate myself. And I have come to the conclusion that some of my seizures are psychological, but there are still some that aren't.

A young professional man with complex partial seizures described his most recent doctor's appointment:

> I just saw him today at one thirty. At first we go through . . . medication and then we go through things which are happening like how many episodes I've had and what happens before and after and how I feel and what kind of activities I've done before and trying to correlate them to find out where the episodes come from . . . which is very fundamental in psychomotor epilepsy, to find out where they came from.

Doctors who encourage a coparticipant relationship draw their patients into determining and administering treatment rather than expecting them simply to take medication, come regularly for checkups, and follow medical regimens. This also provides an opportunity for the physician to understand and appreciate the patient's logic and self-care and treatment (see Schneider & Conrad, 1983, chap. 9, and Trostle et al., 1983), information that for the doctor would be instrumental in providing optimal care. Those patients in our sample who described such coparticipation were the most satisfied with the quantity and quality of information exhanged and also with their doctors (see Segall & Burnett, 1980).

A greater sense of knowledge and understanding may help the patient develop new management strategies that foster greater independence. A woman said:

> I wish they would have told me more, explained to me what epilepsy was because maybe then it could have helped a little more because once they explained the situation to me, and explained to me the differences in seizures . . . I felt I was much more equipped to handle them.

Our respondents wanted their doctors to be allies in the struggle to control not only their seizures, but also the impact of epilepsy on their lives.

CONCLUSION

Controlling epilepsy is not solely the work of medical professionals and their support personnel. In fact, if we seriously consider what epilepsy is beyond a medical diagnosis, it is clear that the people who have it must do most of this work of control, care, coping, and adjustment. We have taken the point of view that the doctor is and should be a source of various kinds of information for patients who have this condition. We have argued that providing this scarce and important resource should go beyond giving the typical medical facts about epilepsy as a neurological condition to include detailed and personally relevant judgments, opinions, affective support, and empathy.

People with epilepsy, as the editors of this volume so well point out, have long been defined as at considerably higher risk for various kinds of "psychopathology." To us, as sociologists of illness and deviance, this proposition itself is an apt subject of study. We see it as a question of how particular kinds of professional labels come to be attached to certain kinds of people under particular conditions. Psychopathology is precisely such a medical moral label that has been so readily attached to people with epilepsy. How such a connection could be made and so easily accepted is a fascinating problem for the sociology of medical science.

Without invoking the psychiatric and psychological concept of psychopathology, we can say that our respondents felt they had a lot of "trouble" with doctors. Whether they "really" did, and even why they did, aside, relationships between our respondents and their pshysicians were in more than a few cases the source of frustration, anxiety, anger, disappointment, and even despair. Patients often felt their doctors failed them precisely where the patients' expectations had been so great, namely, in providing information, answering questions, laying aside misinformation and unfounded fears, or even giving them a clear basis for understanding. Although our data and study certainly do not allow us to conclude either that these people evidence "psychopathology," or that their relationships with doctors "caused" it, unless we are prepared to flatly reject what people told us, it seems clear that for a variety of people we interviewed, relationships with physicians at various points in their experience with epilepsy made coping more rather than less difficult.

At the same time, our respondents did appreciate their doctors and their doctors' concerns with diagnosis, seizure control, and monitoring medications. They also appreciated the sensitivity with which some doctors provided precisely the kind of information described here. But it is important to see that the patients' struggles to control epilepsy and its impact on their lives extends well beyond the clinic. In these everyday, nonmedical settings, doctors can help in limited but very important ways. This struggle to control and cope belongs to the patient. This is as it should be. People with epilepsy ultimately are responsible for managing their own lives. Physicians can (and some do) contribute to this lay management by conveying to patients that the control of epilepsy is their joint project and by encouraging their patients to ask questions about specific problems, worries, and concerns associated with epilepsy. Given the historic imbalance in authority in the patient–physician relationship, doctors have greater responsibility to initiate or continue this change away from the traditional form.

But patients also are responsible for the kind and amount of information exchanged with their doctors. They must distance themselves from the image of the "ideal patient" mentioned earlier. They must take seriously the reciprocity on which the doctor–patient relationship rests. One middle-aged man spoke directly to his own responsibility in not pressing his doctor for the kind of information described. When we asked him what advice he might have for a young person who just discovered he had epilepsy, he said:

> My recommendation would be to find out from a practical standpoint everything about it. To work on learning to accept it. You know, you've got epilepsy, but that isn't the worst thing in the world . . . you just have to learn to live with it and you have to have a doctor who has to help you learn how to live with it. I think you have a right to ask your doctor, "What is this? Why do I have this?" and for him to explain it until you're satisfied, until you have a logical explanation

> of what it is for you. That's what you're going to him for. You know, instead of saying, "Well, I know I have it, but I don't really want to hear about it." 'Cause that's kind of what you do. You get embarrassed and so you don't push the doctor. I didn't ever push him. I just resented the fact that he didn't tell me anything about it.

People with epilepsy must "own" their condition before they can begin to minimize the various social and psychological costs associated with it. Doctors *and* patients owe one another nothing less than this kind of mutual and responsible participation.

If doctors shared more information with patients, and if patients asked for more information from doctors, the result would not, of course, eliminate all the problems people with epilepsy have. It would, however, minimize the degree to which their relationships with doctors contribute to these problems, fears, and frustrations. It would provide sufferers more resources and support, they likely would then feel less overwhelmed or disturbed by their condition, and it in turn no doubt would contribute favorably to their views of doctors as true allies in their joint work to gain greater control over epilepsy.

ACKNOWLEDGMENT

Research for this chapter was funded in part by grants from the National Institutes of Mental Health, Small Grants Section (MH 30818-01), The Epilepsy Foundation of America, and Drake University Research Council.

REFERENCES

Balint, M. (1972). *The doctor, his patient, and the illness* (Rev. ed.). New York: International Universities Press.

Beran, R. G., V. R. Jennings, & T. Read. (1981). Doctors' perspectives of epilepsy. *Epilepsia* 22, 397–406.

Beran, R. G., & T. Read. (1983). A survey of doctors in Sydney, Australia: Perspectives and practices regarding epilepsy and those affected by it. *Epilepsia* 24, 79–104.

Boreham, P., & D. Gibson. (1978). The informative process in private medical consultations: A preliminary investigation. *Social Science and Medicine* 12, 409–16.

Comaroff, J., & P. Maguire. (1981). Ambiguity and the search for meaning: Childhood leukaemia in the modern clinical context. *Social Science & Medicine* 15B, 115–23.

Coombs, R. H. (1978). *Mastering medicine.* New York: Free Press.

Danziger, S. (1978). The uses of expertise in doctor–patient encounters during pregnancy. *Social Science & Medicine* 12A, 359–67.

Davis, F. (1963). *Passage through crisis.* Indianapolis: Bobbs-Merrill.

Dohrenwend, B. S., & B. P. Dohrenwend. (Eds.). (1974). *Stressful life events: Their nature and effects.* New York: Wiley.
Dohrenwend, B. P., & B. S. Dohrenwend. (1976). Sex differences and psychiatric disorders. *American Journal of Sociology* 81, 1447–54.
Dowling, S. J. (1977). Epilepsy in general practice—a general practitioners' view. *Proceedings of the Royal Society of Medicine* 70, 266–69.
Glaser, B. G. (1978). *Theoretical sensitivity.* Mill Valley, CA: Sociology Press.
Glaser, B. G., & A. L. Strauss. (1965). *Awareness of Dying.* Chicago: Aldine.
Glaser, B. G., & A. L. Strauss. (1967). *The discovery of grounded theory.* Chicago: Aldine.
Hilbert, R. (1984). The acultural dimensions of chronic pain: Flawed reality construction and the problem of meaning. *Social Problems* 31, 365–78.
Locker, D. (1981). *Symptoms and illness: The cognitive organization of disorder.* London: Tavistock.
Lofland, J. (1971). *Analyzing social settings.* Belmont, CA: Wadsworth.
Lorber, J. (1979). Good patients and problem patients: Conformity and deviance in a general hospital. In E. G. Jaco (Ed.), *Patients, physicians and illness* (3rd Ed.) New York: Free Press.
Mathews, J. (1983). The communication process in clinical settings. *Social Science and Medicine* 17, 1371–78.
McKinlay, J. B. (1972). Who is really ignorant—physician or patient? *Journal of Health and Social Behavior* 16, 3–11.
Millman, M. (1976). *The unkindest cut.* New York: Morrow.
Molleman, E., P. J. Krabbendam, A. A. Annyas, H. S. Koops, D. T. Sleijfer, & A. Vermey. (1984). The significance of the doctor–patient relationship in coping with cancer. *Social Science and Medicine* 18, 475–80.
Parsons, T. (1951). *The social system.* Free Press: New York.
Quint, J. C. (1965). Institutionalized practices of information control. *Psychiatry* 28, 119–32.
Riessman, C. K. (1983). Women and medicalization. *Social Policy* 14, 3–18.
Roth, J. (1963). *Timetables.* Indianapolis: Bobbs-Merrill.
Schneider, J. W., and P. Conrad. (1983). *Having epilepsy: The experience and control of illness.* Philadelphia: Temple University Press.
Segall, A., & M. Burnett. (1980). Patient evaulation of physician role performance. *Social Science and Medicine* 14A, 269–78.
Spector, M., & J. I. Kitsuse. (1977). *Constructing social problems.* Menlo Park, CA: Cummings.
Speedling, E. J. (1982). *Heart attack: The family response at home and in the hospital.* New York: Tavistock.
Stewart, D. C., & T. J. Sullivan. (1982). Illness behavior and the sick role in chronic disease: The case of multiple sclerosis. *Social Science & Medicine* 16, 1397–1404.
Szasz, T. S., & M. H. Hollender. (1956). The basic models of the doctor–patient relationship. *Archives of Internal Medicine* 97, 585–92.
Tagliacozzo, D. L., & H. Mauksch. (1979). The patient's view of the patient's role. In E. G. Jaco (Ed.), *Patients, physicians and illness* (3rd Ed.). New York: Free Press.
Trostle, J. A., W. A. Hauser, & I. S. Susser. (1983). The logic of noncompliance: Management of epilepsy from the patient's point of view. *Culture, Medicine and Psychiatry* 7, 35–56.

Waitzkin, H., & J. D. Stoeckle. (1976). Information control and the micropolitics of health care: Summary of an ongoing research project. *Social Science & Medicine* 10, 263–70.

West, C. (1983). Ask me no questions . . . : A study of queries and replies in physician–patient dialogues. In S. Fisher & A. Todd (Eds.), *The social organization of doctor–patient communication.* Washington, DC: Center for Applied Linguistics.

West, P. B. (1979a). Making sense of epilepsy. In D. J. Osborne, M. M. Gruneberg, J. R. Eiser (Eds.), *Research in Psychology and Medicine* 2, 162–69.

West, P. B. (1979b). An investigation into the social construction and consequences of the label epilepsy. *Sociological Review* 27, 719–41.

Whitman, S., T. Coleman, C. Patmon, B. Desai, R. Cohen, & L. King. (1984). Epilepsy in prison: Elevated prevalence and no relation to violence. *Neurology* 34, 775–82.

4 / Fear of Seizures

ROBERT J. MITTAN

This chapter is the result of an unexpected discovery that, on hindsight, seems embarrassingly obvious: Persons with epilepsy commonly fear death and/or brain damage due to their seizures. Not only are these fears frequent, but they seem to exert significant disabling effects on a broad range of patients' daily activities. It appears that almost any sphere of patients' daily lives may be affected, including psychological, medical, family, social, and vocational realms of functioning. Based on a study that included 373 epilepsy patients, we will present evidence supporting two related hypotheses. The first is that patients' fears of death and brain damage are common, multiple, and may be a leading cause of psychosocial impairment in epilepsy. The second hypothesis is that the presence or absence of psychopathology in persons with epilepsy may have a strong positive association with the intensity of their fear of death and brain damage due to seizures. Specifically, patients with high levels of fear about seizures are more likely to have significant psychopathology, and patients with low levels of fear are more likely to demonstrate relatively normal psychological functioning. We suspect that patients' fears may prove to exceed the contributions of social stigma or organic impairment in the genesis of psychosocial dysfunction in epilepsy.

Given the intense emotional reactions that commonly surround seizures, it would seem inevitable that at least some patients would fear their attacks. Yet prior to the publication of our preliminary results (Mittan & Locke, 1982; Mittan, Wasterlain, & Locke, 1982), we were unable to find studies that empirically assessed the nature, the incidence, or the effects such fears might have on patients' adjustment. Even the speculative literature rarely discusses this problem. In an exception to this silence, the Commission for the Control of Epilepsy and Its Consequences (1978, Vols. I & II) emphasized that patients' fears of seizures create great emotional stress and significantly impair rehabilitation efforts. The Commission stated that "no matter how well controlled, the fear of seizures is ever-present" (Vol. I, p. 75). This observation was not based on research, but rather on the emphatic testimony of seizure patients. In fact, what little is written appears to be based entirely on clinical observations (Barry, 1971; Thomas & Davidson, 1949), or the personal reports of epilepsy patients (Sullivan, 1981). A substantial portion of this literature came from psychotherapy case studies which, unfortunately, were often laden with archaic Freudian interpretations (Mittleman, 1947; Piatrowski, 1947; Torda, 1977). These studies typically explained that much of a patient's fear derived from his or her preconscious awareness of repressed, explosive, and sometimes murderous hostility, which was symptomatically expressed as seizures.

For the last several decades, epileptologists have been seeking the roots of patients' psychosocial problems in biological and social variables. The biological approach has dominated, with its suggestion that psychopathology and psychosocial impairment in epilepsy are products of cerebral dysfunction (Mittleman, 1947; Sherwin, 1982), and/or the effects of antiseizure medications (Reynolds, 1981; Trimble, 1981a). However, from an empirical standpoint, the contribution of biological factors appears to be disappointingly small, even controversial (Matthews and Klove, 1968; Stevens, Milstein, & Goldstein, 1972; Trimble, 1981a), except for patients with significant underlying brain damage (Dodrill, 1980; Klove & Matthews, 1966; Lennox & Lennox, 1960). Because of the limited ability of organic factors to account for the presence of psychopathology among epilepsy patients in general, interest in such factors was redirected toward psychopathology supposedly consequent to epileptic discharges in the temporal lobe (Geshwind, 1978; Guerrant et al., 1962; Sherwin, 1982). Yet, despite years of research, evidence for this narrowed hypothesis has also proved to be sparse and questionable (Hermann & Whitman, 1984).

The second root of psychosocial problems is presumed to be the intense social stigma to which persons with epilepsy are subjected (Goldin & Margolin, 1975; Lennox & Lennox, 1960). Ironically, for all the speculative attention this explanation has received, there is actually little empirical evidence supporting it (Commission for the Control of Epilepsy and Its Consequences, 1978, Vol. I). The presence of social stigma is implied by some research (Arangio, 1976, 1978; Bagley, 1972; West, 1983), and disputed by the results of others (Caveness & Gallup, 1980; Ryan, Kempner, & Emlen, 1980). The actual role of stigma and other social factors in contributing to psychopathology, either in respect to mechanism or magnitude of effect, has rarely been studied (Hermann & Whitman, 1984). In fact, the chapters in this volume are an attempt to correct this situation. Up to this time, with occasional deference to organic variables, the psychosocial problems of epilepsy have simply, speculatively, and summarily been ascribed to stigma (Commission for the Control of Epilepsy and Its Consequences, 1978, Vols. I, II, part 2; Goldin & Margolin, 1975; Lennox & Lennox, 1960). The general and uncritical agreement on this matter, present for decades, may explain why few have noticed the lack of genuine scientific study of this presumed cause of psychosocial dysfunction in epilepsy.

Despite a history of limited success among the traditional explanations that relate psychopathology and epilepsy, few new models have been proposed. It seems that the lure of discovering brain–behavior relationships that might underpin psychopathology, and the uncritical acceptance of the social stigma model, have impeded new approaches. Most likely this contributed to the neglect of the understanding and of the treatment of patients' fears about epilepsy. There is also a more subtle reason for this neglect: It is the natural concern over alarming the patient—and making the clinician uncomfortable—when one talks about the potential lethality of epilepsy. We have often observed an unspoken and, indeed, unconscious agreement between patient and physician (and between subject and researcher) not to mention the possibility of death or brain damage due to epilepsy. This pervasive "contract" not only has helped to block the study of patients' fears, but has thereby prevented the development of therapeutic measures to help patients cope with their fears.

In this chapter we hope to break this silence by presenting evidence that we believe suggests that patients' fears about their seizures *may* be a key factor in the genesis and maintenance of psychopathology and social impairment in epilepsy. Our findings are presented in two sections that correspond to two hypotheses. First, we will present data in support of our assertion that patients' fears of death and brain damage are frequent, that patients appear to have multiple fears, and that these fears seem to play a significant role in psychosocial impairment. Our evidence is based on three greatly differing patient samples and includes a description of specific fears of death and brain damage, their incidence, and a consideration of the means by which these fears can exert disabling effects on patients' daily lives.

In the second half of this chapter we will present data supporting our hypothesis that the presence of psychopathology among epilepsy patients is

TABLE 4-1. Medicodemographic Characteristics of Patient Samples

	White	*Black*	*Latino*
N	182	110	81
Age in years	45.5	35.0	33.1
% males	81.2	53.8	52.2
Education in years	12.4	11.3	8.4
Avg. per capita income (thousands)	10.6	4.7	4.8
Age at onset	29.4	20.5	18.6
Duration in years	16.0	14.5	14.4
Frequency per year:			
Partial seizures	30.9	30.2	68.4
Generalized seizures	8.3	34.0	34.0

strongly associated with the intensity of patients' fears of death and brain damage due to seizures. This evidence was obtained by pooling our patient samples and dividing them into two groups, those with a "high level of fear" and those with a "low level of fear," as determined by a scale we constructed for this purpose. Scores on three tests measuring psychopathology were compared for these two groups to determine if the "high fear" group would demonstrate a significantly greater amount of psychopathology as predicted.

METHOD

SUBJECTS

For this study, three groups of epilepsy patients were sampled, including 182 suburban white patients, 110 urban black patients, and 81 Spanish-speaking Latino patients, for a total of 373 subjects (see Table 4-1). Our subjects were recruited from the adult outpatient seizure clinics at the Sepulveda Veterans Administration Medical Center, the Martin Luther King, Jr. Medical Center, and the Harbor/UCLA Medical Center, all of which are located in metropolitan Los Angeles. Patients were drawn consecutively from each clinic. Virtually all patients agreed to participate; however, patients who were psychotic, demented, or otherwise severely disturbed, or who had estimated IQs below 85, were not included in the study. Our three patient groups differed from each other in nearly every respect. The white group came from a relatively affluent suburban setting whereas the black and Latino samples came from disadvantaged inner-city urban areas. From a cultural standpoint, the Latino sample differed enormously from the other two. These patients were almost exclusively Spanish-speaking and had recently immigrated from Mexico and other Latin American countries. In terms of demographic characteristics, the white sample was largely male and was much older than the minority samples. Our white patients were also the best educated, averaging 12.4 years of school. The black sample was equally divided between male and female and was 10 years younger than the white group. These patients averaged less than a high school diploma, having completed 11.3 years of school. The Latino sample was also equally divided between male and female. They were the youngest sample and had the lowest educational level, having completed 8.4 years of school.

In regard to seizure-related variables, the white sample had the oldest average age of onset, at 29.4 years, and had had epilepsy the longest, at 16 years. They also had the lowest average seizure frequency per seizure type, including 31 partial seizures and 8.3 generalized convulsive seizures per year. The black sample's average age of onset was 9 years younger (20.5 years) than the white sample and they also had a slightly shorter duration of epilepsy. Our black patients had about the same annual frequency of partial seizures, but a much higher frequency of generalized convulsions (at 34 per year). The Latino group had the youngest age of onset (18.6 years) and the highest frequency of seizures. They averaged twice as many partial seizures (68.4), and had as many generalized convulsive attacks as the black group.

Procedure

All patients were given a structured clinical interview that covered their knowledge about epilepsy and its treatment, their knowledge and opinions regarding their own epilepsy, and their assessment of how epilepsy had affected various aspects of their daily living. The latter included medical, psychological, family, social, and vocational spheres of life. Patients were also given a battery of paper-and-pencil tests, including the Sepulveda Epilepsy Battery (SEB) and the Washington Psychosocial Seizure Inventory (WPSI). The SEB (Mittan & Wasterlain, 1978) is a true–false inventory that contains 18 items related directly to the fears patients have about their seizures. The WPSI (Dodrill, 1977) is also a true–false inventory and has five items relevant to patients' fears. These tests were given in the context of a battery of nine tests. The entire assessment took between 6 and 10 hours spread over several clinic appointments. Because of the time involved, some patients did not complete all of our tests. As a result, the number of patients obtaining scores varied for each instrument. The total *N* for the SEB was 373, including 182 white subjects, 110 black subjects, and 81 Latino subjects. The total *N* for the WPSI was 326, including 156 white, 103 black, and 67 Latino subjects. As part of the assessment battery, patients were also given the Depression Adjective Checklist (DACL), the Hostility and Direction of Hostility Questionnaire (HDHQ), and the Minnesota Multiphasic Personality Inventory (MMPI). Sample sizes and results with respect to these three tests, which are measures of psychopathology, are reported in the second half of this chapter.

Patients' seizure diagnoses were established on the basis of a chart review. An extensive amount of medical information was coded, including EEG, CAT scan, and other neurological results, in addition to historical information. Questionable diagnoses were generally resolved by two neurologists in consultation with project staff, and additional tests sometimes were ordered to assist in this process. If the diagnosis of epilepsy remained questionable, the patient was not included in this analysis. Seizure frequency was established primarily on the basis of patient and family interviews, with reference to historical data in the patient's chart.

RESULTS AND DISCUSSION

NATURE, INCIDENCE, AND CONSEQUENCES OF PATIENTS' FEARS ABOUT SEIZURES

Fear vs. Stigma

We first realized the importance of patients' fears when we asked them whether seizures or social stigma caused them the most emotional stress. Fifty-two percent of our white sample and 54% of our black and Latino samples stated that the fear they felt about their seizures was their greatest problem. All of these patients indicated that stigma never eclipsed the threat of seizures in importance. We were impressed by the fact that a majority of each sample felt this way despite the great differences among them with regard to education, income, cultural background, language, and seizure frequency.

Fear of Death

Based on our surveys, the most common fear among our patients was fear of death due to seizures. Uniformly two thirds of each sample thought that they could die with their next seizure (see Table 4-2). Patients typically thought that death would occur as a result of suffocation from swallowing their tongue during a seizure. However, patients anticipated many other fatal consequences as well. The second most common fear was that they would either die suddenly due to a seizure or that they would die as a result of an accident precipitated by a seizure. Most patients thought that such events were not only possible, but likely. This concern was particularly prevalent among the white sample, including two thirds of these patients. Additionally, patients thought that other events that occur during seizures would be fatal. For example, between 10% and 20% of our patients thought that if they turned blue during a seizure (cyanosis), they would die. A significant number of patients also thought that because they had epilepsy, they necessarily had a brain

TABLE 4-2. Incidence of Patients' Fears about Death Due to Epilepsy (in %)

	White	*Black*	*Latino*
May die with the next seizure	67	69	68
Sudden death, accidents are likely	65	54	53
If patient turns blue during a seizure, he will die	12	19	15
Persons with epilepsy have brain tumors	14	27	33
Persons with epilepsy frequently die from their seizures	22	46	38
Won't live as long as people without epilepsy	20	15	16

tumor. This idea appeared most frequently among our minority samples, where one fourth of blacks and one third of Latinos thought so.

From the foregoing, it is apparent that our patients were concerned about a variety of causes of death from epilepsy, ranging from a fear of vaguely defined sudden death, to more specific causes, such as suffocation. Because we did not realize the importance of these fears at the outset of our study, we did not record the incidence of other frequent concerns, like fear of strokes or of heart attacks during seizures. These also appeared to be common, though seemingly more pronounced among our minority groups. Virtually all our patients expressed multiple fears: Only one patient out of the entire sample of 373 expressed no apprehensions regarding death or brain damage.

From a clinical standpoint, patients' ideas of specific, potentially lethal events only partly reflect the degree of stress they might be experiencing due to their concerns. We were also interested in patients' overall assessment of the likelihood of fatal, seizure-related events. We discovered that a considerable proportion of our patients believed that persons with epilepsy *frequently* die of their seizures. This belief was present among 22% of our white sample, and it rose to nearly half of the black sample (46%) and to over a third of the Latino sample (38%). At this point we encountered a curious paradox. Although nearly every patient was afraid of some specific cause(s) of death due to seizures, and a substantial proportion thought such death was common, a disproportionately small number of patients thought that people with epilepsy do not live as long as other people (20% of white, 15% of black, and 16% of Latino patients).

The contradiction between widespread fears of death as represented by specific concerns about suffocation, sudden death, accidents, and so on and patients' assessment of longevity seemed noteworthy. From clinical interviews, it is our impression that for half of our patients, fear of death posed a significant threat to their psychological homeostasis. Once we "broke the ice" in our interviews, we found it hard to adequately record our patients' sense of urgency regarding these fears, or the amount of day-to-day stress they experienced because of their fears, or how such fears could completely color their world view and dominate their lifestyle. These problems seemed especially common in patients whose seizures were not completely controlled, but they were also present in patients whose seizures had been controlled for years. For many, the psychological alarm created by these fears threatened (sometimes successfully) to overwhelm the emotional concentration and energy needed to cope with the day-to-day requirements of living, requirements already made harder by epilepsy. Many patients made what can only be characterized as heroic efforts to deny their fears of death in order to continue—hence the denial of shortened longevity, at least in part.

The psychological solution that patients seemed to develop was that they could cope with the more immediate threats of specific, and avoidable, causes of death. And, if they exclusively focused on avoiding accidents or various mechanisms they thought triggered their seizures, they would not have to think about the general and unavoidable fear that they might die early. Most patients seemed to circumvent their conscious fear of death by expending a great deal of energy in structuring their lives so as to avoid those specific circumstances that they thought might lead to trouble. Frequently these avoidances were realistic and practical. More often, however, it seemed that these avoidances were phobic or ritualistic in nature. Often patients would not consume certain foods, pursue certain activities, or go certain places, and sometimes they would refuse even to leave their homes except to see the doctor. Frequently these superstitious coping strategies had a real impact on patients' psychosocial lives, as we will describe later. Much less often, counterphobic mechanisms were used. Here, patients would repeatedly place themselves in hazardous situations, and deny the possibility of death by pointedly acting as if epilepsy held no risk at all.

Fewer than 1 in 20 patients said they had ever discussed the possibility of death due to epilepsy with their neurologist. Similarly, few neurologists we have talked with ever broached this subject—except to warn against driving or to threaten a patient who was noncompliant. We found the latter to be a not uncommon practice, one we considered well intentioned, but appalling. There seemed to be a powerful, unspoken, and universal agreement between patient and physician that death from epilepsy was not to be discussed, except for the specific, avoidable causes like auto accidents or drowning. The resulting psychological protection for both sides of the patient–doctor relationship appears to be an important reason why patients' fears were insulated from treatment.

Fear of Brain Damage

We found that patients were not just frightened of death due to seizures. Fears about brain damage were nearly as common, again affecting the great majority of patients (see Table 4-3). Although there was a high frequency of

TABLE 4-3. Incidence of Patients' Fears about Brain Damage Due to Epilepsy (in %)

	White	*Black*	*Latino*
Seizures cause brain damage	56	71	75
Seizures cause loss of intelligence	23	32	60
Seizures cause emotional disorders	34	65	62
Seizures cause memory loss	58	68	62
Seizures cause a loss of ability to think clearly	78	35	33

these concerns among the total sample, we found that the minority patients were selectively more affected. For example, 56% of our white sample were afraid their seizures caused brain damage, but among the minority samples, the proportion leaped to nearly three fourths. Fears of other, more symptomatic forms of brain damage were endorsed by more variable proportions of patients. Nearly a quarter of the white sample thought that their seizures were gradually eroding their intelligence, whereas almost a third of the black sample thought so. Concern over retardation spread to include 60% of the Latino group. One third of the white sample believed that their seizures caused them to be emotionally ill, while nearly two thirds of the black and Latino groups thought so. More than 60% of our patients thought that their seizures were causing progressive memory loss.

There was one exception to the trend of more frequent fear of brain damage among the minority samples. Only about a third of our minority patients complained that they were losing their ability to think clearly as a result of their epilepsy, but this figure ballooned to 78% among our white sample. On the basis of other data, we have speculated that this may be partly due to the greater degree of compliance with antiseizure medication among the white sample (Mittan et al., 1983b, 1983c). This assumes that blood levels of anticonvulsants that are within the therapeutic range can indeed compromise higher cognitive functioning (Reynolds, 1981).

Whatever the phenomenological source of patients' fears of brain damage, these apprehensions were clearly present. It appears that a majority of patients, especially among the minority samples, were afraid either that they were mentally defective now or that they would soon become that way. Our clinical impression is that patients' fears about brain damage are more conscious, though not as acutely overwhelming as their fear of death. However, by virtue of the patients' conscious awareness, fear about brain damage seemed to constitute a more constant psychological stress. Our interview results suggest that fears of brain damage tended to have an insidious effect on patients' long-term adjustment. Patients who believed that they were losing their mental abilities and emotional stability not only suffered losses in self-esteem (as discussed in the second half of this chapter), but were characteristically less motivated to seek employment and overcome social obstacles to prove they were "just as able as anyone else." Instead, many patients saw themselves as "damaged goods," physically and mentally unable to compete on the same level as people without epilepsy.

Psychological Consequences of Patients' Fears

Given the high incidence of patients' fears about death and brain damage due to seizures, it was not surprising that most patients reported a number of disabling psychological consequences (see Table 4-4). For example, between one

TABLE 4-4. Psychological Consequences of Patients' Fears (in %)

	White	*Black*	*Latino*
Continually dread seizures	44	53	33
Afraid to be alone	22	39	27
Always want ambulance called	33	50	53
Worried about health	65	70	46
Become depressed because of epilepsy	79	74	83
Become angry and resentful	61	59	74
Feel they are losing their mind	24	28	28
Suicidal because of epilepsy	25	28	28
Have frequent suicidal thoughts	17	20	18
Often wish they were dead	24	21	24
Persons with epilepsy are suicidal because of their seizures	57	59	51
Psychotherapy would improve seizure control	54	68	67

half and one third of our patients reported that they live in continual dread of their seizures. Specifically, 44% of our white sample, 53% of our black sample, and 33% of our Latino sample said that they exist under a constant siege of psychological threat. Over a quarter of our sample reported that their fears were sufficiently intense that they were uncomfortable being left alone because of the possibility of seizures. Another behavioral indicator of patients' fears of death and/or brain damage was that many wanted an ambulance called *whenever* they had a seizure. This request was present in one third of the white sample and in half of the black and Latino samples.

Given the dread associated with seizures, it was not surprising that patients cited several secondary psychological symptoms. A substantial majority of patients constantly worried about their health, including 65% of whites, 70% of blacks, and 46% of Latinos. Over three fourths reported that they were depressed because of their epilepsy. In fact, depression was the outstanding psychiatric symptom in all three samples. Nearly two thirds reported that their emotional responses had also turned to anger and resentment. Sixty-one percent of whites, 59% of blacks, and three fourths (74%) of Latinos reported that hostile feelings grew out of their experience of being subjected to seizures. The psychological stress of having epilepsy was so great for a quarter of our patients that they felt they were "losing their minds."

Recently epileptologists have discovered that people with epilepsy have a higher rate of suicide than the general population (Barraclough, 1981; Hawton, Fagg, & Marsack, 1980; Mackay, 1979). This trend seemed to be reflected in our patient samples. More than a quarter of our patients said that they had been or currently were suicidal due to their seizures. Nearly one fifth reported that they had frequent thoughts of suicide and nearly one fourth said that they often wished they were dead. Initially, we had expected that the high rate of depression would be the major reason why patients attempted suicide. However, in our study approximately two of every three patients we interviewed who had attempted suicide said that putting an end to the "unpredictable terror" of seizures was the main reason for their attempt (Mittan et al., 1983a). Patients themselves (including 57% of the white sample, 59% of the black, and 51% of the Latino sample) thought that persons with epilepsy became suicidal because of their seizures.

There also appears to be an important interaction between the secondary psychological effects of epilepsy and epilepsy itself. Almost two thirds of our patients thought psychotherapy could reduce their seizure frequency. The number of patients who saw benefit in this nonmedical approach to seizure control is remarkable. We suspect that the connection between stress and seizure occurrence must be so obvious that even patients we might expect to be psychologically naive had made the connection between their emotional states and their seizure frequency. Given the intensity of patients' fears about seizures, it seems possible that such fears could play a significant role in mediating seizure frequency. In any case, the apparent connection of seizure frequency with mental stress suggests that some form of psychotherapy might be a useful adjunct to medical treatment among poorly controlled patients.

Medical Adjustment

In the introduction we noted that the effects of patients' fears about epilepsy are not simply limited to the psyche. Other spheres of functioning, including treatment compliance, appeared to show a relationship to patients' apprehensions. For example, patients' use of antiseizure medications appeared to be commonly influenced by their fear of seizures (see Table 4-5). We found that about a quarter of our patients took extra doses of medication when they were afraid they might have a seizure. Most of these patients explained that they would also take extra medication as "insurance" against having a seizure when they had to leave their homes or when they had to do something important,

TABLE 4-5. Medical Consequences of Fears and Treatment-Related Fears (in %)

	White	*Black*	*Latino*
Should take more medications if you might have a seizure	26	25	19
Should take more medications after a seizure	16	27	31
Antiseizure medications are dangerous	38	40	30
Patients become addicted to medications	24	35	32
Medication side effects become permanent	18	29	21
EEG can tell if you're emotionally ill	20	55	57

usually in social contexts. Nearly as many patients took extra doses of medications after a seizure to ward off the fear of having another one. This practice was less common among our white sample (16%), but rose to 27% in our black sample and 31% in our Latino sample. Patients' rationale for this behavior revealed that they were actually using their antiseizure medications "psychotropically," as a means to quell their fears that a seizure might occur. These self-medication practices are interesting for two reasons: First, they appear to be directly mediated by patients' fears; and second, compliance problems are usually considered ones of undermedication rather than overmedication.

We also encountered some treatment-related fears that appeared to play a role on the other side of the compliance coin. We found that over a third of our patients were afraid of physical and/or mental harm that they thought could be caused by their medications. For example, over one third thought their antiseizure medications were dangerous. Nearly as many thought they were addicted to the medications they took. One fifth were afraid that the side effects of their antiseizure medications would become permanent. Finally, 20% of our white sample and over half of our black and Latino samples thought that the EEG machine could read their minds and could tell if they were emotionally ill. This belief caused many patients to feel that the EEG procedure was an insensitive invasion of personal privacy.

It remains unclear to what extent medication and treatment compliance is affected by patients' concerns about addiction, permanent behavioral or physical changes due to medications, or invasion of privacy. We do know that up to 50% of these patients did not take their medications regularly (Mittan et al., 1983c). We are certain that for some patients, fears regarding medication became a powerful emotional barrier to compliance. In respect to medical treatment overall, it appears that fears about death, brain damage, and treatment itself commonly caused patients to change their medical regimen hazardously to accommodate their emotional needs (Mittan et al., 1983c). The consequences of such practices appear to be decreased seizure control, increased drug toxicity, and impaired compliance with treatment and diagnostic procedures (Mittan, 1982a).

Family Adjustment

Like their medical self-management, patients' family functioning also appeared to be affected by a variety of fears regarding epilepsy. The effect of patients' fears of death or brain damage on family functioning seems largely mediated by the secondary psychological and social effects of those fears, though there are direct effects as well. For example, as a secondary effect of patients' fears, the family is often forced to cope with an anxious, depressed, angry, and/or phobic patient. Both patients and family members reported statistically significant increases in the social expression of such symptoms on the Interpersonal Diagnosis of Personality Test (Mittan, 1982c). The presence of these symptoms in patients often appeared to alter the emotional economy of the family by draining emotional support resources from nonaffected family members (Thomas & Davidson, 1949). Typically, the family was also burdened with a portion of the responsibility for helping the patient cope with his or her fears, such as ensuring that an apprehensive patient was never left alone.

We also found that roles within the family were affected by the secondary social effects of patients' fears. For example, patients who were afraid to leave home for fear of their physical safety (see below) were also unable to shop, to care for children outside the home, or to maintain employment. Family members had to assume these additional responsibilities, and after a time these extra assignments became a source of resentment toward the patient. In previously unreported results, we used the SEB to survey 100 family members without epilepsy from different families. We found that these people were equally afraid that death or brain damage might occur in their relative with epilepsy (Mittan, 1984a). Thus, fear may directly affect family members' adjustment as well.

Our study revealed other epilepsy-related fears that might directly affect family functioning (see Table 4-6). Of primary concern to patients and their spouses was whether children born to a parent with epilepsy would have seizures. Over 10% of our patients thought that the child of a father with epilepsy necessarily would have seizures. If the mother had epilepsy, there was even greater concern. Eighteen percent of our white sample, a quarter of our black sample, and nearly a third of our Latino sample thought that children of mothers with epilepsy necessarily would have seizures. Patients were also afraid that their antiseizure medications could cause birth defects, including 30% of our white and black patients and 42% of Latino patients. This concern has some validity (Niedermeyer, 1983); however, patients overwhelmingly justified their opinions with feelings rather than facts. Because patients were afraid that they might not have healthy children, a considerable number thought that people with epilepsy should adopt children rather than have children themselves, including a quarter of our white sample and a third of our

TABLE 4-6. Family-Related Fears about Epilepsy (in %)

	White	*Black*	*Latino*
Child of father with epilepsy also will have seizures	14	12	11
Child of mother with epilepsy also will have seizures	18	24	31
Antiseizure medications may produce birth defects	31	29	42
Couples with epilepsy should adopt rather than have children	25	32	33

minority samples. The most common family-related fear we were asked about was whether sexual activity would precipitate seizures. Unfortunately, this unanticipated fear was revealed only in our patient interviews and was not assessed systematically in our surveys. However, the concern seemed to be most frequent among our minority patients. In regard to the overall picture of family functioning, epilepsy-related fears appeared to most *directly* interfere with sexual and reproductive functions. However, our interviews and psychological testing suggested that the *indirect* psychological and social effects of patients' fears, such as irritability, depression, and withdrawal, had by far the most toxic effect on the family system (Mittan, 1982b, c).

Social Adjustment

Although most of the social impairments of epilepsy are usually, and perhaps correctly, ascribed to stigma, patients' fears about epilepsy also appeared to play an unexpectedly important role (see Table 4-7). Here the influence of patients' fears seemed to be at a very primary, global level, and the disabling social consequences were a secondary effect. For example, between a third and one half of patients stated that they were afraid of the possibility of accidents. During our interviews, patients let us know that their fear of accidents was a real concern, especially fear of accidents while away from home. We were not surprised, then, to find that more than one fifth of our entire sample reported that they were afraid to go out of their homes because of possible seizures. Thus, fear for their physical safety kept many patients isolated.

This physical withdrawal had little to do with stigma, yet on a practical basis it frequently had the same social effects typically attributed to stigma. By seeking the safety of home, patients' fear of seizures commonly resulted in social withdrawal and its associated consequences. Through this phenomenon, patients' fears appeared to play a significant role in the genesis and maintenance of social isolation. It also appeared that a strong fear of accidents was not a prerequisite for such withdrawal. Many patients who did not report being afraid to leave their home did report spending nearly all their time at home where they felt safe. This included half our white sample, 55% of blacks, and two thirds of the Latino sample.

TABLE 4-7. Socially Related Fears and Their Consequences (in %)

	White	*Black*	*Latino*
Afraid of accidents	36	53	43
Afraid to go out	21	30	18
Mostly stay at home	50	55	67

Overall, the data suggest that patients' fear of accidents or other harm while away from home may play a significant role, and possibly a greater role than social stigma, in keeping persons with epilepsy home and socially isolated (Mittan, 1983). We also observed that such self-isolation often robbed the patient of support networks and led to the additional complications of depression and anxiety that commonly attend an isolated existence. In this way, an understandable and even innocent effect of an epilepsy-related motivation, seeking safety, may have secondarily precipitated significant social and psychological impairment.

Vocational Adjustment

Epilepsy-related fears also appear to create substantial, yet poorly recognized, barriers to employment (Mittan et al., 1983b). We have already noted that over one fifth of our patients were afraid to leave home. Most of these patients reported that they had not sought employment because of this fear. It also appeared that moderate concerns about safety could be sufficient to discourage patients from seeking work. This included several patients from among the 60% who had reported only a preference to remain at home. We found that patients' fears about accidents were commonly and often specifically extended to the workplace. Most of the 36%–53% who were afraid of accidents thought that the workplace was the most hazardous environment for such events. As a result, fear of seizure-related job accidents was frequently given as a reason for not seeking employment.

Besides having general apprehensions regarding accidents, patients also were afraid that specific conditions in the work environment would trigger their seizures (see Table 4-8). For example, because of employment discrimination, people with epilepsy must often accept manual labor. Yet approximately one third of our patients were afraid that physical exertion would cause seizures, including 21% of our white sample, 45% of the black sample, and 37% of the Latino sample. As a result, many patients said that they were unwilling to accept such work. Nearly a third of our patients were also afraid that loud industrial noise, flashing lights, or other triggering mechanisms in the workplace would cause seizures. Many of these patients were reluctant to consider factory work. In our interviews, we found that fear of machinery

TABLE 4-8. Job-Related Fears about Epilepsy (in %)

	White	*Black*	*Latino*
Must avoid physical exertion	21	45	37
Must avoid flashing lights or loud sounds	30	32	32
Stress will cause seizures	80	85	86

was extremely common, even in patients with well-controlled seizures. As a result of this fear, many patients would not consider labor involving any kind of mechanical or electrical equipment.

Possibly the most significant barrier to employment was patients' worry that job stress would precipitate seizures. In excess of 80% of our patients harbored this concern. The psychological imperative of this fear became apparent when we began to add up patients' fears of death, of brain damage, and of harm from industrial accidents to which they believed job stress would subject them. Many patients flatly told us that the money was not worth the risks to their safety or their mental health. In fact, fear that job stress would precipitate seizures was one of the more common explanations our patients gave for their failure to *maintain* employment. Despite stories of how difficult obtaining employment was, we were surprised at the number of patients who reported quitting jobs because they thought the stress was too great. Fear that job stress would precipitate seizures was also offered as a reason for not seeking employment. It should be noted that about half our patients did report job-related seizures, including 55% of whites, 46% of blacks, and 47% of Latinos. For some, fear that job stress will precipitate seizures may not be an excuse to avoid work, but may indeed be valid.

Employment problems of people with epilepsy have typically been ascribed to discrimination, lack of training or education, and to poor seizure control (Sinick, 1975). As with other areas of patient functioning, there has been little consideration of the disabling effects of epilepsy-related fears. Our data suggest that patient fears are a significant barrier to both work readiness and job maintenance. In order to maximize vocational success, we believe that vocational rehabilitation programs must provide patients with enduring skills to cope with fears and job stress (Mittan et al., 1983b).

Summary

The findings from this clinical study lend support to our first hypothesis, namely, that patients' fears of death and brain damage are common and multiple, and may be a significant cause of psychosocial impairment. Despite substantial differences in educational levels, social status, and even culture and language, the reports of our 373 epilepsy patients suggest that fear was nearly universal. Patients typically had more than one fear, and these multiple concerns seemed to play a significant role in how epilepsy affected their lives. Fears about death and brain damage appeared able to engender and enforce dysfunctional behaviors in several spheres of patients' daily functioning, including emotional adjustment, medical self-management, family life, social coping, and employment. Problems such as social withdrawal and unemployment, which are typically blamed on stigma and discrimination, appeared to have significant roots in patients' fears as well. Our findings suggest that a failure to recognize and treat these fears could hinder, or possibly prevent, successful medical treatment and enduring psychosocial rehabilitation.

Possible Association of Patients' Fears About Seizures with Psychopathology

Our clinical findings strongly suggest that patients are commonly and significantly affected by their fears of death and brain damage due to seizures. The central issue is how much effect do these fears actually have on patients' adjustment, and specifically, to what extent do these fears contribute to psychopathology in epilepsy? This question is pivotal since we have seen in the foregoing data that the disabling psychosocial effects of patients' fears often occur as secondary consequences to the psychological impact of these fears on the person. This model of psychosocial impairment in epilepsy led to our second hypothesis: that the presence of psychopathology in epilepsy is positively associated with the intensity of patients' fears of death and brain damage due to seizures. If this hypothesis is correct, patients with relatively high levels of fears should demonstrate significantly higher levels of psychological symptoms than do patients with relatively low levels of fear.

Procedure

In an initial attempt to evaluate this hypothesis, we developed a "Fear of Seizures" scale composed of the 23 true–false items in our battery that appeared to relate directly to patients' fears. These items were judged by the author and three colleagues to reflect patients' apprehensions about death and brain damage due to seizures. Representative items include, "Do people frequently die of seizures?" "Is it likely that an epileptic may swallow his tongue during a seizure and suffocate as a result?" "Do you continually dread the possibility of a seizure?" and "Do seizures usually cause a gradual loss of intelligence?" In order to rate the degree of patients' fearfulness, we assumed that the more items a patient endorsed, the more apprehensive the patient was about his or her seizures.

For this analysis, all subjects were pooled. Scores on the "Fears Scale" were obtained for a total of 321 subjects. We found that the patients' scores on this scale were normally distributed with a slight positive skew, a mean of 8.54, and a standard deviation of 4.06. We divided patients into three approximately equal groups according to their fear scale scores; those with low scores (0–6, $N = 113$), those with middle-range scores (7–10, $N = 109$), and those with high scores (11–23, $N = 99$). Then, to highlight the differences that might exist between patients with low presumed fearfulness and those with high presumed fearfulness, the middle group was discarded and scores on three dependent measures of psychopathology were contrasted for the resulting "low fear" and "high fear" groups.

Our dependent measures were derived from three psychological tests: the Depression Adjective Checklist (DACL) (Lubin, 1967), the Hostility and Direction of Hostility Questionnaire (HDHQ) (Caine, Foulds, & Hope, 1967), and the Minnesota Multiphasic Personality Invensory (MMPI) (Hathaway & McKinley, 1970). Group size varied because not all patients in the two groups completed all of the dependent measures. All patients obtaining a fears scale score completed the DACL (low fear, N = 113; high fear, N = 99) and most completed the HDHQ (low fear, N = 106; high fear, N = 92). However the MMPI was given only to patients seen at the Sepulveda VA Medical Center, resulting in a smaller sample (low fear, N = 49; high fear, N = 27). The t test for independent samples was used to test the significance of differences between group means.

Medicodemographic Characteristics of Low- and High-Fear Groups

We reanalyzed the medicodemographic characteristics of our patient samples according to their distribution between high- and low-fear groups (see Table 4-9) and found several appreciable differences. First, as we would suspect from the foregoing descriptive study, there was a preponderance of minority patients among the high-fear groups. Our overall sample was 49% white, 29% black, and 22% Latino. However, in the DACL/HDHQ sample, the high-

TABLE 4-9. Medicodemographic Characteristics of Patient Samples, "Low-Fear" vs. "High-Fear" Groups, by Measures

	DACL & HDHQ SAMPLE		MMPI SAMPLE	
	Low Fear	*High Fear*	*Low Fear*	*High Fear*
N	113	99	49	27
% White	61.3	29.0	100.0	84.0
% Black	20.8	44.1	0.0	4.0
% Latino	18.0	26.9	0.0	12.0
Age (years)	41.0	38.0	49.5	43.5
Education (years)	12.4	10.1	13.3	11.7
Avg. per capita income (thousands)	9.9	4.8	14.9	7.1
Age at onset (years)	26.4	21.6	34.2	27.8
Duration (years)	14.5	16.3	15.4	15.6
Frequency per year:				
Generalized seizures	23.6	30.4	1.8	13.6
Partial seizures	30.4	75.9	35.8	15.9

fear group included only 29% whites, while blacks represented 44% and Latinos, 27%. In contrast, the low-fear DACL/HDHQ group was composed of twice as many whites and about half as many blacks and Latinos. The MMPI sample was taken at the Sepulveda VA Medical Center, which is primarily composed of white patients. As a result, there was a high percentage of white patients in both the high- and low-fear MMPI groups. However, the few minority patients in this sample all fell within the high-fear group. In the DACL/HDHQ sample, the low-fear group was slightly older than the high-fear group and the same held true for the MMPI sample. The low-fear group was also better educated by about 2 years of school in respect to both test groups. Incomes appeared greatly affected, again in the direction that would be suggested by our previously discussed findings regarding social isolation and impaired job readiness. In both the DACL/HDHQ and MMPI samples, the low-fear group had approximately twice the annual income of the high-fear group. Although other factors are undoubtedly at play in this differential, it remains consistent with our observation that patients' fears may play a role in vocational and economic impairment.

In regard to medical variables, we found that although the low-fear group had a later age of onset, the duration of epilepsy did not differ between groups. The high-fear group did appear to have significantly more seizures than the low-fear groups, as one might expect. Among patients suffering generalized convulsions, the low-fear DACL/HDHQ sample had somewhat fewer seizures annually than the high-fear group. This difference was much greater in the MMPI sample, where the low-fear group averaged only 1.8 generalized convulsions per year compared to 13.6 per year for the high-fear group. In the DACL/HDHQ sample that had partial seizures, the low-fear group had half as many seizures as the high-fear group. There was one notable exception to the high-fear group having more seizures. This occurred in respect to partial seizures in the MMPI sample, where the low-fear group had more than twice as many seizures as the high-fear group.

Depression Adjective Checklist (DACL)

The differences in levels of psychopathology between our low-fear and high-fear groups as measured by the DACL, HDHQ, and MMPI were considerable. The high-fear group obtained scores suggesting significantly greater levels of psychopathology on every scale and subscale that measured such symptoms. There were also two subscales in this battery that were not measures of psychopathology (Direction of Hostility [DIR] on the HDHQ and Masculinity/Femininity [MF] on the MMPI), and these scales did not show significant differences between groups. On the DACL, patients in the high-fear group obtained scores suggesting that they suffered from substantial depression, with a mean score of 16.55 (s.d. = 7.63), compared to a significantly lower mean of 10.17 (s.d. = 6.50 $p < .001$) for the low-fear group. In fact, our high-fear group's mean score exceeded the mean of 14.95 obtained for a normative sample of 100 patients who were psychiatrically hospitalized for depression (Lubin, 1967). These results suggest that patients in the high-fear group were experiencing depression of sufficient intensity to warrant serious psychiatric intervention.

On the other hand, the low-fear group fell substantially below the psychiatric sample, though the mean score still exceeded the mean of 8.10 ($p < .01$) obtained for a normative sample of 856 nonpsychiatric adult subjects (Lubin, 1967). Although the low-fear group's mean score was elevated with respect to normals, from a *clinical* standpoint the degree of elevation was not suggestive of significant depression. This lack of clinical depression among the low-fear group was also reflected in the MMPI depression subscale results (discussed later). We have shown elsewhere (Mittan et al., 1983a) that our patient sample as a whole obtained significantly higher depression scores on the DACL than did normals. However within our sample it now appears that patients who were most fearful about their seizures were at substantial risk of significant depression, whereas patients with low fear obtained scores that were not suggestive of clinical depression.

Hostility and Direction of Hostility Questionnaire (HDHQ)

On the HDHQ the high-fear group also obtained significantly higher scores on all subtests measuring the type and magnitude of hostility present (AH, CO, PH, SC, G, and HOST). Again, the differences between groups were considerable (see Table 4-10). The one HDHQ scale that is not a measure of psychopathology, DIR, did not show significant differences between groups.

TABLE 4-10. Hostility and Direction of Hostility Questionnaire (HDHQ) Scores for "Low-Fear" vs. "High-Fear" Groups

	Low Fear		*High Fear*		
Subtest[a]	*Mean*	*S.D*	*Mean*	*S.D.*	*P*
AH	4.33	1.97	5.91	2.53	.001
CO	4.71	2.50	7.00	2.40	.001
PH	1.57	1.63	3.37	2.26	.001
SC	3.73	2.56	5.89	2.22	.001
G	1.71	1.62	3.65	1.98	.001
HOST	16.89	11.53	25.83	8.64	.001
DIR	−1.36	5.98	−1.02	6.08	NS

[a]AH, urge to act out hostility; CO, criticism of others; PH, projected delusional (paranoid) hostility; SC, self-criticism; G, guilt; HOST, overall hostility; DIR, direction.

In regard to the specific interpretation of subscale scores, the increased AH score obtained by the high-fear group suggests that these patients had a much greater urge to act out their hostility. It should be noted, however, that this scale was not meant to predict whether such urges are more likely to be in the form of verbally oriented acts, such as irritability or argumentativeness, or in the form of physical acts, such as destruction of property or physical assault (Caine et al., 1967; Phillip, 1969). The CO scale (criticism of others) does indicate that the high-fear group was much more critical of persons around them than was the low-fear group. And as might be expected, the elevated PH score (projected hostility) of the high-fear group suggests that they saw others as more hostile toward them. Given the considerable level of hostility the high-fear group was experiencing, it would be surprising if others in their environment were not reciprocating to some extent. We have observed this phenomenon with both family members and medical staff while patients were being seen in the seizure clinic. We feel this may be a major source of impairment in some patients' social functioning.

It is interesting to note that the increased level of hostility among the high-fear group appeared to be a two-edged sword. These patients also seemed to be significantly more hostile in their attitudes toward themselves than were the patients in the low-fear group. The increased SC score (self-criticism) suggests that the high-fear group members were more critical of themselves and of their behavioral performance. As a result, one would anticipate that the high-fear group would have decreased levels of self-esteem, self-acceptance, and social confidence. The G score (guilt) suggests that the high-fear group also felt significantly more to blame for their problems, or at least that they felt more at fault in social contexts. These results agree with our clinical impression that high-fear patients are more self-deprecatory.

Given the significantly increased levels of hostility felt both toward others and toward self, it was not surprising that the high-fear group obtained a very significantly higher overall hostility score (HOST). The difference between groups reflects a considerable clinical magnitude. This provides further evidence for our hypothesis that epilepsy patients who are suffering from a high level of fear regarding their seizures are subject to greater psychopathology. These results also suggest that high levels of fear impair social functioning.

The two groups did not differ on the one HDHQ subtest that does not measure hostility. The direction scale (DIR) does not assess magnitude of hostility, but rather whether the patient's hostility is predominantly directed outward, toward others, or inward, toward self. Both groups obtained negative value scores on DIR, which suggests that patients' feelings of hostility tend to be directed externally rather than internally, regardless of level of fear or hostility. Again, it should be noted that the HDHQ was not meant as a predictor of actual aggression or violence, whether verbal or physical (Phillip,

1973). Rather, it is purported to measure the amount of hostility present in patients' cognitions and subjective feelings (Caine et al., 1967). However, it seems reasonable to assume that such high levels of hostility present in affect and cognition will find their way into behavior, if only in the form of irritability and hypersensitivity. We have shown elsewhere (Mittan et al., 1983a) that unselected people with epilepsy obtain significantly higher hostility scores than normals on the HDHQ. We further suggested that the hostile affects and cognitions reflected in these scores may be important factors in the increased risk of suicide among these patients. If this is correct, it appears that increased fears about seizures may be useful in predicting patients who are at particular risk of suicide, especially considering the apparent association of high fears with increased depression and other psychopathology as well.

Minnesota Multiphasic Personality Inventory (MMPI)
The trend of significantly increased levels of psychopathology in the high-fear group was repeated and expanded with the MMPI (Table 4-11). Among the clinical scales, only Mf measured no significant difference between the high-fear and low-fear group. It is important to note that research regarding

TABLE 4-11. Minnesota Multiphasic Personality Inventory (MMPI), T Scores for Low-Fear vs. High-Fear Groups

	Low Fear		*High Fear*		
Subscale[a]	*Mean*	*S.D.*	*Mean*	*S.D.*	*P*
L	53.04	7.56	48.26	6.24	.01
F	56.49	7.18	71.81	21.56	.001
K	56.67	9.63	46.70	8.93	.001
Hs	62.84	14.17	86.37	17.95	.001
D	64.67	14.25	83.22	12.76	.001
Hy	63.41	11.61	76.11	10.41	.001
Pd	59.96	10.78	71.78	11.99	.001
Mf	58.74	10.50	59.89	10.88	NS
Pa	55.29	8.52	68.89	17.81	.001
Pt	57.33	9.37	74.96	15.14	.001
Sc	63.14	11.54	88.44	19.89	.001
Ma	64.27	12.01	72.59	11.03	.01
Si	51.08	11.74	59.48	11.40	.01

[a]L, Lie; F, Frequency/Confusion; K, Defensiveness; Hs, Hypochondriasis; D, Depression; Hy, Hysteria; Pd, Psychopathic Deviate; Mf, Masculinity–Feminity; Pa, Paranoia; Pt, Psychasthenia; Sc, Schizophrenia; Ma, Hypomania; Si, Social Introversion.

this scale indicates that it is largely a measure of aesthetic and intellectually oriented interests, and not an index of psychopathology (Dahlstrom, Welsh, & Dahlstrom, 1972; Marks, Seeman, & Haller, 1974). On each of the other clinical scales the high-fear group obtained scores suggesting significantly greater psychopathology. In fact, seven of the nine remaining clinical scales in the high fear group exceeded $T = 70$ (Hs, D, Hy, Pd, Pt, Sc, Ma) and three of the seven exceeded $T = 80$ (Hs, D, Sc). These results indicate that the high-fear group as a whole was objectively suffering from severe and clinically significant psychopathology.

The fact that the low-fear group scored well within the normal range on all subscales was just as important. This suggests not only that relatively higher levels of fears about seizures may be associated with an increased risk of psychopathology, but that the reverse may be true as well. Relatively low levels of fears about seizures may be predictive of a significantly decreased incidence of psychopathology and a relatively normal level of adjustment. This latter finding was also present in the DACL and HDHQ results.

The differences between high-fear and low-fear group scores were substantial. Individual *raw* scores for the high fear group typically fell 1 standard deviation above the raw scores for the low-fear group (the s.d. of T scores = 10). In respect to the Hs, Sc, and D scales, raw scores of the high-fear group were nearly 2 standard deviations greater. These differences are notable when one considers the limited success of the MMPI in demonstrating significant differences among groups of people with epilepsy who are partitioned along other factors assumed to be related to psychopathology, including seizure type, duration, and frequency (Hermann & Whitman, 1984; Matthews & Klove, 1968; Stevens et al., 1972).

Interpreting the clinical profile of the high-fear group, it appears that these patients had very significantly increased somatic concerns, to the point of preoccupation with the slightest changes in body function (Hs scale). Such concerns would certainly seem consistent with a high level of fear about death or brain damage due to seizures and with a constant dread that such harm might occur at any moment. The D scale was also greatly elevated, replicating our finding on the DACL, and strongly suggesting that high fear is associated with very significantly increased levels of depression. In contrast, the low-fear group mean fell within normal limits, suggesting that these patients did not suffer from clinically significant depression. This was also consistent with our findings on the DACL.

The high Hy scale supports our earlier impression that patients who are particularly afraid of their seizures attempt to defend themselves against being emotionally overwhelmed through the use of global denial. As a result, high-fear patients may tend to be naive about their psychological states and motivations, and instead present somatic concerns as the focus of their complaints.

The particularly high elevation of this scale necessarily includes the conversion of anxiety into somatic symptoms, suggesting that high-fear patients' psychological defenses may actually exacerbate their fears. This psychological defense would also be consistent with pseudoseizures, which are known to occur in patients with true seizure disorders (Trimble, 1981b).

The remaining highly elevated scale, Sc, suggests that high-fear patients may have difficulty with interpersonal relationships, a tendency toward withdrawal, a damaged self-identity, and individualistic thoughts and behaviors that may border on or include psychotic disturbances. Other researchers have noted that the overall incidence of psychopathology among people with epilepsy is no greater than that of other chronic disability groups. However, when epilepsy patients exhibit psychopathology, it is more serious and tends to be more psychotic than neurotic in nature (Whitman, Hermann, & Gordon, 1984). Since elevations on the Sc scale seem closely associated with level of fear, fear levels may be useful in identifying patients at risk of major disturbances.

The remaining elevated scales, Pt and Ma, suggest increased levels of anxiety and behavioral restlessness in the high-fear group. These scores imply that the high-fear patients were stressed and immobilized in respect to their adaptive functioning, that they had difficulty planning and adhering to a course of action, and that as a result they would appear passive, complaining, yet behaviorally impulsive. This set of symptoms could complicate attempts at social and vocational rehabilitation. The configuration of the validity scales, L, F, and K, suggests that patients in the high-fear group subjectively experienced considerable emotional stress and were asking for help in their test-taking attitude. In contrast, the low-fear group exhibited normal psychological defensiveness and no evidence of being in an emotional crisis.

It should be noted that the clinical interpretation of a group profile is at once representative of everyone and no one. Caution thus should be exercised when applying these results to individual patients. However, from the overall results of the MMPI, it seems clear that patients with relatively high levels of fears of death and brain damage due to seizures have substantially increased levels of psychopathology, whereas those with low levels fall within the normal range of functioning.

Summary

A consistent pattern emerged from the collective results of the DACL, HDHQ, and MMPI. It appears that the presence of psychopathology in epilepsy may be strongly associated with the intensity of patients' fears of death and brain damage due to seizures. On every measure of psychopathology on all three tests, the high-fear group obtained scores indicating substantial impairment. Not only were the differences between low- and high-fear groups statistically significant, but the magnitude of differences was considerable from a clinical standpoint. Thus, the significances obtained were not merely artifacts of large samples. The likelihood of a positive relationship between patients' fears and psychopathology was further reinforced by our finding that patients with low levels of fears scored within the normal range on the MMPI.

Unfortunately, the design of the current analysis does not establish a causal relationship. Our results merely demonstrate a coincidence between high fears and psychopathology, and between low fears and normal functioning. Such a causal relation does appear reasonable, however, and some possible mechanisms to account for it were described in the first part of this chapter. At the same time, certain variables have not been controlled. Our earlier medicodemographic analysis of the high- and low-fear groups suggests that some of these variables may play intervening roles. Certainly it appears that urban minority status, lower educational level, and higher seizure frequency may be associated with both increased fear and increased psychopathology. Earlier age of onset and younger chronological age may also be associated with the presence of psychopathology. Duration of epilepsy seems much less a factor, and the significantly reduced income level of high-fear patients may be more a result than a contributor. There is a chicken-and-egg dilemma with some of these variables as well. For example, both seizure control and educational level may be decreased as a result of patients' high fear levels having caused dysfunctional medical and social-coping responses in the past.

Despite the limitations of our analysis, it is our opinion that the relationship between the level of patients' fears and the incidence of psychopathology in epilepsy is robust. Correlative studies have been done with respect to these and other intervening variables, without succeeding in establishing differences equal in magnitude to those we found in regard to patients' fears (Dodrill, 1980; Guerrant et al., 1962; Hermann & Whitman, 1984; Matthews & Klove, 1968; Stevens et al., 1972). The results presented here appear to support the idea that patients' fears about death and brain damage may be a major factor contributing to psychopathology and psychosocial impairment in epilepsy. It is our view that such fears are positively associated with psychopathology: Patients with high levels of fear appear to be at risk of significant psychopathology, whereas patients with low levels of fear tend to exhibit normal psychological function and a relative absence of impairment.

The current research design also does not preclude the possibility that cause and effect might be the reverse from what we are suggesting, i.e., that psychopathology causes fears about seizures rather than fear causing psychopathology. It seems reasonable that persons already in psychological distress may be at greater risk of developing fears than those who are better adjusted. However, the clinical data in the first half of this chapter lend little support to the notion that patients' fears grew out of preexisting psychopathology. Instead, patients reported anxiety, depression, worry, and withdrawal as a consequence of their concern over the physical and mental harm of seizures.

THE PROBLEM OF PATIENTS' FEARS AND SOME RECOMMENDATIONS REGARDING TREATMENT

For years patients' fears about death and brain damage due to seizures have been neglected as an object of scientific investigation and as an aim of treatment (Mittan et al., 1982). This neglect may have prevented the recognition of one of the more obvious, and possibly one of the more important factors affecting the quality of life of persons with epilepsy. Our results imply that fears of death and brain damage may play a key role in both the formation and maintenance of psychosocial impairment among seizure patients. Such impairments are, of course, multidetermined, and factors such as seizure type, frequency, duration, brain damage, and social stigma are also said to contribute (Goldin & Margolin, 1975; Sherwin, 1982). However, the relative magnitude of the effects of fear, suggested by our findings, indicates that fears about seizures may be a leading cause of disability in epilepsy.

In defense of this assessment, two related hypotheses received empirical support, both directly and indirectly. The first hypothesis was that people with epilepsy commonly fear death and brain damage due to seizures, that they have multiple fears, and that these fears may impair a broad range of daily activities. Among 373 patients, 78 of whom were seizure free, *only one patient* did not report having some fear regarding death or brain damage. Patients reported more than eight specific fears on the average. Over two thirds harbored some fear of death due to their seizures, and more than three fourths were afraid of brain damage. Our clinical findings indicated that these fears created emotional symptoms, impaired family functioning, encouraged social withdrawal, and interfered with job seeking and maintenance.

Our second hypothesis was that the presence of psychopathology in epilepsy was positively associated with the intensity of patients' fears of death and brain damage due to seizures. Patients with high levels of fears obtained significantly higher scores on every one of 16 scales and subscales on the DACL, HDHQ, and MMPI that measured psychopathology. Equally important was our finding that a low level of fear was associated with relatively normal psychological functioning and a lack of clinically significant symptoms.

Our overall pattern of results suggests that the level of a patient's fear may be a useful predictor of his or her overall psychological functioning. In addition, assessing the level of a patient's fear may be helpful in identifying individuals at risk of suicide, depression, social isolation, or impaired job readiness. Traditional variables, such as seizure type or frequency, have been shown to be of limited value with respect to the prediction of such symptoms (Epilepsy Foundation of America, 1975; Guerrant et al., 1962; Hermann & Whitman, 1984).

Our results suggest that neglect of patients' fears in health education and treatment programs may be debilitating and even hazardous to their well-being. We believe that every step of the rehabilitative process, from medical treatment to the development of job readiness, should include the identification and treatment of patients' fears, otherwise the treatment may suffer an appreciable chance of failure. So what can be done to help patients avoid the disabling effects of their fears? We are currently testing a psychotherapeutically oriented educational program for epilepsy patients and their families, called Sepulveda Epilepsy Education (SEE). A major part of this program is designed to help patients and families cope with their epilepsy-related fears. This includes fears of death, brain damage, and the "lesser" epilepsy-related fears, such as apprehensions about medications, childbearing, and so on. Pilot results suggest that the SEE program provides significant short-term relief from fear, and subjective reports from patients and family members are beginning to indicate long-term benefits (Mittan, 1984b). The point is that patients' fears appear amenable to treatment. Our work is carried out in a large group setting (up to 200 participants) and uses a psychoeducational method that employs the following elements.

Educating Patients about Epilepsy

"People are not born knowing how to cope with epilepsy, and understanding does not come with the first seizure." This statement introduces the central premise of our program: Before each patient can learn to cope with his or her fears—or with anything else that might be confronted because of epilepsy—he or she must thoroughly understand the physiological, diagnostic, medication, treatment, and prognostic aspects of the disorder. This effort is thorough, is carefully geared to the patients' level of understanding, makes extensive use of audiovisuals, and takes a full day.

Giving Patients Permission to Be Aware of Their Fears

Patients' fears cannot be effectively treated until they can afford to recognize that they are afraid. We begin by explaining how it is natural to have fears about seizures. Using some of the data presented in this chapter, we show participants that such concerns are common. After patients understand that their fears are normal and to be expected, they are encouraged to acknowledge their own fears by a show of hands, in the presence of other participants. As patients look around the room, they discover that they are not alone in their struggle. The group setting appears necessary to get around the unspoken contract not to discuss lethality in epilepsy. Group support also appears to be effective in modulating the level of anxiety generated by this topic.

Discussing the Variety, Nature, and Incidence of Patients' Fears

Patients typically have not identified their fears because of the psychologically protective denial processes we discussed earlier. As a result, before each fear can be treated, a "shopping list" identifying them is useful. This helps patients recognize which specific fears are operating in their lives, and thereby allows them to begin considering the actual risk of what they fear.

Providing an Honest Account of the Risk Associated with Each Fear

The possibility of death, brain damage, mental deterioration, accidents, and other hazards is reviewed according to the best available scientific evidence. We discuss each fear and its associated risk in an honest, factual, and straightforward manner. Patients are already aware that they are not hearing the "whole story" from the literature generally made available to them. They sense that sources of death and injury have been glossed over. The problem is that without facts, patients' and family members' fantasies regarding the risk of seizures have no constraints and become exaggerated. Accurate information may seem alarming, but it actually helps patients fix their concerns on realistic facts and probabilities. They discover that many sources of morbidity and mortality can be reduced through proper medical and personal self-management, which enhances patients' feelings of being in control. We have found that patients who understand epilepsy, its treatment, and risk management do not have to be threatened or even reminded in order to naturally develop a powerful urge to comply accurately with drug treatment.

Providing Examples of How Fears Affect Day-to-Day Life

Even if patients are now more realistic, they cannot manage the consequences of fear unless they can recognize how their fears actually affect them in their daily lives. Typical maladaptive behavioral responses are described and sometimes acted out with respect to emotional, family, social, and work-related spheres. Patients' maladaptive coping responses are presented as natural and understandable attempts to deal with fear—not a sign of inadequacy, but of inadequate training. Similar to playing a piano, coping with epilepsy is a learned skill.

Providing Instruction in Practical Coping Techniques

Patients are given practical suggestions and concrete examples for the psychological and interpersonal management of fears and stress. We begin by emphasizing the need to get the best medical treatment possible, and the need to understand epilepsy completely, including its treatment and one's proper medical self-management (Mittan, 1982a). It is our impression that accurate knowledge about epilepsy and its treatment and good medical management is primarily responsible for relieving patients of excessive fears. However, we go on to discuss relaxation training, physical exercise, self-help groups, practical strategies to increase safety in and out of the home, and other active and positive techniques patients can use to reduce risk and modulate anxiety.

Encouraging the Patient to Repeat the Entire SEE Course as Often as Possible, Accompanied by Family and Friends

Learning is always partial, and repetitions are necessary. Family members are also quite afraid that the patient may suffer death or brain damage (Mittan, 1984a), and these concerns are often transmitted to the patient. By including the family, we are treating not only the patient, but a significant portion of his or her social context as well. Family involvement also helps provide a greater "pool of knowledge" by the end of the course, and family members encourage productive attitudes and proper medical self-management in the patient. Thus, we maximize the effectiveness of fear-reduction strategies and enhance the therapeutic effect of other SEE program interventions by deliberately designating the unit of treatment as the patient *and* the family.

Fear about seizures cannot be neglected. The clinician interested in treating the whole person must be sensitive to the apprehensions that seizures naturally engender in the epilepsy patient. Service providers must be courageous in helping the patient explore and understand the risks of epilepsy and persistent in helping the patient develop adaptive ways of coping. Such an approach is not only humane, but may be essential to successful medical treatment as well as lasting rehabilitation.

Acknowledgment

This research has been supported in part by the Department of Health and Human Services under contract number NO1-NS-0-2332 and by the Sepulveda Veterans Administration Medical Center.

I wish to express my sincere appreciation for the invaluable support of Claude Wasterlain, MD, George E. Locke, MD, and Mark Goldberg, MD, who opened their clinics to this project and assisted with the medical aspects of the study. Thanks also to Steven Whitman, PhD, and Bruce Hermann, PhD for their thoughtful criticism of this manuscript. I owe a very special thanks to Ms. Maritza Gatica for her compassionate and untiring effort in interviewing patients and their families. Finally, I am most grateful to the 500 epilepsy patients and family members who courageously shared their lives to teach me about their personal experience of epilepsy.

REFERENCES

Arangio, A. (1976). The stigma of epilepsy. *American Rehabilitation* 2, 4–5.

Arangio, A. (1978). A position paper: A systematic examination of the psychosocial needs of patients with epilepsy: The need for a comprehensive change approach. In Commission for the Control of Epilepsy and Its Consequences (Eds.), *Plan for nationwide action on epilepsy* (Vol. II, part 1) (DHEW Publication No. NIH 78-276). Washington, DC: U.S. Government Printing Office.

Bagley, C. (1972). Social prejudice and the adjustment of people with epilepsy. *Epilepsia* 13, 33–45.

Barraclough, B. (1981). Suicide and epilepsy. In E. Reynolds and M. Trimble (Eds.), *Epilepsy and psychiatry.* London: Churchill-Livingstone.

Barry, S. (1971). *The mid career epileptic: Problems of the onset of epilepsy in adulthood.* Boston: Epilepsy Society of Massachusetts.

Caine, T., G. Foulds, & K. Hope. (1967). *Hostility and Direction of Hostility Questionnaire (HDHQ).* London: University of London Press.

Caveness, W., & G. Gallup. (1980). A survey of public attitudes towards epilepsy in 1979, with an indication of trends over the past thirty years. *Epilepsia* 21, 509–18.

Commission for the Control of Epilepsy and Its Consequences. (1978). *Plan for nationwide action on epilepsy* (Vols. I & II, part 2) (DHEW Publication No. NIH 78-276). Washington, DC: U.S. Government Printing Office.

Dahlstrom, W., G. Welsh, & L. Dahlstrom. (1972). *An MMPI handbook: Volume I: Clinical interpretation.* Minneapolis: University of Minnesota Press.

Dodrill, C. (1977). *The Washington Psychosocial Seizure Inventory.* Seattle, WA: Published by the author.

Dodrill, C. (1980). Interrelationships between neuropsychological data and social problems in epilepsy. In R. Canger, F. Angeleri, & J. Penry (Eds.), *Advances in epileptology: XIth Epilepsy International Symposium.* New York: Raven Press.

Epilepsy Foundation of America. (1975). *Basic statistics on the epilepsies.* Philadelphia: Davis.

Geshwind, N. (1978). Behavioral changes in temporal lobe epilepsy. *Psychological Medicine* 9, 217–19.

Goldin, G., & R. Margolin. (1975). The psychosocial aspects of epilepsy. In G. Wright (Ed.), *Epilepsy rehabilitation.* Boston: Little, Brown.

Guerrant, J., W. Anderson, A. Fischer, M. Weinstein, R. Jaros, and A. Deskins. (1962). *Personality in epilepsy.* Springfield, IL: Thomas.

Hathaway, S., & J. McKinley. (1970). *The Minnesota Multiphasic Personality Inventory.* New York: Psychological Corporation.

Hawton, K., J. Fagg, & P. Marsack. (1980). Association between epilepsy and attempted suicide. *Journal of Neurology, Neurosurgery, and Psychiatry* 43, 168–70.

Hermann, B., & S. Whitman. (1984). Behavioral and personality correlates of epilepsy: A review, methodological critique, and conceptual model. *Psychological Bulletin* 85, 451–97.

Klove, H., & C. Matthews. (1966). Psychometric and adaptive abilities in epilepsy. *Epilepsia* 7, 330–38.

Lennox, W., & M. Lennox. (1960). *Epilepsy and related disorders* (Vol. 2). Boston: Little, Brown.

Lubin, B. (1967). *Depression Adjective Checklist (Form D).* San Diego, CA: Educational and Industrial Testing Service.

Mackay, A. (1979). Self-poisoning: A complication of epilepsy. *British Journal of Psychiatry* 134, 277–82.

Marks, P., W. Seeman, & D. Haller. (1974). *The actuarial use of the MMPI with adolescents and adults.* Baltimore: Williams & Wilkins.

Matthews, C., & H. Klove. (1968). MMPI performances in major motor, psychomotor, and mixed seizure classifications of known and unknown etiology. *Epilepsia* 9, 43–53.

Mittan, R. (Speaker). (1982a). *Consequences of inadequate patient education.* (cassette). Gardena, CA: Infomedix.

Mittan, R. (Speaker). (1982b). Differences in psychological symptoms among minority and white epileptics. In G. Locke (Mod.), *Symposium on epilepsy—neurological, neurosurgical, and psychosocial aspects* (cassette). New York: Globecom.

Mittan, R. (1982c, November). *The epileptic personality: New evidence for an old controversy.* Paper presented at the American Epilepsy Society Annual Meeting, Phoenix, AZ.

Mittan, R. (1983, September). *Patients' fear of seizures: A significant psychosocial stressor?* Paper presented at the XV Epilepsy International Symposium, Washington, DC.

Mittan, R. (1984a). [Assessment of family members' knowledge and attitudes regarding epilepsy]. Unpublished raw data.

Mittan, R. (1984b). [Sepulveda Epilepsy Education pre- and posttest program evaluation]. Unpublished raw data.

Mittan, R., & G. Locke. (1982). Fear of seizures: Epilepsy's forgotten symptom. *Urban Health* 11, 30–32.

Mittan, R., G. Locke, & M. Gatica. (1983a, September). *Suicidal impulses among white and minority epileptics.* Paper presented at the XV Epilepsy International Symposium, Washington, DC.

Mittan, R., G. Locke, & M. Gatica. (1983b, September). *Epileptics' attitudes towards finding and maintaining employment.* Paper presented at the XV Epilepsy International Symposium, Washington, DC.

Mittan, R., & C. Wasterlain. (1978). *Sepulveda Epilepsy Battery.* Sepulveda, CA: Published by the authors.

Mittan, R., C. Wasterlain, & M. Gatica. (1983c, September). *Epileptics' medical self-management: A significant source of morbidity?* Paper presented at the XV Epilepsy International Symposium, Washington, DC.

Mittan, R., C. Wasterlain, & G. Locke. (1982). Fear of seizures. In H. Akimoto, H. Kazamatsuri, & M. Seino (Eds.), *Advances in epilepsy—1981*. New York: Raven Press.

Mittleman, B. (1947). Psychotherapy of epilepsy. In P. Hock and R. Knight (Eds.), *Epilepsy*. New York: Grune & Stratton.

Niedermeyer, E. (1983). *Epilepsy guide: Diagnosis and treatment of epileptic seizure disorders*. Baltimore: Urban & Schwarzenberg.

Phillip, A. (1969). The development and use of the Hostility and Direction of Hostility Questionnaire. *Journal of Psychosomatic Research* 13, 283–87.

Phillip, A. (1973). Assessing punitiveness with the Hostility and Direction of Hostility Questionnaire. *British Journal of Psychiatry* 123, 435–39.

Piatrowski, Z. (1947). The personality of the epileptic. In P. Hock & R. Knight (Eds.), *Epilepsy*. New York: Grune & Stratton.

Reynolds, E. (1981). Biological factors in psychological disorders associated with epilepsy. In E. Reynolds & M. Trimble (Eds.), *Epilepsy and psychiatry*. London: Churchill-Livingstone.

Ryan, R., K. Kempner, & A. Emlen. (1980). The stigma of epilepsy as a self-concept. *Epilepsia* 21, 433–44.

Sherwin, I. (1982). Neurobiological basis of psychopathology associated with epilepsy. In H. Sands (Ed.), *Epilepsy: A handbook for the mental health professional*. New York: Brunner/Mazel.

Sinick, D. (1975). Job placement and post placement services for the epileptic client. In G. Wright (Ed.), *Epilepsy rehabilitation*. Boston: Little, Brown.

Stevens, J., V. Milstein, & S. Goldstein. (1972). Psychometric test performance in relation to psychopathology of epilepsy. *Archives of General Psychiatry* 26, 532–42.

Sullivan, M. (1981). *Living with epilepsy*. Modesto, CA: Bubba Press.

Thomas, J. & E. Davidson. (1949). *Social problems of the epileptic patient: Report of a medical-social study*. Montreal: Montreal Neurological Institute.

Torda, C. (1977). On idiopathic epilepsy. *Journal of the American Academy of Psychoanalysis* 5, 107–24.

Trimble, M. (1981a). *The psychopathology of epilepsy*. Horsham, England: Geigy Pharmaceuticals.

Trimble, M. (1981b). Hysteria and other non-epileptic convulsions. In E. Reynolds and M. Trimble (Eds.), *Epilepsy and psychiatry*. London: Churchill-Livingstone.

West, P. (1983). *Acknowledging epilepsy: Improving professional management of stigma and its consequences*. Unpublished manuscript, MRC Medical Sociology Unit, Aberdeen, Scotland.

Whitman, S., B. Hermann, & A. Gordon. (1984). Psychopathology in epilepsy: How great is the risk? *Biological Psychiatry* 19, 213–36.

5 / An Evolving Psychosocial Model of Epilepsy

ROBERT F. DEVELLIS and
BRENDA MCEVOY DEVELLIS

Systematic attempts at understanding functioning in epilepsy have largely ignored the role of psychological and social factors. The most extensively studied conceptual framework has been biomedical, focusing on the neurological causes of seizures and patterns of interictal behavior. Neurological models rarely focus on psychosocial functioning. A second substantial body of work has been descriptive, examining the distribution of mental health problems among people with and without epilepsy and attempting to identify symptom clusters characteristic of the former. Studies of this type have typically been atheoretical, cross-tabulating the presence of convulsive disorders with the appearance of psychiatric symptomatology (e.g., Betts, 1974; Mellor, Lowit, & Hall, 1974; Ramamurthi & Sivaprakasam, 1974), but offering no explanation of causal processes.

Each of these approaches has contributed to knowledge. However, what neither of these research approaches has accomplished is integrating processes across biological, psychological, and social levels of organization.

STAGES OF CONCEPTUALIZATION

Schwartz (1982) has listed four schemata, originally described by Pepper (1942), for conceptualizing health problems or other natural phenomena. These, Schwartz argues, emerge sequentially, reflecting the conceptual and methodological development of a line of scientific inquiry. The first *(formistic)* stage essentially consists of classifying observed events or objects into groups based on similarity. Dividing living things into plants and animals or identifying epilepsy as a distinct phenomenon reflects a formistic conceptual schema. As in these two examples, formistic systems are those applied at the earliest stages of inquiry. This is followed by a *mechanistic* stage in which simple, linear cause–effect relationships are postulated. Positing that events in the brain cause seizures exemplifies this stage. Schwartz's arguments imply that the medical model is essentially mechanistic, and Engel (1982) points out that psychiatry adheres to essentially the same belief system.

The last two stages, *contextual* and *organistic*, share a more complex interpretation of events and characterize the research of more mature scientific disciplines such as Einsteinian physics. Schwartz describes these modes of thinking as rejecting single categories and, instead, viewing events as caused by multiple factors that coexist (contextual) and interact wholistically (organistic).

Epilepsy research has predominantly adopted a mechanistic orientation. It is our position that further advances in understanding psychosocial aspects of epilepsy will be best served by moving away from paradigms predicated on simple single-factor investigations and toward a more complex, multicausal, and transactional view of adjustment and functioning in people with epilepsy. Ultimately, such a paradigm should integrate biological, psychological, and social factors as contributing to functioning in epilepsy. General conceptual models that serve as examples of this paradigm include the public health (e.g., Runyan, DeVellis, DeVellis, & Hochbaum, 1982), biopsychosocial (e.g., Engel, 1982; Schwartz, 1982), transactional (e.g., Dewey & Bentley, 1973), and interbehavioral (e.g., Pronko, 1980) models. It should be noted, however, that these integrative *conceptual* models have not led to the general adoption of equally integrative *research* models in their respective disciplines of public health, medicine, and psychology.

Philosophical adherence to a multideterminate, integrative conceptual schema thus does not automatically provide a useful research framework for studying specific phenomena (e.g., psychosocial factors in epilepsy). What is required is the translation of a broad conceptual paradigm into a series of theoretically derived statements that integrate processes at different levels that are of relevance to the phenomenon and can be empirically tested. In the present case this means a series of hypotheses, based in theory, that relate biological, psychological, and social events and processes and constitute a testable model of functioning in epilepsy. The development of such a model is arduous, requiring theoretical, methodological, and statistical expertise bridging several disciplines. It is not a process completed by a single generation of researchers. However, a failure to meet the challenge posed by this endeavor, to paraphrase H. L. Mencken, binds us to an understanding of psychological factors in epilepsy that is simple, convenient, and wrong.

THEORETICAL PERSPECTIVES

In the following pages we will highlight some of the theoretical perspectives that we believe can help us foster the evolution of a model of psychological aspects of epilepsy. The perspectives we have chosen necessarily reflect our theoretical and disciplinary biases and should be considered examples rather than a comprehensive list of relevant theory. The ideas we present do not encompass the full range of conceptual levels implied by a truly integrative wholistic schema. To do so would carry us far beyond the boundaries of our expertise. We hope, however, that individuals better versed in politics, economics, and other "macro" levels as well as those who study pharmacology, neurology, and similar "micro" levels will find logical points of departure in our ideas.

Sample Psychological Constructs Applicable to Epilepsy

Learned Helplessnes

Epilepsy shares many characteristics with other chronic disorders. Among these characteristics is a degree of uncertainty regarding the disorder. A sense of uncertainty may be especially acute in epilepsy, however, because of the dramatic, unpleasant, and often unpredictable nature of seizures. Individuals with severe and poorly regulated convulsive disorders may subjectively experience seizures as largely independent of their voluntary behavior. Complying with a prescribed treatment regimen may seem not to reduce substantially the likelihood of seizures whereas deviating from the regimen may seem not to increase seizures. When convulsive episodes occur, they do so without warning, often having physically, psychologically, and socially unpleasant consequences. Other individuals whose epilepsy is more tractable may similarly perceive their disorder to be highly uncontrollable and unpredictable, even though their seizures objectively occur less randomly. In both cases, the inevitability and unpredictability of seizures may sap the individual's motivation to respond to life's challenges, leading to a sense of futility and a state of depression.

This account of having epilepsy is strikingly similar to the laboratory operations used to induce learned helplessness. In the laboratory, learned helplessness is induced by exposing subjects to events beyond their control. For example, the subject may be presented with a task of discovering how to avoid an uncomfortable shock or a loud noise. This unpleasant event occurs from time to time in a random fashion. No action on the part of the experimental subject has an effect on whether or not the unpleasant event occurs. That is, the event is noncontingent with respect to the subject's responses. After a number of experimental trials, the subject is typically confronted with a different situation that requires solving the problem or learning a task. As before, the goal is to find a solution that results in avoiding the unpleasant event. Unlike the previous situation, however, the task is now solvable. Nonetheless, these subjects manifest poorer performance on the second task when compared to people who either (a) did not work on the first problem or (b) received contingent (i.e., response-dependent) feedback when attempting to solve the first problem. In addition to demonstrating impaired performance, the subject may report a sense of frustration, futility, and depression.

The mechanism believed to underlie the observed response deficits is as follows: First, an individual confronts a problem (i.e., how to avoid the unpleasant event) to which there is no solution. Nothing the experimental subject does influences the unpleasant outcome's occurrence or nonoccurrence. The subject learns that responses and outcomes are noncontingent. This specific learning situation influences a more generalized expectancy concerning the controllability of events. That is, the subject comes to believe in some more general sense that responses are futile. This belief saps any motivation to respond when confronted with a new problem, and consequently, performance is diminished and depression ensues (Seligman, 1975).[1]

Certain circumstances maximize the state of learned helplessness. From her extensive review of the research literature, Roth (1980) identified seven moderating variables that maximize the behavioral deficits manifested by human research subjects. These are (a) extensive exposure to noncontingent outcomes, (b) occurrence of outcomes that are important and meaningful to subjects, (c) negative rather than positive uncontrollable outcomes, (d) an appraisal by subjects of loss of control as a psychologically threatening event, (e) a subject's prior general expectancy for relatively little control over events, (f) circumstances that cause subjects to attribute undesirable outcomes to enduring personal (as opposed to situational) characteristics, and (g) increased similarity between the situation in which noncontrollable events are initially encountered and the situation in which performance is assessed. The last two moderating factors identified by Roth are consistent with attributional interpretations and reformulations of the learned helplessness phenomenon that have been proposed during recent years (Abramson, Seligman, & Teasdale, 1978; Miller & Norman, 1979). The reformulation asserts that the types of causal attributions made by individuals for their lack of control affect the chronicity and generality of subsequent learned helplessness, as well as self-esteem. However, as Roth and others (e.g., Oakes & Curtis, 1982) have noted, the relationship between types of attributions for a lack of control and the presence, chronicity, and generalizability of learned helplessness has been widely studied with inconsistent results.

Considering once again the experiences of the individual with a seizure disorder clearly reveals the relevance of these variables to epilepsy. Seizures may occur essentially independently of the person's behavior and thus be noncontingent. Their occurrence may be frequent and the condition may have existed for years. Thus, the individual has extensive experience with uncontrollable seizures. Because of their physical and social consequences, the seizures are meaningful and important events in the individual's life. The seizures themselves are clearly negative rather than positive. Although not directly observable and, as yet, untested empirically, it seems possible that the inability to control seizures would be psychologically threatening to the individual. However, the concept of psychological threat is not well developed in the learned helplessness literature and its applicability here is thus more difficult to assess.

With regard to general expectancies for control, research discussed later in this chapter (DeVellis, DeVellis, Wallston, & Wallston, 1980) indicates that individuals with epilepsy do differ from normative groups in their general expectancies for control. Additionally, the seizures are attributed to an enduring factor (epilepsy) that resides within the individual. Finally, because seizures may occur for many individuals at any time and in any place, the experience of being unable to control them probably is not confined to any specific situation. Thus, for individuals with situation-nonspecific seizures, essentially all situations encountered are similar to those in which seizures might have occurred or actually did occur unexpectedly. In short, the experience of having uncontrollable, unpredictable seizures appears to be a nearly perfect blueprint for developing learned helplessness.

If the preceding pattern of events is conducive to the development of learned helplessness, then one would expect certain behavioral deficits to occur more frequently among people with epilepsy. Specifically, poor cognitive performance, passivity, a sense of noncontrol, lack of motivation, and depression are the types of characteristics that should occur. Some authors have reported finding that similar traits characterize epileptic populations. For example, underachievement (Milne, 1974), poor attention span (Stores, Hart, & Piran, 1978), noncompetitiveness (Goldin & Margolin, 1975), isolation (Mellor et al., 1974), a more external locus of control (Matthews, Barabas, & Ferrari, 1982), and depression (Betts, 1974) have been described as characteristics of individuals with epilepsy. Other similarities between helplessness and epilepsy have been noted by Hermann (1979). However, different studies vary with regard to methodological sophistication, variables examined, and the care taken in measuring these variables. The observed manifestations typically have not been linked to specific aspects of experiencing epilepsy.

In a survey of 286 people having epilepsy (DeVellis et al., 1980) we attempted to link manifestations of learned helplessness more directly to the experiences of having epilepsy. The indicators of helplessness we chose were depression and two types of locus of control (LOC) beliefs. The first LOC measure examined general beliefs about how much control people perceived themselves as having and to what degree they perceived chance as determining the course of events. The second measure of LOC was specific to health beliefs and included perceptions of powerful other people (e.g., health professionals) in addition to oneself and chance as potential determinants of events or outcomes such as becoming ill or remaining well. Compared to people without epilepsy, individuals in our sample believed less in their ability to influence events, believed that the state of their health was more a matter of chance, and were more depressed. We also tested a regression model consisting of predictors measuring three types of variables: perceived seizure predictability, perceived seizure controllability, and seizure frequency. This model significantly predicted the extent of beliefs in personal control over both general outcomes (e.g., becoming a leader, making friends) and health-related outcomes (e.g., avoiding illness), belief in chance as a determinant of general outcomes, and level of depression. Thus, respondents' expectancies for control and level of depression were significantly related to their experiences with seizures. Describing seizures as less controllable, less predictable, and more frequent was associated with more helpless control beliefs and greater depression. It should be noted, however, that these findings are preliminary and that the relationships are weak (explaining about 5% of variance) although statistically significant and consistent with one another.

Peterson (1982) has argued that many investigators of health-related learned helplessness have observed apparent manifestations of helplessness and thus assumed that uncontrollability must have preceded these manifestations. He has suggested that it is essential to establish that uncontrollable events have in fact occurred. This criticism seems less applicable in the case of epilepsy than with other disorders. As we discussed earlier, the experience of having epilepsy certainly is consistent with developing helplessness. For many people the very nature of their disorder implies that they experience response-independent events, namely seizures. Also, descriptions of people with epilepsy often include characteristics similar to those found in helplessness. Finally, specific relevant aspects of seizures have been linked to the level of control beliefs and depression in people with epilepsy. Thus the antecedents (events uninfluenced by behavior), cognitions (relatively strong beliefs in chance and weak beliefs in their own efficacy), and symptoms (e.g., depression) of learned helplessness have been documented in individuals with epilepsy. Collectively, these sources of evidence strongly suggest that learned helplessness is an important process in epilepsy. However, future research might profitably control for alternative causes of passivity, depression, and other symptoms of helplessness. Medications and specific neurological impairments are examples of potential confounders.

Social Support

Learned helplessness theory promises to increase our understanding of how and why people adjust to epilepsy. However, by itself this approach provides an extremely incomplete picture. What other factors help to explain the variance not accounted for by learned helplessness? What factors potentially influence the helplessness process? What role do factors outside the individual play in adjustment?

One body of work relevant to each of these questions is the literature pertaining to social support. Defined as "the comfort, assistance, and/or information one receives through formal or informal contact with individuals or groups" (Wallston, Alagna, DeVellis, & DeVellis, 1983, p. 369), social support is widely recognized as a variable of potential importance to health outcomes (see Broadhead et al., 1983, and Wallston et al., 1983, for recent reviews). The bulk of research in this area suggests that social support is beneficial, although some investigators have reported negative effects (e.g., McLeroy, DeVellis, DeVellis, Kaplan, & Toole, 1984).

One of the ways in which social support might influence health is by influencing beliefs regarding the predictability and controllability of outcomes, that is, by influencing the degree of learned helplessness (Schulz & Decker, 1982; Wallston et al., 1983). Indirect evidence supports this line of reasoning. An animal study by Conger, Sawrey, and Turrel (1958) demonstrated that social contact could mitigate the effects of uncontrollable shock. Food-deprived animals were placed in a conflict situation that allowed them access to food only if they crossed an electrified grid. Although not a learned helplessness paradigm, this procedure exposed the animals to a stressor (i.e., conflict) that was beyond their control. Half of the animals in this study were exposed to the conflict situation in the presence of littermates and the rest were exposed to it alone. Whereas animals who received uncontrollable shock in isolation developed peptic ulcers (Seligman, 1975), animals shocked in the presence of littermates did not. This finding implies that the presence of "significant others" serves as a safeguard against the adverse consequences of potentially helplessness-producing stimulation.

Research with humans also indirectly suggests that social support may disrupt or avert helplessness. Caplan, Robinson, French, Caldwell, and Shinn (1976) conducted a study whose primary purpose was to examine the relationship of social support to compliance with hypertension regimen. Among the people they studied, social support had no *direct* effect on compliance. Rather, the effect of social support on compliance was mediated by a series of intervening variables. Relative unavailability of support was associated with attenuated perceptions of the instrumentality of compliance in producing desired outcomes, attenuated motivation to comply, attenuated perceptions of competence, and increased depression. This pattern of variables is nearly identical to the pattern of cognitive, motivational, and affective deficits that characterizes learned helplessness (Seligman, 1975). Thus, by inference, access to social support in the Caplan et al. study appears to have reduced learned helplessness, which in turn influenced compliance.

A study by Schulz (1976) provides another interesting perspective on the relationships between social support, learned helplessness, and health. Schulz studied the effects of different types of social contact on the well-being of nursing home residents. Consistent with many social support studies, he found that interpersonal contact was beneficial to his older subjects. However, these benefits accrued only when social contact was predictable and controllable. Receiving visits was associated with improved health status among residents who were told when visits would occur or who scheduled visits themselves. Those receiving visits in an identical pattern without prior knowledge of visitation scheduling did not manifest improved health status. Schulz concluded that, as in laboratory experiments of learned helplessness, the ability to control outcomes was a vital part of his interventions.

These studies collectively suggest an important link between social support and helplessness. Effects (i.e., ulcers) commonly found in animals in helplessness studies did not occur when animals endured inescapable stress in the presence of littermates. In humans, the presence of support was associated with a sense of competence, enhanced perceptions of an ability to influence events, decreased depression, and greater motivation—characteristics incompatible with helplessness. The provision of social support was beneficial only when it occurred in a manner that was antagonistic to helplessness, that is, when it was predictable or controllable. Although the evidence is circumstantial, it certainly suggests that social support and helplessness are related.

A number of mechanisms might account for an attenuating or buffering effect of social support on helplessness. Helplessness was first investigated in laboratory animals that came to manifest extreme passivity following uncontrollable shock. Physically forcing these animals to make correct, adaptive responses was the only means of reversing the helplessness effect (Seligman, 1975). By analogy, supportive others who cajole or push a helpless individual into making adaptive responses might reverse the effects of previous uncontrollable events. This suggestion is consistent with the observation that not all support is equally beneficial (e.g., Schulz, 1976). Some authors (see Silver & Wortman, 1980) have implied that support that encourages mastery is superior to support that encourages dependence. Lewis (1966), for example, found that social support had an adverse effect on heart patients' returning to work when their families were overprotective. This finding is consistent with the notion that pushing someone toward independence is a potentially critical component of beneficial social support.

Alternatively, social support might disrupt helplessness in other ways. For example, contact with others may provide information confirming that one's actions do, in fact, produce desired consequences (e.g., Satariano & Syme, 1981), a circumstance incompatible with a belief in inefficacy. Or, others may help an individual to interpret available information in ways that clarify when various beliefs or attributions of causality are appropriate or inappropriate (e.g., Rodin, 1980), yet another circumstance potentially incompatible with helplessness.

In addition to its effects on learned helplessness, social support might influence psychological functioning in other ways. Broadhead et al. (1983) suggest that social support theory is congruent with biological processes. For example, they point out that evolutionary forces have created needs for human contact and that biochemical events (e.g., hormonal balance) beneficial to the organism may be traceable to social support, particularly in the presence of environmental stressors. These ideas are provocative, but they remain speculative. What is known, however, is that social support can exert a powerful positive influence.

Social support has not been widely or systematically studied, to our knowledge, in epilepsy. This is unfortunate in light of the physical and psychological benefits from social support that have been documented for other disorders. Especially in light of its relevance to learned helplessness, social support appears to be an important variable for linking interpersonal to intrapersonal phenomena in epilepsy.

Neurological Theories

Obviously, epilepsy is a neurological disorder and psychological functioning in individuals with seizure disorders may thus be influenced by atypical brain activity. We are neither qualified nor inclined to review the neurology of epilepsy. Rather, we wish to illustrate how neurological processes can be integrated with psychological and social variables as part of a multidimensional view of epilepsy. To illustrate this point we will discuss briefly a specific set of research findings concerning laterality of epileptic focus in temporal lobe epilepsy.

Laterality of temporal lobe seizures frequently has been linked to specific behavioral characteristics. For example, Flor-Henry (1969) reported that, among cases of temporal lobe epilepsy accompanied by psychosis, thought disorders tended to be associated with a left hemisphere focus and affective disorders with the right hemisphere. However, several authors have challenged these findings (e.g., Sindrup & Kristensen, 1979; Springer & Deutsch, 1981). Bear and Fedio (1977) note that the global personality assessments such as those based on the MMPI or Rorschach have not consistently identified a set of personality traits that reliably differentiate temporal lobe epilepsy from other conditions. As an alternative to this more global approach, they developed a 90-item questionnaire tapping 18 specific characteristics that have been attributed to temporal lobe epilepsy. These include affective (e.g., sadness, anger, euphoria), behavioral (e.g., dependence, aggression), and cognitive (e.g., paranoia, perseveration) items.

Bear and Fedio administered their questionnaire to 27 temporal lobe epilepsy patients with clearly lateralized foci and to 21 control subjects. At the same time, informants who were familiar with the subjects (e.g., family members) rated them on the same set of characteristics. Thus, for each subject there were self-ratings and informant ratings. Scores on the 18 characteristics clearly differentiated epileptic from nonepileptic groups. There were also differences based on laterality among people with epilepsy. One of the most interesting findings is that, compared to the view of presumably more objective informants, left temporal lobe patients saw themselves as feeling more sad, having less self-worth, finding less meaning in their suffering, and acting less appropriately. Right temporal lobe patients, in contrast, tended to evaluate themselves more favorably than did their acquaintances and relatives who served as informants. The self-perceptions among left temporal lobe patients exaggerate their sense of depression, dependency, anger, meaninglessness, and diminished self-worth. This cluster of characteristics also is reminiscent of those associated with helplessness, namely, depression (e.g., Abramson et al., 1978; Seligman, 1975), dependency and lowered self-esteem (e.g., Rodin & Langer, 1980), and a sense that events are determined by fate or chance (e.g., DeVellis et al., 1980).

Bear and Fedio's findings are based on a small sample and one could argue that the self-perceptions exaggerated by left temporal lobe epilepsy patients are an imperfect match to manifestations of helplessness. The more important point for the present discussion, however, is that factors operating at the biological (e.g., site of epileptic focus), psychological (e.g., experience with uncontrollable, unpredictable events), and social (e.g., social supports) levels all can effect common phenomena (e.g., depression) of relevance to epilepsy. The precise mechanisms linking these phenomena are unknown. However, it is possible to speculate about relationships, using theory as a basis, and to test these speculations. Unless the linkages among variables at different levels are explored systematically in this way, we are unlikely to increase our understanding of them.

A Tentative Model of Psychosocial Functioning in Epilepsy

Thus far, we have argued in favor of a multivariate view of epilepsy and provided examples of variables of potential relevance to epilepsy and to each other. To illustrate these points jointly, we now will present an example of a model (Figure 5-1). This model follows the theoretical perspectives we have discussed and is consistent with the relevant data available, but has not been tested as an overall model. Furthermore, many variables important to a full understanding of seizure disorders (e.g., attitudes of others toward people with epilepsy) have been excluded for the sake of clarity and as a necessity of the limits to existing knowledge. For purposes of simplicity, the model is limited to temporal lobe epilepsy. At a minimum, the model is an example of how one might hypothesize relationships among social, psychological, and biological variables of relevance to epilepsy. At a maximum, the model is a starting point for the evolution of a progressively more complex and integrative conceptualization and line of research.

Diagrammatic Conventions

Each single-headed arrow in the model represents a causal assumption with a variable at the arrow's origin seen as the cause of the variable at its head. Curved, double-headed arrows represent noncausal association between variables. That is, two variables joined by a double-headed arrow are presumed to be correlated but no presumption is made concerning direction of causality or the possibility of a third variable causing both. The absence of arrows also has an explicit meaning, namely, that no associations are assumed. For example, perceived predictability/controllability of seizures is seen as having no influence on functioning that is not mediated by learned helplessness.

Specification of Interrelationships

The largest obstacle to overcome in developing a model is ignorance concerning the true relationship among all variables of interest. A full understanding obviates the need for a model whereas gaps in knowledge can lead us to incorrect conclusions. Theory, past research, and common sense must be used in building a model. The presence of a causal relationship between every pair of variables in the model must be considered. Some examples of how these choices are made follow.

In our model, some specified relationships are based on a substantial amount of past research; others are more speculative. For example, Seligman (1975) has argued that early experience with noncontingency enhances helplessness but that early experience with controllable outcomes inoculates against helplessness. Thus, early onset of seizures should increase a sense of learned helplessness. Learned helplessness and social support both have been studied extensively. Enough is known about their effects to rule out certain types of interrelationships and to make others more plausible. For example, the relationship between perceived uncontrollability and helplessness is well established (Abramson, Garber, & Seligman, 1980). Similarly, the possibility of social support being an antagonist to helplessness is consistent with pre-

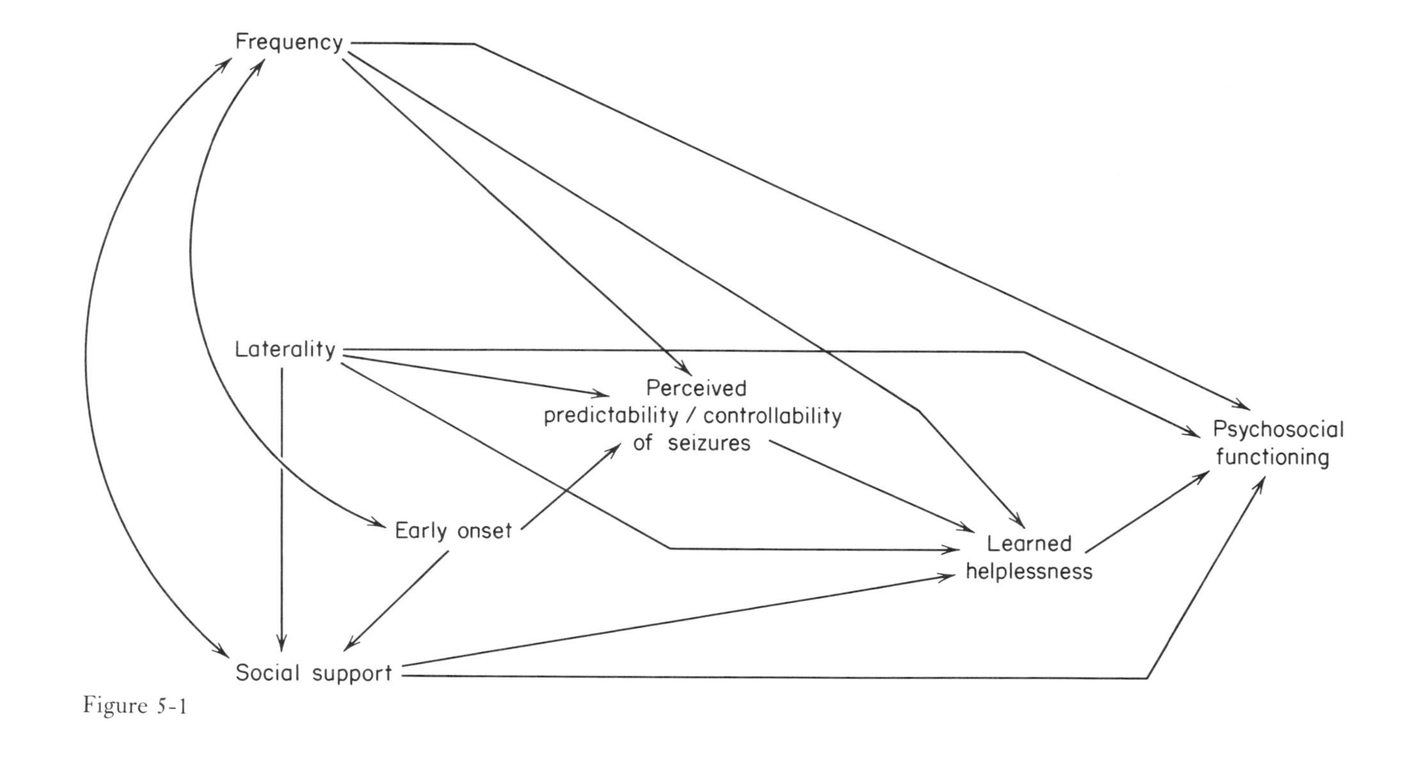
Frequency
Laterality
Perceived
predictability / controllability
of seizures
Psychosocial
functioning
Early onset
Learned
helplessness
Social support

Figure 5-1

vious research (e.g., Caplan et al., 1976) and with theory (Schulz & Decker, 1982; Wallston et al., 1983). Thus it is reasonable to hypothesize that at least part of the effect of social support on functioning may be mediated by learned helplessness.

DeVellis et al. (1980) found that reported seizure frequency was related to learned helplessness but did not resolve the issue of how they were related. Patients might see frequent seizures as inherently less controllable and these seizures might thus contribute to helplessness by influencing perceived controllability. Alternatively, frequency and perceived uncontrollability of seizures might independently contribute to helplessness. That is, frequent seizures may have an adverse impact on psychosocial functioning even if the individual believes that the seizures are influenced by behavior. Accordingly, we have hypothesized both a direct route from frequency to helplessness and an indirect route mediated by perceived controllability. Frequency is also related to early onset in our model. The curved arrow linking these in Figure 5-1 indicates that they are hypothesized to be correlated, but not necessarily related in a direct causal way. Although we are unsure of the exact nature of their relationship, we are willing to say that one exists.

In contrast, Bear and Fedio (1977) found that frequency of seizures was unrelated to the patterns of characteristics that differentiated left from right temporal lobe epilepsy patients in their research. Consequently, we have explicitly specified no direct relationship between frequency and laterality, even though both variables jointly influence other common variables.

As we noted earlier, social support has not, to our knowledge, been studied systematically in epilepsy. Nor is theory sufficiently well developed to guide our thinking concerning certain aspects of epilepsy and social support. Specifically, we cannot say with confidence what the relationship of social support to seizure frequency would be. Both seizure frequency and laterality have social consequences that might influence relationships with others and thus access to support. We also know that social support is associated with reductions in stress and with improved health status (Broadhead et al., 1983; Wallston et al., 1983) and that emotional stress can influence seizures (e.g., Gumnit, 1981). Thus, social support might influence seizure frequency just as seizure frequency might influence support. Because we are unwilling to say with confidence that an empirical relationship between the two variables would represent one or the other of these options, we have linked these variables with a double-headed arrow to indicate correlation without specifying causality. Laterality, in contrast, seems unlikely to shift with changes in social support and thus we are more willing to assert a causal direction between these variables.

As in the preceding examples, much of the task in determining which relationships are correct is deciding which of two correlated variables is cause and which is effect or if both reflect a common cause. In addition to recourse to theory, a longitudinal research strategy may resolve this issue since temporal precedence is necessary for causality. Thus, an association between early onset and later helplessness can have one causal direction. It is worth noting that, as in this example, design need not be prospective to be longitudinal, as long as accurate retrospective data are available.

Some aspects of our model, as we have noted, are better established than others. This is often the case. Most models typically will consist of both more firmly and less firmly established components. The better established relationships provide a framework for evaluating the less certain relationships. Testing the model may support the latter's existence or point to a need for model revision. In this way, a progressively more accurate, complex, and inclusive model can be built up over successive cycles of theoretical speculation, empirical testing, and model revision. This is, of course, merely an extension of the process followed in the development of simpler mechanistic models. In either instance, early versions of a model are likely to be incomplete or somewhat incorrect representations of reality that require progressive refinement.

Measurement

Assuming that the relationships among variables specified by a model are substantially correct, a second requirement is that the variables be measured accurately. Rather than discuss in detail how one might operationalize these variables in the example model presented, we will discuss measurement issues more generally. These issues are more complex than many investigators realize. Our theories concern relationships among hypothetical constructs such as learned helplessness and social support yet our data consist of statistical relationships among measured phenomena such as questionnaire responses. We need some assurance that the correspondence between hypothetical and measured variables is adequate.

With some variables such as sex or age our accuracy of measurement may be extremely high even if only a single question or information source (e.g., medical record) is used. With others such as learned helplessness or social support we must take steps to assure data quality. One method is to use multiple indicators of variables. If several indicators of the same hypothetical variables are used, then the information from these can be combined into a more reliable estimate of the hypothetical variable of interest. For example, factor analytic procedures can be used to arrive at a score that is theoretically error free (Long, 1983a; Nunnally, 1978). The researcher has three options: (a) use a measure of proven reliability (e.g., a standardized instrument), (b) use an essentially infallible indicator (e.g., birth records as an indicator of age), or (c) combine multiple measures that are individually weak (e.g., by factor analysis) into a composite score that is a more reliable estimate of the underlying variable of interest.

Failing to measure variables reliably can introduce substantial distortions into the model-development process. One specific problem can arise from mixing reliable and unreliable measures. When using analytic procedures such as regression analysis, highly reliable measures of variables such as age, race, or sex may mask theoretically more important but less reliably measured variables. For example, if age is correlated with age at seizure onset, as one would expect, then only one of the two variables might make a significant contribution to the prediction of some aspect of functioning. By virtue of being more reliably measured (i.e., measured with less error), age might overshadow age at seizure onset. However, in a given model, age at seizure onset might be far more theoretically relevant and interesting than the subject's age at the time of filling out the questionnaire. Blalock (1982) thus cautions investigators to avoid the use of highly reliable but theoretically barren variables. In the extreme, including demographic variables in models without theoretical justification can lead to this type of problem.

Another common measurement pitfall is inadvertantly defining causes and effects in terms of the same operations. This is especially likely to be a problem with social and psychological variables related to health. Many of these variables were originally seen as health status outcome measures by health researchers. For example, measures of general well-being (e.g., Ware, Johnston, Davies-Avery, & Brook, 1979) often include items tapping depression. If such a measure were used to operationalize psychosocial functioning and a depression scale were also used as a part of a helplessness assessment (e.g., DeVellis et al., 1980), some of the items defining the dependent and independent measures might be nearly identical. A significant correlation between these variables would be all but guaranteed irrespective of the true association between the underlying constructs. A similar problem might arise if social support were a predictor and an outcome measure included items concerning social contact or activities. (See McLeroy et al., 1984, for a discussion of this issue and an example of how to circumvent it.) As theory advances, many social and psychological variables such as these are seen as causes, and not merely indicators, of functioning status. Including them in models as causes while failing to recognize their inclusion in outcome measures can produce grossly erroneous and misleading results.

Another measurement issue often overlooked is the specificity versus generality of measurements. All other things being equal, two measurements that are at the same level on a continuum of specificity are likely to correlate more highly than two comparable measurements that are not comparable with respect to specificity (Fishbein & Ajzen, 1975). Thus, a very global measure of beliefs about control may be a weaker predictor than a measure of health-specific beliefs if the outcome of interest is specific to health. Or, to use another example, perceptions of seizure controllability may be a better predictor of adjustment to epilepsy than of adjustment in general. This issue may become especially important in model building. Certain elements of a conceptual model that is being tested may inadvertently start off at a disadvantage because they are measured at a different level of specificity than other key variables in the model.

Analytic Strategies

Analytic procedures that simultaneously address both the nature of the relationship among variables and their measurement have become more common in the social sciences (see Bentler, [1980] and Carmines & McIver [1981] for discussions and examples). The LISREL computer program (Jöreskog & Sörbom, 1981) is the analytic tool most commonly associated with this approach. Horn and McArdle (1980) have discussed some of the advantages and disadvantages of using procedures such as LISREL. Structural equation modeling techniques of this type are extremely powerful and permit the simultaneous consideration of an entire network of relationships rather than necessitating a series of sequential comparisons (e.g., Long, 1983b). However, their complexity often necessitates surrendering a full understanding of the analytic procedures to the computer. Heise (1975) and Kenny (1979) describe alternative methods based on ordinary least squares procedures (such as regression analysis) for testing causal models. These are both less cryptic and less powerful. Irrespective of the analytic method chosen, one's ability to test a model is only as good as the theory and measurement underlying the model. If confidence in major components of a model is low, then results must be interpreted cautiously irrespective of how elegant the analytic procedure may be.

CONCLUSIONS

The purpose of this chapter has been to state the importance of viewing epilepsy from a multideterminate, theory-based conceptualization and to describe an example model reflecting such a perspective. The model presented in Figure 5-1 represents a compromise between the true complexity of biological, psychological, and social aspects of epilepsy on the one hand and the poverty of extant knowledge concerning their interrelationships on the other. Many potential influences on the psychosocial functioning of people with epilepsy (e.g., employment discrimination) have been omitted. Similarly, potentially useful elaborations of theoretical constructs (e.g., the role of attributions in helplessness) have not been included. Psychosocial functioning, the outcome measure depicted in the model, is obviously not a unitary entity. We have avoided a lengthy discussion of these issues in the interest of simplicity. Our model is fully recursive (e.g., Kenny, 1979); that is, it contains no feedback loops or instances of explicit mutual causality. This constraint carries with it a host of assumptions that future research may prove to be unwarranted. However, at present it greatly simplifies the model. Similarly, the model in Figure 5-1 implies measurement at only a single point in time. A full understanding of many of the relationships among biological, psychological, and social variables related to epilepsy will eventually require multiple measurements across time.

Despite these and other limitations, we believe that our model is useful. First, despite its simplicity, it does suggest how variables at different levels—namely, biological, psychological, and social—can be related to one another and viewed as interconnected elements that jointly influence functioning in epilepsy. In addition, we believe that our model provides a reasonable starting point for considering how some specific variables might be related to epilepsy and to one another. The model suggests empirically testable hypotheses that can clarify our understanding of epilepsy. Finally, our model is a potential catalyst to critical, creative, and integrative thinking. We hope that readers will see both strengths and weaknesses in the specific conceptual framework we have depicted and that any uneasiness they may feel with our model will stimulate the development of testable alternatives.

NOTE

1. An extensive review of the learned helplessness literature is beyond the scope of this chapter. For a discussion of theoretical and research issues related to learned helplessness and reviews that are both supportive and critical of this approach, the reader is referred to Abramson et al. (1978), Alloy (1982), Levis (1976, 1980), Maier (1980), Maier and Seligman (1976), McReynolds (1980a, b), Miller and Norman (1979), Oakes (1982), Oakes and Curtis (1982), Peterson (1982), Roth (1980), Silver, Wortman, and Klos (1982), Tennen (1982), Tennen, Gillen and Drum (1982), Tennen, Drum, Gillen, and Stanton (1982), Winefield (1982), Wortman & Brehm (1975), and Wortman and Dintzer (1978). Points worth noting in these reviews include the recent emphasis on the role of attributional mediators in predicting the degree to which helplessness will generalize (e.g., Abramson et al.), the subsequent criticisms of invoking cognitive and attributional mediators to explain deficits resulting from noncontingency (e.g., Oakes; Tennen) and the trend over time to more tests of learned helplessness in applied and nonexperimental contexts (e.g., Silver et al.).

REFERENCES

Abramson, L. Y., J. Garber, & M. E. P. Seligman. (1980). Learned helplessness in humans: An attributional analysis. In J. Garber & M. E. P. Seligman (Eds.), *Human helplessness*. New York: Academic Press.

Abramson, L. Y., M. E. P. Seligman, & J. D. Teasdale. (1978). Learned helplessness in humans: Critique and reformation. *Journal of Abnormal Psychology* 87, 49–74.

Alloy, L. B. (1982). The role of perceptions and attributions for response-outcome noncontingency in learned helplessness: A commentary and discussion. *Journal of Personality* 50, 443–79.

Bear, D. M., & P. Fedio. (1977). Quantitative analysis of interictal behavior in temporal lobe epilepsy. *Archives of Neurology* 34, 454–67.

Bentler, P. M. (1980). Multivariate analysis with latent variables: Causal modeling. *Annual Review of Psychology*, 31, 419–56.

Betts, T. A. (1974). A follow-up study of a cohort of patients with epilepsy admitted to psychiatric care in an English city. In P. Harris & C. Mawdsley (Eds.), *Epilepsy*. Edinburgh: Churchill-Livingstone.

Blalock, H. M. (1982). *Conceptualization and measurement in the social sciences*. Beverly Hills, CA: Sage.

Broadhead, W. E., B. H. Kaplan, S. A. James, E. H. Wagner, V. J. Schoenbach, R. Grimson, S. Heyden, G. Tibben, & S. H. Gehlbach. (1983). The epidemiologic evidence for a relationship between social support and health. *Journal of Epidemiology* 117, 521–37.

Caplan, R. D., E. A. Robinson, J. R. French, J. R. Caldwell, & M. Shinn. (1976). *Adhering to medical regimens: Pilot experiments in patient education and social support*. Ann Arbor: University of Michigan, Institute for Social Research.

Carmines, E. G. & J. P. McIver (1981). Analyzing models with unobserved variables: Analysis of covariance structures. In G. W. Bohrnstedt & E. F. Borgatta (Eds.), *Social measurement: Current issues*. Beverly Hills: Sage Publications.

Conger, J. J., W. L. Sawrey, & E. S. Turrel. (1958). The role of social experience in the production of gastric ulcers in hooded rats placed in a conflict situation. *Journal of Abnormal Psychology* 57, 214–20.

DeVellis, R. F., B. M. DeVellis, B. S. Wallston, & K. A. Wallston. (1980). Epilepsy and learned helplessness. *Basic and Applied Social Psychology* 1, 241–53.

Dewey, J., & A. Bentley. (1973). Knowing and the known. In R. Handy & E. C. Harwood (Eds.), *Useful procedures of inquiry*. Great Barrington, MA: Behavior Research Council.

Engel, G. L. (1982). The biopsychosocial model and medical education. *New England Journal of Medicine* 306, 802–805.

Fishbein, M., & I. Ajzen. (1975). Belief, attitude, intention and behavior: An introduction to theory and research. Reading, MA: Addison-Wesley.

Flor-Henry, P. (1969). Schizophrenic-like reactions and affective psychoses associated with temporal lobe epilepsy: Etiological factors. *American Journal of Psychiatry* 26, 400–403.

Goldin, G. J., & R. J. Margolin. (1975). The psychological aspects of epilepsy. In G. Wright (Ed.), *Epilepsy rehabilitation*. Boston: Little, Brown.

Gumnit, R. J. (1981). *Epilepsy: A handbook for physicians* (4th ed.). Minneapolis: University of Minnesota Comprehensive Epilepsy Program.

Heise, D. R. (1975). *Causal analysis*. New York: Wiley.

Hermann, B. P. (1979). Psychopathology in epilepsy and learned helplessness. *Medical Hypotheses* 5, 723–29.

Horn, J. L., & J. J. McArdle. (1980). Perspectives on mathematical/statistical model building (MASMOB) in research on aging. In L. Poon (Ed.), *Aging in the 1980s: Psychological issues*. Washington, DC: American Psychological Association.

Jöreskog, K. G., & D. Sörbom. (1981). *LISREL: Analysis of linear structural relationships by the method of maximum likelihood*. Version V User's Guide. Uppsala, Sweden: University of Uppsala, Department of Statistics.

Kenny, D. A. (1979). *Correlation and causality*. New York: Wiley.

Levis, D. J. (1976). Learned helplessness: A reply and an alternative S–R interpretation. *Journal of Experimental Psychology: General* 105, 47–65.

Levis, D. J. (1980). The learned helplessness effect: An expectancy, discrimination deficit, or motivational-induced persistence? *Journal of Research in Personality* 14, 158–69.

Lewis, C. E. (1966). Factors influencing the return to work of men with congestive heart failure. *Journal of Chronic Disease* 19, 1193–1209.

Long, J. S. (1983a). *Confirmatory factor analysis*. Sage University Paper series on Quantitative Applications in the Social Sciences, Series No. 07-033. Beverly Hills, CA: Sage.

Long, J. S. (1983b). *Covariance structure models: An introduction to LISREL*. Sage University Paper series on Quantitative Applications in the Social Sciences, Series No. 07-034. Beverly Hills, CA: Sage.

Maier, S. F. (1980). Learned helplessness and the schedule-shift hypothesis. *Journal of Research in Personality* 14, 170–86.

Maier, S. F., & M. E. P. Seligman. (1976). Learned helplessness: Theory and evidence. *Journal of Experimental Psychology: General, 105*, 3–46.

Matthews, W. S., G. Barabas, & M. Ferrari. (1982). Emotional concomitants of childhood epilepsy. *Epilepsia* 23, 671–81.

McLeroy, K. R., R. F. DeVellis, B. M. DeVellis, B. Kaplan, & J. Toole. (1984). Social support and physical recovery in a stroke population. *Journal of Social and Personal Relationships*, 1, 395–413.

McReynolds, W. T. (1980a). Learned helplessness as a schedule-shift effect. *Journal of Research in Personality* 14, 139–57.

McReynolds, W. T. (1980b). Theories, research, and evidence of learned helplessness: A reply to Levis and Maier. *Journal of Research in Personality* 14, 187–95.

Mellor, D. H., T. Lowit, & D. J. Hall. (1974). Are epileptic children behaviourally different from other children? In P. Harris & C. Mawdsley (Eds.), *Epilepsy*. Edinburgh: Churchill-Livingstone.

Miller, I. W., & W. H. Norman. (1979). Learned helplessness in humans: A review and attribution theory model. *Psychological Bulletin* 86, 93–118.

Milne, A. (1974). The epileptic child in school. In P. Harris & C. Mawdsley (Eds.), *Epilepsy*. Edinburgh: Churchill-Livingstone.

Nunnally, J. C. (1978). *Psychometric theory*. New York: McGraw-Hill.

Oakes, W. F. (1982). Learned helplessness and defensive strategies: A rejoinder. *Journal of Personality* 50, 515–25.

Oakes, W. F. & N. Curtis. (1982). Learned helplessness: Not dependent upon cognitions, attributions or other such phenomenal experiences. *Journal of Personality* 50, 387–408.

Pepper, S. C. (1942). *World hypotheses.* Berkeley: University of California Press.

Peterson, C. (1982). Learned helplessness and health psychology. *Health Psychology* 1, 153–68.

Pronko, N. H. (1980). *Psychology from the standpoint of an interbehaviorist.* Monterey, CA: Brooks/Cole.

Ramamurthi, B., & R. Sivaprakasam. (1974). Psychological adjustment among epileptics. In P. Harris & C. Mawdsley (Eds.), *Epilepsy,* Edinburgh: Churchill-Livingstone.

Rodin, J. (1980). Managing the stress of aging: The role of control and coping. In S. Levine & H. Ursin (Eds.), *Coping and health.* New York: Plenum Press.

Rodin, J., & E. J. Langer. (1980). Aging labels: The decline of control and the fall of self-esteem. *Journal of Social Issues* 36, 12–29.

Roth, S. (1980). A revised model of learned helplessness in humans. *Journal of Personality* 48, 103–33.

Runyan, C. W., R. F. DeVellis, B. M. DeVellis, & G. M. Hochbaum. (1982). Health psychology and the public health perspective: In search of the pump handle. *Health Psychology* 1, 169–80.

Satariano, W. A., & S. L. Syme. (1981). Life changes and disease in elderly populations: Coping with change. In J. McGough, S. B. Kiesler, & J. C. March (Eds.), *Biology, behavior and aging.* New York: Academic Press.

Schulz, R. (1976). Effects of control and predictability on the psychological well-being of the institutionalized aged. *Journal of Personality and Social Psychology* 33, 563–73.

Schulz, R., & S. Decker. (1982). Social support, adjustment, and the elderly spinal cord injured: A social psychological analysis. In G. Weary & H. L. Mirels (Eds.), *Integrations of clinical and social psychology.* New York: Oxford University Press.

Schwartz, G. E. (1982). Testing the biopsychosocial model: The ultimate challenge facing behavioral medicine? *Journal of Consulting and Clinical Psychology* 50, 1040–53.

Seligman, M. E. P. (1975). *Helplessness: On depression, development and death.* San Francisco: Freeman.

Silver, R. L. & C. B. Wortman. (1980). Coping with undesirable life events. In J. Garber & M. E. P. Seligman (Eds.), *Human helplessness: Theory and applications.* New York: Academic Press.

Silver, R. L., C. B. Wortman, & D. S. Klos. (1982). Cognitions, affect, and behavior following uncontrollable outcomes: A response to current human helplessness research. *Journal of Personality* 50, 480–514.

Sindrup, E. H., & O. Kristensen. (1979). Psychomotor epilepsy and psychosis: Electroencephalographic findings. *Epilepsia* 20, 187.

Springer, S. P., & G. Deutsch. (1981). *Left brain, right brain.* San Francisco: Freeman.

Stores, G., J. Hart, & N. Piran. (1978). Inattentiveness in school children with epilepsy. *Epilepsia* 19, 119–75.

Tennen, H. (1982). A review of cognitive mediators in learned helplessness. *Journal of Personality* 50, 526–41.

Tennen, H., P. E. Drum, R. Gillen, & A. Stanton. (1982). Learned helplessness and the detection of contingency: A direct test. *Journal of Personality* 50, 426–42.

Tennen, H., R. Gillen, & P. E. Drum. (1982). The debilitating effect of exposure to noncontingent escape: A test of the learned helplessness model. *Journal of Personality* 50, 409–25.

Wallston, B. S., C. W. Alagna, B. M. DeVellis, & R. F. DeVellis. (1983). Social support and physical health. *Health Psychology* 2, 367–91.

Ware, J. E., A. Johnston, A. Davies-Avery, & R. H. Brook. (1979). *Conceptualization and measurement of health for adults in the Health Insurance Study: Vol. III. Mental health.* Santa Monica, CA: Rand.

Winefield, A. H. (1982). Methodological difficulties of demonstrating learned helplessness in humans. *Journal of General Psychology* 107, 255–66.

Wortman, C. B., & J. W. Brehm. (1975). Responses to uncontrollable outcomes: An integration of reactance theory and the learned helplessness model. In L. Berkowitz (Ed.), *Advances in experimental social psychology* (Vol. 8). New York: Academic Press.

Wortman, C. B., & L. Dintzer. (1978). Is an attributional analysis of the learned helplessness phenomenon viable? A critique of the Abramson-Seligman-Teasdale reformulation. *Journal of Abnormal Psychology* 87, 75–90.

6 / The Perceived Psychosocial Consequences of Having Epilepsy

PAUL ARNTSON, DAVID DROGE,
ROBERT NORTON, and ELLEN MURRAY

Ordinarily when people become ill they have very little difficulty integrating their "sick roles" into their interpersonal relationships. An appointment or two may be missed, there may be frequent coughing or sneezing, and allowances may be made for the increased irritability of the affected person. Others may do a few extra things for the person if the sick role is not too overplayed. With more acute illnesses and disorders, patients, their families, friends, and co-workers still expect only a short period of disruption of normal social interaction. However, expectations can shift radically when a person is diagnosed and labeled as having a chronic, life-changing condition. The sick and patient roles can then stigmatize the individual, seriously disrupting and distorting interpersonal communication.

A stigma is an "attribute which is deeply discrediting" in a social relationship (Goffman, 1963, p. 3). An attribute becomes stigmatized when it "interrupts the flow of everyday interaction" (Friedson, 1966, p. 79). According to Goffman (1963, pp. 8–9), a stigma disrupts the process of identity negotiation that underlies most informal social interaction.

> Those who have dealings with [the stigmatized individual] fail to accord him the respect and regard which the uncontaminated aspects of his identity have led them to anticipate extending, and have led him to anticipate receiving.

Epilepsy is both a medical diagnosis and a social label that can stigmatize individuals with the disorder. Medically, epilepsy is a category of neurological disorders characterized by recurrent seizures. Epilepsy is considered a symptom of some underlying brain dysfunction, which may or may not be identified in each case. The stigma surrounding epilepsy is to a large extent based on seizure occurrence. The seizure is an "attack of altered consciousness"

(Taylor, 1969, p. 109) whose occurrence is unpredictable. Because the disorder is seated in the brain, the epileptic seizure "touches a deep dread" in others (Taylor, 1969). David Kahn maintains that this fear centers around the "loss of control, occurring unpredictably and for reasons that are ill understood" (Bakal, 1979, p. 170).

The perception of control may be very difficult for some people with epilepsy to maintain. In addition to the ever-present dread of losing control over one's own body, feelings and cognitions, other aspects of epilepsy may make the perception of being in control tenuous. The cause of the disorder may not be explainable in individualistic terms. "Why me?" is usually not answerable. People do not take well random events that can so profoundly affect their lives (Silver & Wortman, 1980). Dependency on anticonvulsant drugs and health professionals may make the perception of control even more difficult. Many of the drugs can have side effects that may seem to appear randomly. However, it may be the social and economic restrictions placed on some people who have epilepsy that contribute the most to a diminished sense of control. Several researchers (Garber & Seligman, 1980; Langer & Rodin, 1976; Schulz, 1980; Seligman, 1975; Silver & Wortman, 1980) have found that an individual's diminished sense of control has serious physiological and psychological consequences in the general population, including feelings of helplessness, depression, anxiety, and low self-esteem.

Socially, seizure occurrence means that epilepsy "constantly impinges, continuously threatens to express a deviance, and repeatedly demands renegotiation of personal status" (Taylor & Harrison, 1976, p. 30). The social disruptiveness of seizures, when coupled with a generalized fear and misunderstanding of epilepsy, may frequently lead to the social isolation of people with epilepsy (Arangio, 1975). Schlesinger and Frank (1974, p. 99) contend that the person with epilepsy frequently "is caught in a negative feedback cycle in which his functioning stimulates rejection by society, which results in further deviation by the client and intensified rejection." Rejection and social isolation can lead to stigmatization, depression, anxiety, and somatic symptoms (Norton, Murray, & Arntson, 1982).

The social label "epileptic" is thus considered a major cause of the psychosocial problems of people with epilepsy (Goldin & Margolin, 1972). Graham (1958) and many others have attributed the incidence of personality disturbances among people with epilepsy to the prejudice and stigma associated with the label "epileptic." Falk and Gorman (1972, p. 56) contend that

> a central aspect of epilepsy is the status-role of being epileptic and that this status-role is the consequence of definitions concerning epilepsy and epileptics rather than the inevitable result of the physical condition known as epilepsy.

Finally, the Commission for the Control of Epilepsy and Its Consequences concluded that the psychological and social problems surrounding epilepsy are "more difficult to handle than the actual seizure problem itself" (1978, p. 133).

Our recent national study of epilepsy self-help groups has reaffirmed the importance of these issues. At the same time, it has presented us with a unique data set that would allow empirical investigation into the hypothesized relationship between the psychosocial ramifications of epilepsy and their effects on the mental health of individuals with epilepsy.

In the study reported here, we examine the relationships between psychopathology and reported seizure occurrence, perceptions of control, stigmatization, and psychosocial measures of health. More specifically, we do the following: First, we document the nature of several psychosocial problems and concerns in individuals with epilepsy. Second, we show that self-reported rates of depression, anxiety, and other indicators of psychological distress are significantly elevated in epilepsy relative to healthy controls. Both of these points replicate and extend previous findings. Third, we document the association between the social ramifications of epilepsy and the individual's psychological problems—a step very rarely taken in the epilepsy/psychopathology literature. Finally, we demonstrate how seizure frequency also affects measures of psychopathology and suggest that the relevance of this neuroepilepsy variable, along with the social variables, indicates the need for multietiologic models for this field.

METHOD

The data for this study were derived from a national survey developed by researchers from the Self-Help Institute at Northwestern University and by self-help group leaders in the greater Chicago area. For about 2 years an epilepsy self-help group workshop was held in which over 20 leaders of Chicago self-help groups met with researchers on a monthly basis. The workshop also brought in leaders from other parts of the country for presentations and discussions. In addition, researchers and group leaders from the Self-Help Institute were sent on site visits to epilepsy self-help groups in other states. As a result of these activities we decided to poll the members of epilepsy self-help groups to learn more about their perceptions of epilepsy, relationships between biological and social aspects of the disorder and mental health problems, and the reasons for and dynamics underlying self-help group participation. To that end we developed a relevant questionnaire, which we now describe.

QUESTIONNAIRE

Questions were generated by the workshop's activities and were added to items adapted from an extensive study of self-help groups conducted at the University of Chicago by Lieberman and Borman (1979). Also added to our survey was a series of open-ended questions that were initially utilized in an interview-based study conducted at the University of Illinois Epilepsy Clinic (Arntson & Montgomery, 1980). The initial version of the survey was then revised based on the suggestions obtained from self-help group leaders from around the country, and it was subsequently pilot tested on individuals attending epilepsy self-help groups in the Chicago area.

The final version of the survey contained 15 separate sections that covered the following topics: seizure activity, general health, health attitudes, perceived causes of epilepsy, medication, employment, education, life management, attitudes toward epilepsy, interpersonal relationships, attitudes toward self, professional services, the Hopkins Health Checklist, information-seeking behaviors, and demographic information. Six additional sections dealt with issues surrounding self-help groups for people with epilepsy. The questionnaire was 29 pages long and generated 377 data points. Details concerning the major sections of our questionnaire follow.

Seizure Activity

Respondents were asked to indicate what kind of seizures they experienced and the rate for each type on a per-day, per-week, per-month, or per-year basis. They were then asked "How severely does your seizure activity currently affect your life?" They were asked to respond on a seven-point scale that ranged from "very severely" to "not at all severely," and this measure was used to indicate the perceived impact of seizure activity on the lives of the respondents.

Open-Ended Questions

The following open-ended questions were taken from a previous interview-based investigation of epilepsy (Arntson & Montgomery, 1980). Subjects were asked:

- What is the single greatest problem you experience because of your epilepsy?
- How would your life be different if you did not have epilepsy?
- What is the best advice you could give to a person who has just found out that he or she has epilepsy?
- What have others done to be helpful?
- What have people done who have given you trouble?

- What are the positive aspects of having epilepsy?
- What advice would you give to the family and friends of a person with epilepsy?

These questions had been used in our previous studies to give patients with epilepsy an opportunity to share with us how they managed their lives and interacted with other people. Previous responses were very informative and we therefore felt these questions were pertinent for our national survey and would give us insight into the social aspects of epilepsy as described by the respondents.

Categories for the responses were developed with the first 140 returned questionnaires. Each respondent's reply to each question was typed on an index card and three coders independently sorted the cards for each question into categories. Coders were instructed to follow two general criteria in grouping responses into logical categories (Weick, 1968): The categories for each question were to be mutually exclusive and exhaustive, and the categories should occur at a similar level of abstraction. The coders then met to resolve differences and develop the "final" category system. During the coding of the entire data set adjustments were made to category systems and then reapplied to previously coded responses. Periodic checks were made between coders during the analyses of the responses.

Psychosocial Measures

The 11 measures used in this study assessed perceptions of control, social isolation, and psychological state. For all the items the respondents were asked to indicate how much they agreed or disagreed with each statement by circling one of five choices. The responses were then transformed into a five-point scale for analysis. The 11 measures are as follows.

The *stigma* scale consisted of 10 items taken from Lieberman and Borman (1979) that were reworded for epilepsy. The respondents were asked to agree or disagree with statements describing their relationship with employers and co-workers, how people treated them because of their epilepsy, their looks and sex appeal, and their willingness to disclose their epilepsy to others.

Self-esteem was measured by taking five items from Coopersmith's Self-Esteem Inventory (1967). All of the statements asked respondents to indicate either what significant others thought of them or how they compared themselves to their peers.

Helplessness was measured by summing the responses to four items taken from Lieberman and Borman (1979) that were reworded for epilepsy. Items measured the respondents' attributions of control as either internal or external (external being largely a function of the patient's epilepsy).

Health locus of control was measured by taking two items from each dimension of the Multidimensional Health Locus of Control Scale (Wallston, Wallston, & DeVellis, 1978) and adding to them two items that measured external family control. Four dimensions of control were therefore assessed with this instrument: *internal* (the individual believes that he or she primarily determines his or her own state of health), *fate* (things beyond human control accidently affect one's health), *doctor external* (dependence on doctors is the best way to maintain one's health), and *family external* (the family has a great deal of influence on one's state of health).

Three dimensions from the Hopkins Symptom Checklist (Derogatis, Lipman, Rickels, Uhlenhuth, & Covi, 1974) were used. Nine items from the *somatic* scale reflected distress arising from perceptions of body dysfunction, e.g., complaints focused on cardiovascular, gastrointestinal, and respiratory systems. Headaches, pain, and discomfort also were represented. Eight items subsumed under the *depression* scale reflected a broad range of the concomitants of a clinical depressive syndrome. Symptoms of dysphoric mood and affect were represented as were signs of withdrawal of life interest, lack of motivation, loss of vital energy, and feelings of hopelessness. Six items from the *anxiety* scale comprised a set of symptoms and behaviors associated clinically with high manifest anxiety. General indicators such as restlessness, nervousness, and tension also were represented.

The last measure, *life satisfaction*, consisted of three items taken from Robinson and Shaver (1972). We incorporated these items because we wanted some overall measure of the respondents' perceptions of their life situations.

Procedure

The survey was distributed through a number of channels to people with epilepsy throughout the United States. Via an article in our Epilepsy Workshop Newsletter (a publication we distributed nationally to all known epilepsy self-help groups in the United States), survey plans were announced and interested individuals and self-help groups were invited to participate in the survey. An announcement of this project also appeared in *The Spokesman*, the national newsletter of the Epilepsy Foundation of America. Finally, medical and social service professionals in a number of locations were asked to distribute questionnaires to their clients. In total, 3,000 survey forms were printed and sent out to group leaders, professionals, and directly to individuals with epilepsy. We have no idea how many of the surveys were actually distributed to appropriate individuals, but 357 completed questionnaires were returned to us. Twenty-six states, the District of Columbia, and Puerto Rico are represented in this survey, with the largest proportion of respondents (19%) living in Illinois.

RESULTS

SOCIODEMOGRAPHIC CHARACTERISTICS

Table 6-1 presents a profile of our survey sample and contrasts it with demographic characteristics of the entire U.S. population. On the average the respondents were slightly older than the general population and had roughly the same levels of education. The survey sample contained a higher proportion of women and single individuals. One particularly noteworthy difference was the discrepancy between educational achievement and household income. Although the respondents completed roughly the same amount of schooling as the rest of the population, the respondents' reported level of income was far below the national average. Part of the difference may be attributable to the higher proportion of women in our survey. However, this discrepancy between educational achievement and household income may also be an indicator of the persistence of chronic unemployment and underemployment as significant problems for people with epilepsy. Indeed, only 48% of the survey sample held a full-time job.

TABLE 6-1. Demographic Characteristics of Survey Respondents

Characteristic	*Survey Profile*	*U.S. Population Profile**
Mean age	32.7 years	30.0 years
Median education	12.4 years	12.5 years
Sex		
Male	141 (40%)	48.5%
Female	214 (60%)	51.5%
Marital status		(18 years and older)
Single	168 (48%)	20%
Married	122 (35%)	66%
Divorced	37 (11%)	6%
Separated	15 (4%)	(not available)
Widowed	6 (2%)	8%
Household income		
$0– 5,000	139 (43%)	7%
5,001–10,000	63 (19%)	14%
10,001–15,000	51 (16%)	16%
15,001–20,000	28 (9%)	16%
20,001–25,000	15(5%)	14%
25,001–30,000	11 (3%)	19%
over 30,000	17 (5%)	14%

*From Statistical Abstracts of the United States, 1981.

Unfortunately we do not have a similar national profile for patients with epilepsy so that we could examine the demographic representativeness of our sample for epilepsy in particular. A crude approximation can be gleaned by comparing a sample of 157 patients from the University of Illinois epilepsy clinics, gathered as part of a prior research project (Arntson & Montgomery, 1980). The individuals from the epilepsy clinics may be slightly more representative of the general population of people with epilepsy seeking medical care than our national survey sample, which consisted mainly (67%) of people who had attended epilepsy self-help groups. In comparing the two samples, we found that the survey respondents were slightly more likely to be employed (48% vs. 40%) and more likely to be women (60% vs. 40%) than the clinic sample and equally likely to be married (36% vs. 37%). In summary, in spite of the obvious selection factors involved in the generation of this study sample, the respondents to this survey were demographically similar to a typical clinic population.

Although these two epilepsy samples may not be representative of the *general* population of people who have epilepsy, the available sociodemographic data indicate that people with epilepsy experience chronic unemployment and underemployment, and are not as likely to be married and hence have a family of their own in adult life (Commission for the Control of Epilepsy and Its Consequences, 1978). Most of the unmarried people in both the survey and clinic samples were living with their parents, a sibling, or alone. For an adult, being unemployed and living alone or with one's parents can disrupt and distort interpersonal relationships.

Seizure Frequency

The reported rate of seizure activity in our survey sample varied widely. For the 77% of the respondents who reported current seizure activity, the rate ranged from 1 seizure every 2 years to 14 seizures a day. Computed in seizures per week, this is a range of .01 to 98 per week. The distribution was skewed toward lower seizure activity, with the median rate being 2 seizures a month.

Most of the survey respondents reported that their seizure activity did not severely affect their lives. The mean for the seven-point scale (ranging from a "1" if "not at all severely" to a "7" if "very severely") was 2.96 with 39% circling "1" and other 12% circling "2." For purposes of further analyses, we split the respondents into those who had circled the first two responses and those who had circled the remaining five. Severity changed significantly with seizure frequency; as the rate of seizure activity increased, perceived severity also increased.

TABLE 6-2. Answers Given to the Question: "What is the Single Greatest Problem You Experience Because of Your Epilepsy?" (N = 328)

Answer	*Percent*
Emotional problems (worry, lack of confidence)	24
Job-related problems (unable to find work, trouble on the job)	22
Lifestyle restrictions (not socially active, restricted)	14
Driving (inability to obtain license)	13
Marriage and family	4
No problems	3
Other problems	20
Total	100%

OPEN-ENDED QUESTIONS

The responses to the open-ended questions presented in Tables 6-2 through 6-6 indicate that the respondents felt their opportunities for social interaction were restricted, that social support from others was very important in their lives, and that they wanted to maintain as much control over their lives as possible. Their opportunities for social interaction were restricted by their employment situations, by not being active socially, by being single or living by themselves, and by negative social reactions they may have received (Table 6-2).

Yet the respondents indicated that understanding and social support were essential for the situations they found themselves in. We all need social support, and this need is made even more salient for the respondents given the social disruptions and distortions they experienced. In response to the question "How would your life be different if you did not have epilepsy?" 83% mentioned having employment, educational, social, family, and/or driving

TABLE 6-3. Answers Given to the Question: "How Would Your Life Be Different If You Did Not Have Epilepsy?" (N = 312); (More Than One Answer Is Possible; Proportions Total More Than 100%)

Answer	*Percent*
Improved employment or educational opportunity	37
More active (improved social life)	22
Driving (could obtain license)	17
Emotional improvement (more self-confidence, less worry)	15
No difference	11
Family and marriage	7
Could smoke or drink	1

TABLE 6-4. Answers Given to the Question: "What Is the Best Advice You Could Give to a Person Who Has Just Found Out That He or She Has Epilepsy?" (*N* = 327; More Than One Answer Is Possible; Proportions Total More Than 100%)

Answer	*Percent*
Maintain self-esteem (avoid self-pity)	70
Seek medical help you can trust (follow medical advice)	37
Educate yourself and others about epilepsy	27
Take medication regularly	26
Live normally, maintain independence	23
Find a support source	23
Respond to others honestly and assertively (e.g., be open, ignore negative reactions)	15
Take care of yourself physically	11
Maintain religious feelings	5
Avoid drugs, including alcohol	4
Don't tell anyone	1

restrictions removed from their lives (Table 6-3). Seventy percent said that the best advice they would give someone who has just found out that he or she has epilepsy is to maintain self-esteem, whereas 23% suggested a normal and independent life (Table 6-4). When asked what others had done to be helpful, 27% indicated that others had encouraged independence or normal living (Table 6-5). This corresponds to the advice some respondents would give to the family and friends of a person with epilepsy. Thirty-three percent suggested that the person be treated normally, and 10% warned against overprotecting the person (Table 6-6). Again, everyone wishes to be independent, but the economic and social restrictions and social reactions experienced by some people with epilepsy make the perception of control even more salient in their lives.

TABLE 6-5. Answers Given to the Question: "What Have Others Done to Be Helpful?" (N = 325; More Than One Response Is Possible; Proportions Total More Than 100%)

Answers	*Percent*
Provided emotional support	67
Encouraged independent or normal living	27
Shared knowledge	18
Gave advice or help on medical treatment	17
Helped when seizures occur	14
Offered general assistance (transportation, home care)	5
Gave professional counseling	3
Helped with job, financial, or legal problems	2

TABLE 6-6. Answers Given to the Question: "What Advice Would You Give to the Family and Friends of a Person with Epilepsy?" (N = 319)

Answer	*Percent*
Treat the person normally (don't pity the person)	33
Support the person (love and understand)	31
Learn about epilepsy	14
Don't overprotect the person	10
Get good medical care	3
Keep open communication (listen, share feelings)	2
Find a support group	1
Other	6
Total	100%

What is just as interesting to note about their answers to all the open-ended questions is what was *not* mentioned by the respondents. Issues concerning actual seizure occurrence, medications, side effects, or relationships with health care professionals were almost never mentioned. This is the case even though our sample represents people who are currently experiencing seizure activity.

In summary, much of these data substantiate again the widespread psychosocial problems experienced by individuals with epilepsy. We next document the oft-reported finding of increased psychopathology in epilepsy relative to healthy controls.

ATTITUDE MEASURES

Of the 11 measures reported here, the three subscales from the Hopkins Symptoms Checklist provide normative data that can be used in making epilepsy/health control comparisons as to reported psychopathology. Table 6-7 shows the results. All the items from the epilepsy sample differ from the normative data. Overall, anxiety is the most frequently reported problem. On average, 39% of the epilepsy respondents indicated symptoms of anxiety versus 9% of the normative sample. This suggests that the reported incidence of anxiety is about four times greater among this sample of people with epilepsy than the norm group. On average, 33% of the respondents with epilepsy indicated somatic symptoms as compared to 10% of the norm sample. In general, the epilepsy group reported incidences of somatic symptoms about three times more frequently than the norm group. Finally, on average 25% of the epilepsy group indicated symptoms of depression as opposed to 9% of the norm sample. Again, the reported incidence of depression in the epilepsy group is about three times greater than in the norm group.

TABLE 6-7. Comparison of the Hopkins Symptom Checklist between Normative Data and Data from People Who Have Seizure Activity

Health-Related Variables	*Reporting Symptom* *Epilepsy Sample*	*Norm Sample*	*Number of Standard Deviations Greater Than Norm*[a]
DEPRESSION VARIABLES			
I lack enthusiasm for doing things	28%	22%	1.2
I feel hopeless about the future	23%	9%	1.0
I feel downhearted or blue	37%	11%	2.0
I feel lonely	38%	10%	2.0
I feel bored or have little interest in doing things	25%	6%	2.0
I have thoughts of possibly ending my life	15%	1%	4.0
I lose sexual interest or pleasure	21%	4%	2.7
I have a poor appetite	16%	9%	1.0
ANXIETY VARIABLES			
I feel nervous or shaky inside	38%	18%	1.7
I feel tense or keyed up	54%	20%	2.0
I feel fearful or afraid	27%	5%	3.0
I cry easily or feel like crying	41%	5%	3.0
I notice my hands trembling	43%	3%	6.0
I have to avoid certain things, places, or activities because they frighten me	34%	3%	5.0
SOMATIC VARIABLES			
I have trouble getting to sleep or staying asleep	41%	5%	3.0
I have noticed my heart pound or race when I'm not physically active	31%	6%	2.3
I have trouble getting my breath	18%	3%	2.0
I sweat when not working hard or overheated	29%	13%	1.0
I have headaches or head pains	46%	17%	1.7
I feel faint or dizzy	31%	4%	2.7
I have an upset or sour stomach	Information not available for comparison		
I have tightness or tension in my neck, back, or other muscles	There is no comparable item in the original HSCL work		
I feel low in energy or slowed down	34%	22%	1.7

[a]This comparison is made by using the following formula:

$$\text{Standard deviation difference} = \frac{\text{(Mean from epilepsy sample} - \text{Norm mean)}}{\text{(Norm standard deviation)}}$$

TABLE 6-8. Intercorrelations of Measures of Psychological Well-being

Measure	*1*	*2*	*3*	*4*	*5*	*6*	*7*	*8*	*9*	*10*	*11*
1 Stigma (alpha = .72)	X	−.35[a]	−.27[a]	.39[a]	−.06	.17[a]	.12[b]	.17[a]	.30[a]	.30[a]	.30[a]
2 Self-esteem (alpha = .65)		X	.60[a]	−.56[a]	.05	−.15[a]	−.17[a]	−.13[a]	−.52[a]	−.62[a]	−.42[a]
3 Life satisfaction (alpha = .83)			X	−.61[a]	.15[a]	.00	−.02	−.06	−.38[a]	−.68[a]	−.28[a]
4 Helplessness (alpha = .60)				X	−.19[a]	.17[a]	.14[a]	.23[a]	.39[a]	.55[a]	.39[a]
5 Internal control					X	.00	.15[a]	−.12[b]	.03	−.07	−.05
6 External professional control						X	.19[a]	.35[a]	.29[a]	.17[a]	.25[a]
7 External family control							X	.11[b]	.16[a]	.08	.21[a]
8 External fate control								X	.24[a]	.16[a]	.25[a]
9 Anxiety (alpha = .80)									X	.63[a]	.68[a]
10 Depression (alpha = .85)										X	.49[a]
11 Somatic symptoms (alpha = .77)											X

[a] $p < .01$
[b] $p < .05$

In summary, the epilepsy group reported significantly more physiological and psychological problems than the normative sample. These findings are, again, consistent with the bulk of the epilepsy/psychopathology literature in demonstrating that rates of self-reported psychopathology are elevated in patients with epilepsy relative to healthy controls.

Table 6-8 presents perhaps the most important part of this chapter—the intercorrelations between the 11 psychosocial measures. The standardized alpha reliability coefficients are also presented as are the significance values of each coefficient. The correlation coefficients show that the stigma scale is positively and significantly related to perceived helplessness ($r = .39$), depression ($r = .30$), anxiety ($r = .30$), and somatic symptoms ($r = .30$). Stigma is also negatively and statistically significantly related to self-esteem ($r = -.35$) and life satisfaction ($r = -.27$). Therefore, the respondents' perceptions of the stigmatizing effects of epilepsy were significantly associated with indexes of psychological and physiological well-being.

The respondents' feelings of helplessness (i.e., success being attributed to the self and failure to having epilepsy) were significantly related to self-esteem ($r = -.56$), life satisfaction ($r = -.61$), anxiety ($r = .39$), depression ($r = .55$), and somatic symptoms ($r = .39$).

The three external subscales of the Multidimensional Health Locus of Control Scale were for the most part significantly and positively related to the anxiety, depression, and somatic symptoms variables (Table 6-8). The more the respondents believed that doctors, their families, and fate controlled their health, the more anxious, depressed, and ill the respondents felt. The three

TABLE 6-9. Perceived Severity and Psychological Well-Being

Measure	*Low Severity Mean*	*High Severity Mean*	*t Value*
Stigma	29.34	32.77	4.92[a]
Self-esteem	20.09	17.66	5.53[a]
Life satisfaction	11.09	10.52	3.86[a]
Helplessness	7.01	9.15	6.30[a]
Internal control	8.19	7.74	2.38[c]
External professional control	5.20	6.14	3.76[b]
External family control	5.88	6.67	3.03[b]
External fate control	5.10	6.01	3.90[a]
Anxiety	10.09	12.92	5.89[a]
Depression	18.01	21.84	4.39[a]
Somatic symptoms	23.84	29.68	5.77[a]

[a] $p < .001$
[b] $p < .01$
[c] $p < .05$

external locus of control measures were also marginally significantly related to the respondents' stigma and self-esteem scores.

The 11 psychosocial measures were subsequently compared to the respondents' reported seizure frequency and the impact of seizures on their lives. Of the 11 measures, the anxiety, depression, and somatic symptoms dimensions of the Hopkins Symptoms Checklist were significantly related to seizure rate ($p < .05$ for each measure).

The perceived impact of the seizure activity variable was collapsed into two categories ("low" and "high") and also compared to all 11 psychosocial measures. Table 6-9 shows the mean differences for each measure between the low- and high-impact categories. Although the absolute differences in means are small, they are large compared to the pooled standard errors, and all differences are thus statistically significant.

DISCUSSION

Any generalizations drawn from this survey must take into consideration three qualifications. First, it is difficult to specify the nature of the population from which the sample was drawn. Two-thirds of the people in the sample were at one time in epilepsy self-help groups. The remaining third were recruited primarily from Epilepsy Foundation of America chapters, university hospital seizure clinics, friends who have epilepsy, and so on. The respondents were activists in the sense that they were participating in epilepsy self-help groups or EFA chapters. Thus, it perhaps should not be surprising that the respondents primarily brought up social problems, were depressed and anxious, and strongly endorsed statements about how epilepsy had stigmatized their lives. If their only difficulties with having epilepsy were medical, they might not be in self-help groups or associated with an EFA chapter. The people who filled out this 29-page questionnaire may be that part of the epilepsy population who both experience social problems associated with being "epileptic" and are attempting to do something about it.

Second, and a more serious qualification in our minds, is that one cannot infer causality from correlational analyses such as the ones presented here. Are the social restrictions and isolation causing helplessness, depression, and so forth, or is it the other way around? Is it the seizure activity or the negative reactions of others that lead to learned helplessness with its concomitant depression, anxiety, and loss of self-esteem? Or is it people's psychological characteristics that affect their seizure management and feedback from significant others? These kinds of questions must await longitudinal research preferably with individuals who have been newly diagnosed as having epilepsy.

The third qualification is the least worrisome, yet it must be mentioned. It is entirely possible that the respondents' reported seizure rates do not necessarily correspond to reality. Nor can respondents' epilepsy or negative social reaction be blamed for every problem in their lives. Such attributions are constantly being worked on in the self-help groups with which we cooperated. Yet, the perceptions held by our sample are real to them, as are the perceptions of every other human being. Based on these perceptions, our respondents manage their daily lives, interact with health professionals and others, and understand the meaning of having epilepsy for their personal lives. We must start with the perceptions of the people experiencing epilepsy and then move into their social environments to get other perspectives.

Given these qualifications, three generalizations can be made from the data reported here. First, consider those measures that reflect aspects of the respondents' social-psychological environment (i.e., perceived stigma, helplessness, locus of control, self-esteem, life satisfaction, and responses to the open-ended questions). The results of our analyses would suggest that our respondents' social-psychological environments seem more important than the physical characteristics of seizure activity. In the open-ended questions, the respondents identified social and economic restrictions, negative social reactions, and the loss of personal and social control as disrupting and distorting their lives. They rarely mentioned their actual seizure activity or its immediate consequences.

Further, actual seizure frequency was not significantly associated with the measures of stigma, helplessness, external locus of control, life satisfaction, and self-esteem. Conversely, the patients' perception of the severity of the seizure disorder was highly associated with these measures. It appears that for these psychosocial indices actual seizure frequency is less important to a person with epilepsy than the perception of how severely the seizures affect one's life. Someone who has seizures about twice a year could feel out of control and in some psychological and social difficulty, whereas another person whose seizures are much more frequent may have a much greater sense of control and report that he or she is doing reasonably well. This is one plausible explanation for the lack of any significant relationship between actual seizure rate and stigma, self-esteem, helplessness, life satisfaction, or health locus of control. On the other hand, the perceived seizure impact variable was significantly related to all of these measures. This is not to say that actual seizure rate is not important. When there are sudden changes in either the frequency or intensity of a person's seizure activity, real problems may occur until the individual recalibrates his or her seizure expectations.

Second, consider the measures of psychopathology derived from the Hopkins Symptom Checklist, i.e., depression, anxiety, and somatic symptoms. Here, actual seizure frequency is found to be significantly associated with psychopathology. Additionally, most of the psychosocial variables are also significantly correlated with depression, anxiety, and somatic symptoms. (Table 6-8). The implication here is that a full understanding of the determinants of psychopathology in epilepsy requires a multietiologic approach encompassing neuroepilepsy factors (such as seizure frequency), psychosocial factors (such as those utilized in this study), and medication factors.

The third generalization we can draw from this data set concerns the applicability of the reformulated learned helplessness model to epilepsy. Given the size of the interrelationships between helplessness, depression, anxiety, and self-esteem, the model may provide a theoretical framework for understanding the psychosocial problems associated with epilepsy. The model posits that people who become helpless are likely to be depressed and anxious, and have diminished self-esteem.

However, our data set also raises a number of issues concerning the relationship between learned helplessness and seizure activity. First, based on our data, the origins of the respondents' perceived helplessness seem to reside more in their social situations than in their seizure activity. The quantity and intensity of the social restrictions and reactions to having epilepsy as measured in the stigma scale were significantly related to the helplessness measure while perceived seizure rate was not. Additionally, the lack of a strong relationship between helplessness and external health locus of control may confirm the assertion of Abramson, Garber, and Seligman (1980) that helplessness and external locus of control are orthogonal. At least that may be the case for epilepsy where individuals may attribute their degree of seizure activity to external causes ("medications control my seizures" or "no one else can control my seizures either") without becoming helpless. Of the respondents in our study, 93% indicated that taking medications regularly was the most important thing they could do to control their seizures. Finally, given the number of respondents who did not make global, internal, and/or stable attributions about how epilepsy was affecting their lives in the survey's open-ended questions, and the number of respondents who reported that they could predict (67%) and even control (45%) an upcoming seizure, we should also study "the process by which individuals move from helplessness or depression to recovery or resolution" (Silver & Wortman, 1980, p. 294). The viability of the learned helplessness model for understanding the psychosocial problems associated with epilepsy will require in-depth attributional analyses and longitudinal studies.

CONCLUSION

One of the major aims of this chapter was to investigate the relationship between the psychosocial consequences of epilepsy and interictal psychopathology. This study demonstrated, we think for the first time, a statistically significant and meaningful relationship between a social aspect of epilepsy (stigma), attitudinal variables (helplessness, self-esteem, and life satisfaction), and measures of psychopathology (depression, anxiety, and somatic symptoms). Although causality has not yet been established, we hypothesize that it exists and does so in the direction implied here. Although this is an open matter to be examined empirically, the finding of relationships between social factors and psychopathology clearly implies that greater attention and research deserve to be focused on these possible precursors of psychopathology.

Acknowledgment

This research was sponsored by the Epilepsy in the Urban Environment Project of Northwestern University's Center for Urban Affairs and Policy Research.

REFERENCES

Abramson, L. Y., J. Garber, & M. E. Seligman. (1980). Learned helplessness in humans: An attributional analysis. In J. Garber & M. E. Seligman (Eds.), *Human helplessness: Theory and applications*. New York: Academic Press.

Arangio, A. (1975). *Behind the stigma of epilepsy*. Washington, DC: Epilepsy Foundation of America.

Arntson, P. H., & B. Montgomery. (1980). *The antecedent conditions and social consequences of epilepsy*. Paper presented at the annual meeting of the International Communication Association, Acapulco, Mexico.

Bakal, C. (1979). *Charity USA*. New York: New York Times Books.

Commission for the Control of Epilepsy and its Consequences. (1978). *Plan for nationwide action on epilepsy* (DHEW Publication No. NIH 78–276). Washington, DC: U.S. Government Printing Office.

Coopersmith, S. (1967). *The antecedents of self-esteem*. San Francisco: Freeman.

Derogatis, L., R. Lipman, K. Rickels, E. Uhlenhuth, & L. Covi. (1974). The Hopkins symptom checklist (HSCL): A self-report symptom inventory. *Behavioral Science* 19, 1–15.

Falk, G., & J. Gorman. (1972). The epileptic: A study in status-role relationships. *Australian Journal of Social Issues* 7, 56–66.

Friedson, E. (1966). Disability as social deviance. In M. Sussman (Ed.), *Sociology and rehabilitation*. Washington D.C.: American Sociological Association.

Garber, J., & M. Seligman. (Eds.). (1980). *Human helplessness: Theory and applications*. New York: Academic Press.

Goffman, E. (1963). *Stigma: Notes on the management of spoiled identity*. Englewood Cliffs, NJ: Prentice-Hall.

Goldin, G., & R. Margolin. (1972). *The psychosocial aspects of epilepsy*. Paper presented at Western Institute on Epilepsy, San Diego.

Graham, L. (1958). Personality factors and epileptic seizures. *Journal of Clinical Psychology*, 14, 187–88.

Langer, E. J., & J. Rodin. (1976). The effects of choice and enhanced personal responsibility for the aged: A field experiment in an institutional setting. *Journal of Personality and Social Psychology* 34, 191–98.

Lieberman, M., & L. Borman. (1979). *Self-help groups for coping with crisis.* San Francisco: Jossey-Bass.

Norton, R., E. Murray, & P. Arntson. (1982). *Communicative links to health.* Paper presented at the annual meeting of the International Communication Association, Boston, MA.

Robinson, J., & P. Shaver. (1972). *Measures of social psychological attitudes.* Ann Arbor, MI: Institute for Social Research.

Schlesinger, L., D. Frank. (1974). From demonstration to dissemination—gateways to employment of epileptics. *Rehabilitation Literature* 35, 98–109.

Schulz, R. (1980). Aging and control. In J. Garber & M. E. Seligman (Eds.), *Human helplessness: Theory and applications.* New York: Academic Press.

Seligman, M. E. P. (1975) *Helplessness: On depression, development and death.* San Francisco: Freeman.

Silver, R., & C. Wortman. (1980). Coping with undesirable life events. In J. Garber & M. E. Seligman (Eds.), *Human helplessness: Theory and applications.* New York: Academic Press.

Taylor, D. C. (1969). Some psychiatric aspects of epilepsy. In R. Herrington (Ed.), *Current problems in neuropsychiatry.* Ashford, KY: Hardley.

Taylor, D., & R. Harrison. (1976). On being categorized in the speech of others: Medical and psychiatric diagnosis. In R. Harre (Ed.), *Life sentences.* London: Wiley.

Wallston, K. A., B. S. Wallston, & R. DeVellis. (1978). Development of the multidimensional health locus of control (MHCL) scales. *Health Education Monographs* 6, 160–70.

Weick, K. (1968). Systematic observational methods. In G. Lindzey & E. Aronson (Eds.), *The handbook of social psychology* (2nd ed.). Reading, MA: Addison-Wesley.

7 / Perceptions of Control Among Children with Epilepsy

WENDY S. MATTHEWS and
GABOR BARABAS

The many psychosocial issues that invariably arise during the development of children with epilepsy pose a major challenge to treatment. Health care professionals must find ways to handle both the minor and profound psychological problems that might impede a child's social, emotional, and intellectual growth. Identifying the key stumbling blocks to the child's optimal adjustment is the first step in intervention and toward developing ways to guide the child toward healthy means of adapting to his or her medical condition, evolving sense of self, and social environment.

Past research has described a wide range of emotional, behavioral, and social concomitants of childhood epilepsy. These studies, which are reviewed in this chapter, help us recognize the breadth of the problems experienced by children with epilepsy. But the questions arise: To what extent are the problems unique to epilepsy, rather than characteristic of chronic illnesses generally? What quality of the condition of epilepsy might evoke the sorts of psychological disturbances that those studies describe? By considering the distinguishing features of childhood epilepsy in the light of social-learning theory, a specific hypothesis has evolved. Briefly, this hypothesis states that children with epilepsy might generalize the feeling of a lack of control over their medical condition to other aspects of their lives. Having confirmed this hypothesis, in an investigation that we will describe later in this chapter, we discuss the possible psychopathological ramifications of perceptions of a lack of control for various aspects of the child's functioning (e.g., academic, social, emotional), and whether these perceptions derive from the affected children themselves, their parents, their teachers, or others with whom the children interact.

EMOTIONAL, BEHAVIORAL, AND SOCIAL ASPECTS OF CHILDHOOD EPILEPSY

Many clinical reports cite a high risk of psychological disturbances among children with epilepsy. Livingston (1972), for example, has written that children with epilepsy may be "more susceptible to the development of emotional difficulties" than children without epilepsy. He noted that the manifestations of disturbance often included severe anxiety and depression, as well as fears and feelings of insecurity. Hughes and Jabbour (1958) observed worrying and brooding, anxiety, embarrassment, and feelings of rejection, frustration, and helplessness in some of their young patients with epilepsy. Although Bridge (1949) emphasized that no set "epileptic personality" exists, he too found that some of his patients with epilepsy showed a great deal of fearfulness, dependence, demandingness, and anxiety, which he described as a "common pattern of reaction."

Some investigators have utilized surveys in a systematic search for the emotional concomitants of epilepsy in childhood. For example, Breger (1975) sent a questionnaire to parents of 60 patients evaluated and diagnosed as having epilepsy. The survey focused on the child's current medical status and level of general functioning, the effect of epilepsy on the child and family, and the long-term value of the earlier evaluation and recommendations. On the basis of 26 returns (43%), Breger identified impairments in academic functioning and peer relationships, poor self-esteem and a "deterioration in emotional development" in a population that was generally medically improved, or at least stable. (The remaining 57% of his patients might have been unmotivated to reestablish contact with the clinic due to positive adjustment or unable to respond due to medical complications. Breger's poor response rate makes it difficult to interpret the findings.)

Surveying the teachers of 85 children with epilepsy in regular public schools, Holdsworth and Whitmore (1974) reported that in 42% of the cases, teachers noted that the children were apathetic or "just not with us." Deviant behavior was said to characterize 18 (21.1%) of the children, 14 (16.4%) were described as being aggressive, objectionable, truculent, spiteful, or bullying, and attention seeking, and 4 (4.7%) as isolated or withdrawn.

Past reports such as these have raised the issue of psychological maladjustment, but have failed to demonstrate that the adjustment difficulties found among children with epilepsy differ in frequency or in kind from those seen in children with other chronic maladies or those with no known health problems.

Controlled investigations comparing the psychological functioning of children with epilepsy have begun to appear only in the past decade or so. For example, Hackney and Taylor (1976), using a version of Rutter's Teachers' Questionnaire for assessing teachers' perceptions of pupils, found that school children with epilepsy (N = 30) were perceived as generally more disturbed than their healthy peers (N = 30) (as indicated by mean scores). However, further analyses revealed equal frequencies of neurotic and antisocial behaviors, hyperactivity, and psychosis in both groups. Only 1 of the 26 specific behaviors tapped by the questionnaire, "unresponsiveness or apathy," differentiated the groups, with teachers reporting that it occurred more frequently among children who had epilepsy.

Using the same questionnaire, Mellor, Lowit, and Hall (1974) solicited responses from another group of teachers who were unaware that they were participating in a study involving epilepsy. They did not know that one of the groups of targeted children was part of a group of 295 children with epilepsy whereas the other was part of an age- and sex-matched control group of 295 children with no known health problems. Twenty-seven percent of the children with epilepsy, compared with 15% of the control children, were reported to have behavioral problems. Those with epilepsy were more frequently described as appearing miserable and having a short attention span as well as being fidgety and not liked by the other children. Complaints of aches and pains, destructive behavior, nail biting, solitariness, speech difficulties, restlessness, and disobedience were also reported more commonly among the children with epilepsy.

In the oft-cited Isle of Wight study (Rutter, Graham, & Yule, 1970), various groups of chronically ill children, alike in terms of age, sex, and socioeconomic status but differing in terms of medical status, were compared. A higher prevalence of psychiatric disorder was found among the group of children with uncomplicated epilepsy (28%) compared with blind (17%), deaf (15%), and healthy (7%) children. (The highest prevalence was found among children with structural abnormalities of the brain with or without seizures: 58% and 38%, respectively.) Among the psychiatrically disturbed children, the distribution of disorders across the general categories of neurosis, antisocial conduct, mixed disorders, hyperactivity, and psychosis was indistinguishable between the medically healthy children and those with epilepsy. The only specific problems differentiating these two groups involved greater fidgetiness and poorer concentration reported by teachers and parents (but not interviewers) in children who had epilepsy.

Methodological differences may account for the wider range of disturbance seen in the Isle of Wight and the Mellor et al. studies, as compared with Hackney and Taylor's. For example, Hackney and Taylor's teachers, unlike those in the other studies, were aware of the research interest in the pupils with epilepsy, and consequently may have been particularly sympathetic in their responses. The discrepancies may also derive from the fact that Hackney and Taylor separated out all children who had ever been inpatients at a children's neuropsychiatric hospital. Thus, their sample probably represented a better functioning group. In any case, these studies reveal that children with epilepsy, compared with their healthy peers, manifest a medley of affective and behavioral difficulties within the school setting.

Within the home setting, Long and Moore (1979) found a series of additional problems reported by parents to characterize the child with epilepsy. For example, the youngsters with epilepsy were perceived by their parents as having more emotional problems and as being more unpredictable and higher strung than their siblings. The children with epilepsy were expected to perform less well in school, to play in fewer sports, to concentrate poorly, and to have a narrower range of occupational choices than their healthy siblings, despite the fact that all of the children involved in the study were free of associated disabilities and were attending regular school. Unlike most investigators, Long and Moore also obtained data directly from the children. To document earlier reported characteristics of children with epilepsy (Winston & Chilman, 1964), and to test their own hypothesis related to the possible effects of feeling "different" from peers, Long and Moore examined the children's feelings of self-esteem using the Coopersmith Self-Esteem Inventory. They found the children to have significantly lower levels of self-esteem than their unaffected siblings.

In another study using measures derived from children, Hartlage, Green, and Offut (1972) focused on dependency as a particular problem area in the psychosocial development of children with epilepsy. Their objective was to attribute the academic and social underachievement found in an earlier study (Hartlage & Green, 1972) to inappropriate dependency in childhood epilepsy. Comparing patients with epilepsy with groups of cystic fibrosis and tonsillectomy patients, these investigators substantiated higher dependency levels, as measured by the Children's Dependency Scale, but not the Parental Attitude Research Inventory, among the children with epilepsy. Since there was no difference in the attitudes of parents of children with epilepsy when compared to those of the parents of children in the other diagnostic groups, they speculated that the overdependency seen in childhood epilepsy might in some unspecified manner stem from the "direct impact" of the illness or its treatment.

Work in the area of psychosocial functioning in childhood epilepsy, whether through clinical report, survey, or empirical investigation, has identified an array of factors commonly found in epilepsy. However, without a conceptual basis, contributions to the literature provide little more than an ever-growing checklist of the possible problem areas. Scant progress has been made in the 25 years since Deutsch and Wiener (1948) lamented that a "recognized lack of a common denominator has greatly hampered understanding."

PERCEPTION OF A LACK OF CONTROL: A POSSIBLE DETERMINANT OF ADJUSTMENT DIFFICULTIES IN CHILDHOOD EPILEPSY

The failure of past investigations to explain the pervasive emotional concomitants of childhood epilepsy derives primarily from the descriptive, atheoretical nature of their approach. By considering the factors entailed by the epileptic condition, however, one can speculate on specific social and psychological sequelae. For example, a distinctive feature of epilepsy is its unpredictability, with respect to the time, place, and social circumstances in which a seizure might occur. It has been suggested that the episodic, unforeseeable nature of a seizure, in contrast to symptoms of other chronic illnesses, is particularly handicapping since it deprives the child of the "constant opportunity to develop adaptive reactions to the disability" (Goldin & Margolin, 1975). Since the individuals present during a seizure may differ at each occurrence, the people who make up the child's social environment may also lack sufficient opportunity to develop appropriate ways of responding to the child's condition.

Another factor unique to epilepsy is the overt manifestation of the symptom in a manner often described by the child and by others as frightening and grotesque. Thus, the "unpracticed" reaction of others to a seizure is likely to be negative rather than positive—awkward, inept, and even cruel, rather than smooth, helpful, and supportive. Last, the convulsive seizure represents a loss of control to the child and may also be perceived as such by those around him or her.

Focusing on these distinguishing features of epilepsy, we can formulate a number of congruous hypotheses. For example, children might generalize the feeling of a lack of control over their seizure activity to other aspects of their lives. Social learning theorists explain the generalization phenomenon in terms of individuals developing an expectancy that specific experiences (such as seizures, school reports, or popularity) are within or beyond one's control. Rotter (1966) defines a "locus of control" as follows:

> When a reinforcement is perceived by the subject as following some action of his own but not being entirely contingent upon his action, then, in our culture, it is typically perceived as the result of luck, chance, fate, as under the control of powerful others, or as unpredictable because of the great complexity of the forces surrounding him. When the event is interpreted in this way by an individual, we have labeled this a belief in external control. If the person perceives that the event is contingent upon his own behavior or his own relatively permanent characteristics, we have termed this a belief in internal control. (p. 1)

Because children with epilepsy are likely to perceive that the occurrence of a seizure is not contingent on their actions, we hypothesized that they also would attribute other events in their lives to external sources of control. Second, we hypothesized that the sense of lack of control and its public disclosure via the overt seizure manifestation would adversely affect children's self-concept. Third, we hypothesized that the unpredictability of the seizure occurrence and the associated difficulty in developing consistent and reliable strategies to cope with their condition would be manifested by high levels of anxiety among children with epilepsy.

Although our concern centered primarily on the child with epilepsy, these issues can also be viewed from a wider perspective. For example, one can also hypothesize that other individuals, observing or contemplating the child's loss of control during a seizure, might generalize this perception in such a way that they come to view the child as lacking control over a variety of situations. Second, the overt manifestation of the seizure might detract from others' views of the child as controlled, competent, attractive, lovable, or worthy. Third, one can hypothesize that the unpredictability of the seizure occurrence and the lack of preparedness on the part of others would increase their anxiety levels as well as those of the child with epilepsy. Research on the wider social constellation of the child with epilepsy would help us to distinguish the extent to which a child's perception of lack of control derives from self versus others.

A STUDY OF PERCEPTIONS OF CONTROL IN CHILDHOOD EPILEPSY

METHOD

Subjects

To test these hypotheses, 45 children between the ages of 7 and 12 ($\bar{x} = 9.9$ years) were selected as subjects. Of these, 15 children with epilepsy composed the experimental group (E). All were identified from the records of the Pediatric Seizure Control Center, Middlesex General-University Hospital in New Brunswick, New Jersey. All were diagnosed as having idiopathic epilepsy. Seizure type was variable: Eight children had complex partial seizures, two had primary generalized tonic–clonic seizures, four had elementary partial seizures, and one had classical absence. All children with associated disabilities such as cerebral palsy or mental retardation were excluded from the study.

Fifteen children with diagnosed diabetes mellitus served as a chronically ill control group (D). They were recruited from a variety of sources including practicing local physicians, specialized groups within the community, and informal social networks. Diabetes is a systemic condition that, when well controlled, has relatively stable symptomatology. By utilizing the diabetic group, the effects of the episodicity, unpredictability, and lack of control seen in epilepsy can be separated from the effects of chronic illness in general. At the same time, the effects of daily administration of medication on a child's psychological functioning can be ruled out.

For baseline data, 15 healthy children served as an additional control group (H). They were found primarily through informal social networks such as friends of parents with chronically ill children. By utilizing a third control group, detrimental effects associated with having a chronic illness, irrespective of specific symptomatology, could be assessed.

All three groups were matched for age, sex, socioeconomic status, general intellectual level, and family status as depicted in Table 7-1. All children were pupils in primary public schools. Both chronically ill groups of children were matched for age of onset and for duration of illness as well. Socioeconomic status was determined according to the Hollingshead scale (Hollingshead, 1975) and found to be equivalent for all groups.

Procedure

An investigator, initially blind to the diagnosis of the subjects, visited the homes of healthy children and children with epilepsy and with diabetes, usually in the early evening hours. The investigator first administered an assortment of instruments (described later in this section) to the child, and then extensively interviewed the parent. Because of the salience of a chronic illness within a family, the diagnosis was invariably made known to the investigator in the course of the 2–3-hour session. Objectively scorable tests and reliability measures, however, served to minimize experimenter bias.

Measures

Multidimensional Measure of Children's Perception of Control. To determine the degree to which the child feels that events in his or her life are

TABLE 7-1. Subject Characteristics

Group	*Age*	*Sex*		*SES*	*Mental Age*[a]	*Family Status*	*Age of Onset*	*Duration of Illness*
		M	*F*					
Epileptic	9.87	7	8	2.88	10.34	13 Intact 2 Separated	6.89	3.05
Diabetic	9.82	8	7	2.93	9.91	14 Intact 1 Separated	6.96	2.86
Healthy	9.96	7	8	2.98	9.99	14 Intact 1 Separated	—	—

[a]As determined by the Goodenough criteria for Draw-a-Person scoring.

controlled by external or internal sources, the Multidimensional Measure of Children's Perception of Control (MMCPC) (Connell, 1980) was administered. The scale consists of 48 statements. The child must indicate how true he or she believes each statement to be: very true, sort of true, not very true, or not at all true. The test was designed to tap (a) perceived source of control (internal, powerful others, or unknown); (b) competency areas within which the belief is held (cognitive, social, physical, and general skills); (c) the relation of the outcome (success or failure) to the child's notion of the source of control (e.g., some children might view success as resulting from luck or external factors while regarding failures as stemming from within themselves, i.e., from some inadequacy of their own); and (d) the realm of reference (i.e., whether the children are referring to the way life is for them versus the way it is for other children). To illustrate, the statement "When I do well in school, it's usually because I've worked hard on my school assignments" taps an internal locus (" . . . because I've worked hard. . ."), refers to a success outcome (" . . . do well in school . . ."), cites an event in the cognitive competency area (" . . . in school . . ."), and is in the personal realm ("when I do well . . .").

Piers-Harris Self-Concept Scale. Self-esteem was measured by the Piers-Harris Self-Concept Scale (Piers & Harris, 1969). It consists of 80 items concerned with children's attitudes toward themselves in six major areas; behavior, intellectual and school status, physical attributes, anxiety, popularity, and happiness and satisfaction. Each of the 80 items requires a yes or no response to brief positive and negative statements dealing with each of these areas; for example, "I am among the last to be chosen for games," and "my classmates think that I have good ideas." The inventory is suitable for use with children in grades 2 through 12 and has been shown to have high concurrent validities with other children's self-concept rating instruments (e.g., Mayer, 1965). It is one of the more highly reliable and valid self-report questionnaires (Quay & Werry, 1979).

Draw-a-Person. The Draw-a-Person test was utilized in two manners: first, as a measure of mental maturity, and second, as a projective test of children's concerns. Used as an intelligence measure, Goodenough's standardized and validated scoring method provided a mental age for each of the subjects from which the groups could be matched according to general level of intellectual functioning. As a projective instrument, Koppitz's Emotional Indicators served as objectively scorable indexes of psychological difficulty. The 38 indicators have been shown to have clinical validity, i.e., to differentiate children with and without emotional problems, to occur infrequently in the drawings of normal children (among 15% or less), and to be independent of age and maturation (Koppitz, 1968).

Scored independently by two investigators, a high reliability coefficient was found. Perfect agreement occurred 88.2% of the time on exact item-per-item analysis, and the overall number of emotional indicators assigned by each rater for each drawing was in exact agreement 92.2% of the time.

Rochester Adaptive Behavior Inventory (RABI). The Rochester Adaptive Behavior Inventory was used to assess the general adaptive functioning of the children. It was administered to the parents while both were present. The RABI consists of a series of five age-appropriate parallel forms designed to examine the social competence of children from early childhood through adolescence. On the 7- and 10-year forms utilized in the present study, 119 of the 123 items were parallel; only these items were considered in the analysis. The format of the RABI involves a series of questions related to the child's behavior and adjustment in home, school, and peer settings. The questions were posed in a conversational manner permitting the parents the freedom to elaborate on their responses as needed. Responses were categorized by the interviewer, who was trained in the RABI scoring procedure. The RABI yields scores in a number of general content areas including school behavior, sociability, atypical behavior, communications, home behavior, and sexual awareness (Jones, 1977). Interrater reliability of scoring between two investigators was high, with exact agreement occurring on 88.4% of the items, and a 10.4% incidence of disagreements of a single point on the five-point RABI scales.

Results

Multidimensional Measure of Children's Perception of Control.

Results of analyses of variance for children's perceptions of control are summarized in Table 7-2. Regardless of the outcome, the competency domain, or the realm of the reference, children with epilepsy invariably displayed the greatest perception of an external source of control relative to other children. The likelihood that the children with epilepsy perceived the source of control over events in their lives to be unknown was significantly greater than that found among the diabetic or healthy children in every subcategory except "general" competency.

Outcomes. With respect to outcome, children with epilepsy differentiated themselves from their diabetic and healthy peers. All children were equally likely to perceive powerful others as responsible for their failures, and both groups of chronically ill children were equally likely to perceive unknown sources as responsible for failures. However, the children with epilepsy exceed both their diabetic and their healthy peers in the tendency to attribute even their own successes to unknown sources [$F(2, 42) = 7.24, p < .002$].

Competency domains. The competency domain over which children with

TABLE 7-2. Multidimensional Measure of Children's Perceptions of Control

	Source of Control: Unknown			*Source of Control: Powerful Others*		
	Epileptic (E)	*Diabetic (D)*	*Healthy (H)*	*Epileptic (E)*	*Diabetic (D)*	*Healthy (H)*
Overall means	2.50 A[a]	2.21 A	1.77 B	2.38 A	2.26 A	2.02 A
Outcome						
Success	2.53 A	2.14 B	1.74 C	2.46 A	2.29 A	1.93 A
Failure	2.49 A	2.26 A	1.81 B	2.31 A	2.23 A	2.13 A
Competence domain						
Cognitive/academic	2.52 A	2.23 A	1.68 B	2.08 A	2.03 A	1.88 A
Social	2.63 A	2.13 B	1.80 B	2.47 A	2.05 AB	1.77 B
Physical	2.38 A	2.13 AB	1.70 B	2.38 A	2.38 A	2.20 A
General	2.48 A	2.50 A	2.03 A	2.49 A	2.46 A	2.13 A
Realm of reference						
Personal (self)	2.53 A	2.24 A	1.80 B	2.49 A	2.46 A	2.13 A
Maxim (others)	2.49 A	2.16 A	1.75 B	2.28 A	2.07 A	1.94 A

[a]In each row, means with different letters are significantly different at the .05 level. (Higher numbers imply greater Unknown perception of control over a particular set of events.)

epilepsy were more likely to attribute control to external sources was the social domain. Their social functioning was significantly more likely to be perceived as controlled by unknown sources than that of their diabetic or healthy peers and more likely to be perceived as controlled by powerful others than was that of their healthy peers. The degree to which the children with epilepsy are differentiated from their peers in the social domain underscores the significance of the social dimension for individuals with epilepsy.

Realm of reference. Whether the children with epilepsy were focusing on their own personal functioning or on any child's functioning did not alter their attributions of internal control or control by powerful others. However, when they were considering events in their own lives, particularly their successes and their social experiences, they were significantly more likely to attribute control to unknown sources than when they were considering events in other children's lives. In fact, the source of their own success appears to be unknown to them in every one of the competency domains, without exception.

Piers-Harris Self-Concept Scale

Piers-Harris self-concept scores significantly differentiated the groups as well. An analysis of variance with a significant group effect [$F(2, 39) = 11.92$,

$p < .0001$] was followed by post hoc comparisons revealing that the children who have epilepsy had lower overall self-concept scores. As indicated in Table 7-3, their self-esteem on matters related to intellectual and academic functioning, anxiety, and popularity was significantly lower than that of their peers.

Draw-a-Person

The higher level of anxiety that emerged on the Piers-Harris measure among children with epilepsy was substantiated by the anxiety scores derived from the Draw-a-Person. Using the Koppitz scoring procedure for emotional indicators, there was a significant group effect [$F(2, 39) = 6.89, p < .03$], with Duncan tests revealing the anxiety levels among children with epilepsy to exceed those of their healthy peers. (The diabetic group's score fell between the two and did not differ significantly from either group.)

Rochester Adaptive Behavior Inventory

Parental reports substantiated many of the findings reported earlier. The RABI analysis revealed that parents' perceptions of the child's school behavior [$F(2, 39) = 4.82, p < .01$], sociability [$F(2, 39) = 4.79, p < .01$], and atypical behavior [$F(2, 39) = 4.93, p < .01$] differed according to the child's medical status. Duncan tests showed that the parents of children with epilepsy discerned problems with sociability and atypical behavior, whereas parents in both groups of chronically ill children saw problems with school and home behavior. Focusing on those items that differentiated the children who have epilepsy from both their diabetic and healthy peers, the analysis revealed that their parents are significantly less likely to perceive them as initiating activities ($p < .02$), as leading rather than following other children ($p < .0001$), and as sticking up for themselves ($p < .02$). The children with epilepsy were

TABLE 7-3. Piers-Harris Children's Self-Concept Scale

	Epileptic	*Diabetic*	*Healthy*
Overall self-concept	53.2 A[a]	60.3 B	67.1 C
Domains			
Behavior	7.2 A	7.8 A	8.3 A
Intellectual/ academic	4.1 A	4.7 AB	5.3 B
Physical	4.0 A	3.8 A	4.1 A
Anxiety	2.3 A	3.5 B	4.1 B
Popularity	1.9 A	3.1 B	3.7 B
Happiness/ satisfaction	3.5 A	3.3 A	3.7 A

[a]In each row, means with different letters are significantly different at the .05 level.

also reported to be more likely to complain that everyone is picking on them ($p < .003$), to laugh or smile at serious events such as death or illness ($p < .004$), to behave immaturely or babyishly ($p < .03$), to have periods of emotional upset ($p < .05$), to behave assaultively toward the parents ($p < .05$) and to have a variety of school-related problems. In addition, the parents of children with epilepsy describe their family as less close ($p < .02$) and note that their discussions tend to focus more on specific than general issues ($p < .003$). The academic and family functioning of children with epilepsy has been discussed fully elsewhere (Ferrari, Matthews, & Barabas, 1983; Matthews, Barabas, Ferrari, 1983).

DISCUSSION

To the extent that the children with epilepsy might perceive the events in their lives as resulting from forces outside themselves, failing to recognize the role of their own behavior in bringing about certain outcomes, they are at risk of maladapting. By denying themselves an appreciation of their personal effectiveness, they can become less motivated, less flexible in their problem-solving strategies, less receptive to evaluative feedback and incentives, and more helpless in their interactions with the environment. These maladaptive response patterns affect their behavior in a number of domains ranging from interpersonal to academic. It is to these more general issues that we now turn in an effort to put our results in a broader perspective.

Social Functioning and External Locus of Control

Children's perceptions of control could affect their readiness to approach other individuals, to expend effort to maintain a friendship, and to alter or terminate an unconstructive relationship. Among children with epilepsy, we found that external attributions were more pronounced in the social sphere than in any other. Many of the children saw themselves as unpopular, but were unable to explain why. (They would tend to agree with statements such as "A lot of times, kids have a lot of friends for no reason at all" or "If somebody doesn't like me, there is probably nothing I could do about it.") If the children do not feel in control of interpersonal relationships, why not? Are their external attributions based exclusively on their generalized perception of not being in control of themselves? Or are they based, in part, on fact? How much are children with epilepsy actually in control of their social environment?

To the extent that the children's social interactions are influenced by other individuals' stereotypes and misconceptions of epilepsy, they do lack control over the course of their potential or developing social relationships. The effect of social stigma is profound and is discussed at length throughout this volume. Of interest at present, however, is the extent to which the social cognition of children with epilepsy leads them to view their social world as beyond their control. The processes by which children form expectations and beliefs about interpersonal events are not unlike the processes by which children form ideas about nonsocial events. They involve, first, the recognition of a problem requiring a solution; second, the consideration of possible problem-solving strategies; third, a decision about which solution to use; and last, action. The internal cognitive processes that lead to successful social problem solving are akin to and influenced by the same sort of cognitive strategies that mediate nonsocial problem solving. The child must recognize that a social interaction has an implicit contractual aspect that requires some negotiation and problem solving; he or she must have a notion of some possible strategies for negotiating the interaction and must decide on an approach. Then, the child must act on the preferred social strategy, consider its effectiveness in achieving the sought-after social goal, and revise the approach accordingly. As these different steps are tried and evaluated, children develop a set of expectations about how social interactions will proceed for them and, it is hoped, come to understand their role in the outcome of social interaction. As social learning theory proposes, a child's prior responses and their consequences are the best determinants of the perspective the child will form about the degree of his or her control over life events.

Children with epilepsy must deal not only with the feedback that they derive from their bodies (e.g., "I did nothing, yet I suffered a seizure") or from their own cognitions (e.g., "This trophy shows that I practiced hard"), but also from the feedback they derive from others. Because it is often influenced by societal misconceptions about epilepsy, the feedback others give to children with epilepsy might vary significantly from that they give to individuals without epilepsy. For example, the implicit social contract may begin to evolve on less than equitable grounds because the other person ascribes an "inferior" status to the child with epilepsy. Interpersonal strategies that might work well for ordinary children may backfire when the child with epilepsy confronts an irrational fear or superstition in his or her prospective playmate. As the child with epilepsy tries alternate strategies in an effort to accommodate, he or she might realistically come to attribute the social failure to an unknown cause. In a study by Ritchie (1981), families of children with epilepsy were observed in an interactive, decision-making situation. Found to be somewhat domineering and autocratic, these families apparently did not give the child a chance to participate fully in the proceedings, possibly on the assumption that the child was in some way "limited". It is not inconceivable that the cumulative effect of depriving a child of active, participatory status in a variety of situations would be to shift his or her attributions of control from the self to powerful others or to unknown sources as the child becomes increasingly aware of his or her powerlessness.

Looking further at the specific family-related variables that differentiate children with epilepsy from those with another chronic illness or from those with no medical problems, we found a significant number of areas in which families with a child with epilepsy are uniquely affected (Ferrari et al., 1983). For example, it appears that they are inclined to perceive the child as immature and relatively unassertive. The families saw themselves as less close than other families and as characteristically having poor intrafamilial communication. The children perceived themselves as problematic with regard to their families. They were more likely to feel that they caused trouble for and disappointed their families, in spite of the fact that they saw themselves as behaving obediently. Our results suggest that the presence of a chronic illness such as epilepsy in a young family member places the family at risk for problems with communications, cohesion, and integration, and places the child at risk for developing a sense of helplessness. Further research, focusing on specific dynamics that might account for these effects within families with children who have epilepsy, is needed. Until then, parents can be advised that they can probably promote their child's. psychosocial adjustment by refraining from protecting the child from all harm and from making all the child's decisions. Rather, parents might encourage children to take responsibility for their own actions, to make some mistakes and learn from them, and to suffer some hurts and adapt to them. By encouraging independence and a recognition and acceptance of its consequences, parents can encourage children to view themselves as a source of control over their own actions. Research indicates that positive parental behavior, such as nurturance, warmth, affection, and independence training, is associated with internality in children. The greater perception on the part of children that they are accepted by their parents, the stronger their perception is of an internal locus of control (Rohner, Chaille, & Rohner, 1980).

Psychopathology and Locus of Control

The locus-of-control orientation most commonly thought to be associated with psychopathology is externality (Lefcourt, 1976). Individuals who believe their actions have little effect on their environment are expected to take a more passive stance, to be less willing to assume personal responsibility for events in their lives, and to exhibit less initiative or flexibility in the ways in which they choose to cope. These response styles would be more apt to lead to mental illness. Individuals with an internal orientation, believing that reinforcements are contingent on their own actions, would be expected to take a more active stance toward life, to accept responsibility for their acts, and to develop effective strategies for assuring that their needs are met. Thus, they would be less prone to mental illness (Lefcourt, 1976). Investigations of the relationship between psychopathology and locus of control, usually involving adults, generally substantiate a greater degree of maladjustment among individuals with an external orientation, particularly with respect to depression and anxiety.

In children, the belief that one's outcomes or reinforcements are not contingent on one's actions is thought to be associated with decreased motivation and negative affect, particularly after the preschool and early elementary school ages (Rholes, Blackwell, Jordan, & Walters, 1980). In adults, perceived uncontrollability over events has been recognized as a significant contributor to depression (Seligman, 1975) and is discussed more fully by DeVellis and DeVellis in this volume (chap. 5). This finding has also been substantiated in children (Lefkowitz, Tesiny, & Gordon, 1980).

Although our investigation of the emotional concomitants of childhood epilepsy did not mention depression, it highlighted the tendency toward an external orientation, a poor self-concept, and a high level of anxiety among many of the children with epilepsy. The clinical significance of these and related findings is considerable, especially insofar as suicide is concerned. Reviewing the literature on suicide and epilepsy (Matthews & Barabas, 1981), we found an inordinately high rate of suicide for which the variables targeted in our research and outlined in the present chapter—feelings of helplessness and lack of control, low self-esteem, and anxiety—are taken to be significant risk factors. The clinician who sees these conditions in children should be aware that they might be precursors of later suidical behavior. A longitudinal study in which children with a highly external orientation, low self-esteem, and high anxiety are followed through adolescence and early adulthood would add to our understanding of the development of the psychological vulnerability underlying suicide among some individuals with epilepsy. In the meantime, routine mental status examinations that include questions about perceptions of control, self-concept, and anxiety would help physicians identify young patients at risk. Specifically, the physician can monitor the child's emotional status, expressed in unhappiness or weepiness, look for any changes in behavior, particularly involving an impairment in social or family relationships or a decline in school performance, and inquire about symptoms such as sleep disturbance, change in appetite, loss of energy or interests, reduction in activity, expression of self-deprecatory ideas, suicidal threats or behavior, increased irritability, new somatic complaints, wandering behavior, and depressive delusions and hallucinations, as outlined by Birleson (1981).

Academic Functioning and External Locus of Control

An inability to appreciate one's personal responsibility for failures as well as for achievements in an academic setting can lead to chronic underachievement. Research studies confirm that children who perceive control as external tend to have lower achievement test scores than children who have an internal orientation (Duke & Nowicki, 1974; Tesiny, Lefkowitz, & Gordon, 1980). This finding is explained by the fact that children must have some expectation about success; and without this, they are unlikely to look at themselves as responsible agents for the achievement of success and unlikely to strive for accomplishment (Midlarsky & McKnight, 1980).

Children with specific learning disabilities appear to be particularly vulnerable to the view that their actions are unrelated to the consequences that befall them, perhaps because their efforts are, in fact, often to no avail. Bosworth and Murray (1983) compared dyslexic learning-disabled children with average school children and found that the dyslexic children believed themselves to have less control over events occurring both in the academic setting and in general life situations. They did not differ from their peers in the degree to which they felt they were responsible for their own mistakes, but differed significantly in the degree to which they believed their successes were not of their own making. The authors summarized: "Dyslexic children lack conviction in their ability to affect successful outcomes." This perception, in turn, adversely affects their motivation to achieve. Likening this response to the behavioral patterns seen in learned helplessness, the authors note that the children are likely to exhibit (1) a decrease in motivation to control events, and (2) difficulties in learning when a response has actually succeeded. The analogy to the learned helplessness model comes from the fact that the repeated frustration, frequent failures, and decreased ability to master academic skills experienced by the children can elicit a "state of learned helplessness" in the dyslexic children. The investigators caution that this situation might lead to depression, disruptive behavior, and academic difficulties beyond those directly related to the learning disability. They suggest the recovery, or the construction, of the belief that "effort produces desirable consequences" would alleviate it. A remediation program that facilitates a sense of self-mastery in the children is recommended to encourage self-determined academic achievement and to prevent the development or maintenance of maladaptive attributions or behaviors.

In our study of academic achievement and perceptions of control among children with epilepsy (Matthews et al., 1983), we found the same tendency to believe that one's outcomes are related to external factors such as luck, chance, fate, or powerful others, that other researchers have found among learning disabled children. Although the majority of children with epilepsy do not differ from their classmates in general intelligence, many pupils with epilepsy do experience subtle learning problems. Thus, it is not surprising that their pattern of response in an academic setting would be similar to that of healthy learning-disabled children. The variables underlying learning disabilities in epilepsy are complex, however. They may stem from the association between learning and a variety of neuroepileptic phenomena such as overt seizures or subconvulsive epileptiform discharges, from the effects of the anticonvulsant medication, or from the psychosocial environment of the child. Like learning-disabled children who do not have epilepsy, children with seizures are likely to agree with the statement "If I get a bad grade in school, I usually don't understand why I got it," thus reflecting their attributions of their performance to some unknown source of control. Our investigation found this to be true whether the final outcome of the performance was failure (a poor grade) or success (a good grade). Like children with dyslexia, those with epilepsy might be missing out on an important mediator of good school performance, namely, an expectancy for success following effort.

A child's achievements also depend to some degree on the teacher's expectancy of his or her success. In a classic study by Rosenthal and Jacobson (1968) entitled *Pygmalion in the Classroom,* those children who had randomly been identified to teachers as "late bloomers" did well. Apparently attentive to signs of progress in these children, the teachers acted in a way that enhanced the children's functioning, and they bloomed.

A teacher's classroom behavior can specifically influence a child's perceptions of control. Buriel (1981) reviewed the findings of several recent studies indicating that children's feelings of internal responsibility in various problem situations can be increased and maintained over time through the use of social reinforcement and structural techniques by their teachers (Andrews & Debus, 1978; Dweck, 1975), that feelings of internal control among hyperactive boys were enhanced using self-control techniques (Bugenthal, Collins, Collins, & Chancy, 1978), and that students experience greater feelings of personal control when teachers' classroom behavior is positive and rewarding (DeCharms, 1976). They then emphasize that a teacher's instructional practices can have a profound effect on the children's achievement-related causal attribution.

In our work with schools having pupils with epilepsy, we recommend that instances of success following effort, or failure following a lack of effort (e.g., inattention, noncompliance), should be pointed out to the child in order to help the child recognize the causal relationship between his or her activity and school achievement. A number of studies have pointed to the necessity of a highly structured reinforcement situation for pupils with learning disabilities (Bendell, Tollefson, & Fine, 1980; Pascarella & Pflaum, 1981). For example, to improve the performance of learning-disabled children with an external locus of control on tasks requiring them to learn 15 new spelling words,

Bendell et al. presented the children with a highly specific instruction: "For each word you missed, trace the word with your finger, write it three times on your paper, say the word and the letters to yourself in a whisper each time you write the word." They found that under these conditions the external-locus-of-control children did significantly better than when they were told merely to "study the words for 15 minutes." In the Pascarella and Pflaum study, the investigators found that students with an external locus of control tended to improve their oral reading most dramatically when the teacher provided highly specific feedback about their performance. The directive approach involved the teacher's saying "No, the correct answer is *dishes*" in order both to indicate the child's mistake and to identify the correct answer. Another example of the directive approach would be "your guess does not fit the sentence meaning; a better guess is *want*." This is in contrast to a less directive approach (e.g., "What do you think? Does *want* fit the sentence?"), a method by which the students themselves must determine the correctness or incorrectness of their response and adjust it accordingly. Those students who ascribed their success or failure in the classroom to themselves fared better with the nondirective approach.

CONCLUSION

Many children with epilepsy perceive the source of control over events in their lives to be unknown. Their apparent lack of recognition of their control over outcomes can impede their motivation to learn, to interact, and to pursue happiness. It can also lead to anxiety and depression. Given the extreme clinical importance of the psychosocial effects of feelings of lack of control, we recommend that children with epilepsy routinely be encouraged to exercise personal responsibility and to recognize personal effectiveness. The correlation between one's actions and their outcomes can be underscored in numerous contexts. In a medical setting, one can point out that compliance with a medical regime leads to a greater chance of reduction of seizures, and noncompliance to a greater risk of increased seizure frequency. In an academic setting, completing one's homework assignments can be recognized as leading to a greater chance of improvement on a report card. In a social situation, social initiative can be recognized as leading to further social interaction. The greater the children's awareness of their effectiveness in determining consequences, the greater their motivation toward initiative and personal growth.

On a social level, the specificity of loss of control during seizure activity can be underscored, and the wrongness of generalizing to situations other than seizures can be resolutely declared. Parents, siblings, teachers, friends, and others with whom children with epilepsy share their social world must view them as responsible, effective individuals who happen to manifest an intermittent, time-limited, neurological symptom that need not affect other aspects of their lives.

REFERENCES

Andrews, G. R. & R. I. Debus. (1978). Persistence and causal perception of failure: Modifying cognitive attributions. *Journal of Educational Psychology* 70, 154–66.

Bendell, P., N. Tollefson, & M. Fine. (1980). Interaction of locus of control orientation and the performance of learning disabled adolescents. *Journal of Learning Disabilities* 13, 32–35.

Birleson, P. (1981). The validity of depressive disorder in childhood and the development of a self-rating scale: A research report. *Journal of Child Psychology and Psychiatry* 22, 73–88.

Bosworth, H. T., & M. E. Murray. (1983). Locus of control and achievement motivation on dyslexia children. *Developmental and Behavioral Pediatrics* 4, 253–56.

Breger, E. (1975). Psychiatric consultation to the epileptic child and his family: A study of 60 cases. Part 3: Follow-up study. *Maryland State Medical Journal,* 47–50.

Bridge, E. M. (1949). *Epilepsy and convulsive disorders in childhood.* New York: Irvington (distributed by Halsted Press).

Bugenthal, D. B., S. Collins, L. Collins, & L. A. Chancy. (1978). Attributional and behavioral changes following two interventions with hyperactive boys: A follow-up study. *Child Development* 49, 247–50.

Buriel, Raymond. (1981). The relation of Anglo- and Mexican-American children's locus of control beliefs to parents' and teachers' socialization practices. *Child Development* 52, 104–13.

Connell, J. P. (1980). *A multidimensional measure of children's perceptions of control* (manual). Denver, CO: University of Denver.

DeCharms, R. (1976). *Enhancing motivation in the classroom.* New York. Irvington (distributed by Halsted Press).

Deutsch, L., & L. L. Wiener. (1948). Children with epilepsy: Emotional problems and treatment. *American Journal of Orthopsychiatry* 18, 65–72.

Duke, M. P., & S. Nowicki. (1974). Locus of control and achievement: The confirmation of theoretical expectation. *Journal of Psychology* 87, 263–67.

Dweck, C. S. (1975). The role of expectations and attributions on the alleviation of learned helplessness. *Journal of Personality and Social Psychology* 31, 674–85.

Evans, R. G. (1981). The relationship of two measures of perceived control to depression. *Journal of Personality Assessment* 45, 66–70.

Ferrari, M., W. S. Matthews, & G. Barabas. (1983). The family and child with epilepsy. *Family Processes* 22, 56–59.

Goldin, G. J., & R. J. Margolin. (1975). The psychosocial aspects of epilepsy. In G. N. Wright (Ed.), *Epileptic rehabilitation.* Boston: Little, Brown.

Hackney, A., & D. C. Taylor. (1976). A teachers' questionnaire description of epileptic children. *Epilepsia* 17, 275–81.

Hartlage, L. C., & J. B. Green. (1972). The relation of parental attitudes to academic and social achievement in epileptic children. *Epilepsia* 13, 21–26.

Hartlage, L. C., J. B. Green, & L. Offut. (1972). Dependency in epileptic children. *Epilepsia* 13, 27–30.

Holdsworth, L., & K. Whitmore. (1974). A study of children with epilepsy attending ordinary schools. 1. Their seizure patterns, progress, and behavior in school. *Developmental Medicine and Child Neurology* 16, 746–57.

Hollingshead, A. B. (1975). *Four factor index of social status.* Unpublished manuscript, P.O. Box 1965, Yale Station, New Haven, CT 06520.

Hughes, J. G., & J. T. Jabbour. (1958). The treatment of the epileptic child. *Journal of Pediatrics* 53, 66–68.

Jones, F. H. (1977). The Rochester Adaptive Behavior Inventory: A parallel series of instruments for assessing social competence during early and middle childhood and adolescence. In J. S. Strauss, H. M. Babigian, & M. Roff (Eds.), *The origins and course of psychopathology: Methods of longitudinal research.* New York: Plenum Press.

Koppitz, E. M. (1968). *Psychological evaluation of children: Human figure drawings.* New York: Grune & Stratton.

Lefcourt, H. M. (1976). *Locus of control: Current trends in theory and research.* Hillsdale, NJ: Erlbaum.

Lefkowitz, M. M., E. P. Tesiny, & N. H. Gordon. (1980). Childhood depression, family income, and locus of control. *Journal of Nervous and Mental Disease* 168, 732–35.

Livingston, S. (1972). *Comprehensive management of epilepsy in infancy, childhood, and adolescence.* Springfield, IL: Thomas.

Long, C. G., & J. R. Moore. (1979). Parental expectations for their epileptic children. *Journal of Child Psychology and Psychiatry* 24, 299–312.

Matthews, W. S., & G. Barabas. (1981). Suicide and epilepsy: A review of the literature. *Psychosomatics* 22, 515–24.

Matthews, W. S., G. Barabas, & M. Ferrari. (1983). Achievement and school behavior among children with epilepsy. *Psychology in the schools* 20, 10–12.

Mayer, L. C. (1965). A study of the relationship of early special class placement and the self-concepts of mentally handicapped children. *Dissertation Abstracts International* 27, 143A.

Mellor, D. H., I. Lowit, & D. J. Hall. (1974). Are epileptic children behaviorally different from other children? In P. Harris, C. Mawdsley, (Eds.), *Epilepsy: Proceedings of the Hans Berger centenary symposium.* Edinburgh: Churchill-Livingston.

Midlarsky, E., & L. B. McKnight. (1980). Effects of achievement, evaluative feedback, and locus of control on children's expectations. *Journal of Genetic Psychology* 136, 203–12.

Molinari, V., & P. Khanna. (1981). Locus of control and its relationship to anxiety and depression. *Journal of Personality Assessment* 45, 314–17.

Pascarella, E. T., & S. Pflaum. (1981). The interaction of children's attribution of level of control over error correction in reading instruction. *Journal of Educational Psychology* 73, 533–70.

Piers, E. V., & D. B. Harris. (1969). *The Piers-Harris children's self-concept scale.* Nashville, TN: Counselor Recordings and Tests.

Quay, H. C., & J. S. Werry. (1979). *Psychopathological disorders in childhood* (2nd ed.). New York: Wiley.

Rholes, W., J. Blackwell, C. Jordan, & C. Walters. (1980). A developmental study of learned helplessness. *Developmental Psychology* 16, 616–24.

Ritchie, K. (1981). Research note: Interaction in the families of epileptic children. *Journal of Child Psychology and Psychiatry* 22, 65–71.

Rohner, E. C., C. Chaille, & R. P. Rohner. (1980). Perceived parental acceptance-rejection and the development of children's locus of control. *Journal of Psychology* 104, 83–86.

Rosenbaum, M., & N. Palmon. (1984). Helplessness and resourcefulness in coping with epilepsy. *Journal of Consulting and Clinical Psychology* 52, 244–53.

Rosenthal, R., & L. Jacobson. (1968). *Pygmalion in the classroom.* New York: Holt, Rinehart & Winston.

Rotter, J. B. (1966). Generalized expectancies for internal versus external control of reinforcement. *Psychology Monograph,* 80 (609).

Rutter, M., P. Graham, & W. A. Yule. (1970). *A neuropsychiatric study in childhood* (Clinics in developmental medicine no. 35/36). London: SIMP Heinemann Medical.

Seligman, M. E. P. (1975). *Helplessness: On depression, development and death.* San Francisco: Freeman.

Tesiny, E. P., M. M. Lefkowitz, & N. H. Gordon. (1980). Childhood depression, locus of control, and school achievement. *Journal of Educational Psychology* 72, 506–10.

Winston, E., C. Chilman. (1964). Epilepsy, some social, psychological, educational, economic, and legal aspects. *Welfare Review* 2, 1–9.

III / *Stigma and Epilepsy*

Historically, stigma and discrimination have been the defining social responses to epilepsy. Reviews of the history of the disorder, best illustrated in the work of Temkin, have described in detail the myths and superstitions associated with epilepsy as well as the adverse social consequences that have developed as a result of these beliefs (e.g., institutionalization, sterilization). In these "enlightened" times pernicious social reactions to individuals with epilepsy continue. These reactions include social isolation, decreased social support, and vocational and educational discrimination. Although considerable attention has been paid to these problems by groups such as the Epilepsy Foundation of America and the National Commission for the Control of Epilepsy and Its Consequences, the stigma and discrimination associated with epilepsy persist.

The four chapters in this section directly address the nature and extent of the relationship between the adverse social reactions to epilepsy and their effects on the psychological state of the patient. In chapter 8 Jade Dell provides us with a comprehensive conceptual overview of the literature concerned with the problems of stigma and discrimination associated with epilepsy and reviews the difficult problems that pertain to this field of inquiry. For example, what is the prevalence of stigma and discrimination attached to epilepsy, and how does one best measure such concepts? These are fundamental issues addressed by subsequent chapters in this section.

Two longitudinal studies from Great Britain report the results of their attempts to ascertain the behavioral effects of these social factors on people with epilepsy. In chapter 9 Christopher Bagley reviews the results obtained from the National Child Development Study, which examines data on children born in one week in 1958, and in chapter 10 Nicky Britten, Michael Wadsworth, and Peter Fenwick report findings from the National Developmental Study, which originated in 1946. In addition to their emphasis on measuring the behavioral effects of stigma, these two investigations provide much needed longitudinal information on the academic, behavioral, and occupational outcomes of childhood epilepsy.

Finally, in chapter 11 Patrick West analyzes the results of his careful studies of the effects of parental perceptions of epilepsy on childrearing practices, and their further effects on the psychological and social development of the child with epilepsy.

All in all, these papers provide considerable information about the processes associated with epilepsy that generate stigma and discrimination and, most important, their relevance for the epilepsy/psychopathology literature.

8 / Social Dimensions of Epilepsy: Stigma and Response

JADE L. DELL

A recent government commission has maintained that the social problems of people with epilepsy can be more damaging than the medical difficulties they face (Commission for the Control of Epilepsy and Its Consequences, 1978). This is a helpful formulation since it gives prominence to the social dimensions of the lives of people with epilepsy in a world that has described their lives only in terms of abnormal neurons. Future research in the area of naming and measuring these social dimensions is vital. But before such research can meaningfully proceed, it will be necessary to address several important questions.

Three questions seem especially central. First, how are the many dimensions of the social problems faced by people with epilepsy interconnected? Second, who or what is responsible for these problems? Third, given an estimate of the source of these problems, what are the available and optimal solutions?

Although there exists a substantial literature about the social dimensions of the lives of people with epilepsy, it is widely scattered and divergent in terms of methodology and theoretical construct. The purpose of this chapter is to critically review the literature in this area and to delineate what is suggested about potential answers to the three questions posed above.

Five specific tasks are undertaken to address this purpose. First, stigma in general is discussed. How is it manifested in the interrelationship of society and the person with epilepsy? Second, the issue of stigma ideology in epilepsy is analyzed. What are the factors that underlie the stigmatization of epilepsy? Third, the social factors that influence the functioning of people with epilepsy in their relationships with their families and society are analyzed. Fourth, the question is asked, "What needs to be done?" Two strategies are discussed: education of persons about epilepsy; and political organization of people with epilepsy. Fifth, some of the problematic issues concerning the measuring of stigma, the problems with research, and the current ideology operative in contemporary society are noted.

WHAT IS STIGMA AND HOW IS IT MANIFESTED?

In his classic work, *Stigma: Notes on the Management of Spoiled Identity*, Erving Goffman (1963), a well-known sociologist, states:

> The special situation of the stigmatized is that society tells him he is a member of the wider group, which means he is a normal human being, but that he is also "different" in some degree, and that it would be foolish to deny this difference. This differentness itself of course derives from society, for ordinarily before a difference can matter much it must be conceptualized collectively by the society as a whole. (p. 123)

In other words, Goffman maintains that society initiates the context in which stigma can thrive. Howard Becker (1963), the sociologist who wrote the most central work on deviance, *The Outsiders*, concurs:

> Social groups create deviance by making the rules whose infraction constitutes deviance and by applying those rules to particular people and labeling them as outsiders. From this point of view, deviance is *not* a quality of the act the person commits, but rather a consequence of the application by others of rules and sanctions to an "offender". (p. 9)

Stigma can thus be defined as the relationship between the differentness of an individual and the devaluation society places on that particular differentness.

But there is another aspect that must occur for stigma to exist: The devaluation society ascribes to a person must be internalized in the individual with the difference. The stigmatized person must believe that she or he is discreditable. As Schneider and Conrad (1983) note, "A discreditable attribute or performance becomes relevant to self only if the individual perceives it as discreditable" (p. 152).

What is the genesis of the devaluation of epilepsy? There seems to be a whole mythology that undergirds the taintedness of epilepsy. It is ancient, founded on early superstitions and fears, and is based partly on the perception that a person with epilepsy is severely diseased or insane and that the disease or insanity is either contagious or inheritable (Temkin, 1971). This devaluation is reflected in the laws of our society as well as in the perceptions of people and has resulted in both legal and social discrimination against the individual with epilepsy. Some examples suggest the dimensions of the problem.

Legal Issues

Historically in legal documents and statutes it was common to see the term *epileptic* in a series of words like *idiotic, epileptic, feebleminded, and imbecile* (Commission for the Control of Epilepsy and Its Consequences, 1978, p. 647). These word associations bolstered prejudice against persons with epilepsy that resulted in decades of legal abuses in the areas of marriage, sterilization, adoption, and institutionalization.

Prohibition Against Marriage

The first eugenics law in the United States that forbade the marriage of people with epilepsy was enacted in 1895 in Connecticut, and by 1956 there were still 17 states whose laws prohibited the marriage of a person with epilepsy (Barrow & Fabing, 1956). The 1943 North Dakota statute #14-0307 says:

> Marriage by a woman under the age of forty-five years or by a man of any age, unless he marries a woman over the age of forty-five years, is prohibited if such a man or woman in an habitual criminal, an epileptic, an imbecile, a feebleminded person, an idiot, an insane person, a person who has been afflicted with hereditary insanity, or a person afflicted with pulmonary tuberculosis in its advanced state or with any contagious venereal disease. (Barrow & Fabing, 1956, p. 12)

In fact, until 1965, prohibitions against people with epilepsy marrying were still operational in some states (Schneider & Conrad, 1983). It was not until 1980 that Missouri finally struck its law forbidding such marriages (*National Spokesman*, 1980).

Sterilization

In 1907, Indiana passed the first eugenic sterilization law in the United States (Barrow & Fabing, 1956; Chase, 1977). Included under this law were criminals, idiots, rapists, imbeciles, and people with epilepsy. One by one, other states followed suit: a total of 21 states by 1928 (Chorover, 1979); and 30 states by 1931 (Chorover, 1979; Ludmerer, 1972). Between 1907 and 1964, 63,678 people were sterilized under these state laws (Chase, 1977, p. 16).

Most of the compulsory sterilization laws were based on the Model Eugenical Sterilization Law that was the early creation of Harry H. Laughlin, who later published his views in the 1922 book, *Eugenical Sterilization in the United States.* Laughlin advocated compulsory sterilization for persons in the "socially inadequate classes," defined by him as follows:

> (1) Feeble-minded; (2) Insane (including the psychopathic); (3) Criminalistic (including the delinquent and wayward); (4) Epileptic; (5) Inebriate (including drug-habitués); (6) Diseased (including the tuberculous, the syphilitic, the leprous, and others with chronic, infectious, and legally segregable diseases); (7) Blind (including those with seriously impaired vision); (8) Deaf (including those with seriously impaired hearing); (9) Deformed (including the crippled); and (10) Dependent (including orphans, ne'er-do-wells, the homeless, tramps, and paupers). (p. 446–447).

In the context of the increasing waves of immigrants entering the United States in the early part of the 20th century, the idea of eugenic sterilization became a popular and acceptable ideology. In 1927, Supreme Court Justice

Holmes proclaimed the constitutionality of these laws with the words, "Three generations of imbeciles are enough" (Barrow & Fabing, 1956, p. 29).

Exhibitions at fairs and expositions in the 1920s and 1930s exacerbated peoples' concern about the inheritance of bad or evil traits. Exhibits at the 1929 Kansas Free Fair featured posters and charts claiming to illustrate how the genetic laws of Mendel regulated inheritance in the human species. One chart proclaimed, "Unfit human traits such as feeblemindedness, epilepsy, criminality, insanity, alcoholism, pauperism, and many others run in families and are inherited in exactly the same way as color in guinea pigs" (Kevles, 1984, p. 57).

Compulsory sterilization gained more respectability when in 1934 the American Neurological Association appointed a special committee "to evaluate in a critical manner both the facts and the theories which constitute the subject-matter of the inheritance of the mental diseases, feeblemindedness, epilepsy, and crime" (Committee of the American Neurological Association for the Investigation of Eugenical Sterilization, 1936). Out of the study and report of this committee, a book entitled *Eugenical Sterilization* was approved by the American Neurological Association and published in 1936. There are nine entries in the subject index referring to issues related to epilepsy.

This important work, funded through a grant from the Carnegie Foundation, reinforced the legal devaluations of epilepsy already extant. The committee recommended that "selective sterilization be considered in cases of the following diseases" (Committee of the American Neurological Association, 1936, p. 179):

1. Huntington's chorea, hereditary optic atrophy, familiar cases of Friedreich's ataxia and certain other disabling degenerative diseases recognized to be hereditary.
2. Feeblemindedness of familial type.
3. Dementia praecox (Schizophrenia).
4. Manic-depressive psychosis.
5. Epilepsy.

By 1956, 18 states still had eugenic sterilization laws applicable to people with epilepsy.

Adoption laws

The devaluation of persons with epilepsy did not apply only to adults of marriageable or procreative age. Children with epilepsy too have been stigmatized. As recently as 1978, Arkansas and Missouri allowed the annulment of an adoption if the child developed epilepsy within 5 years (*National Spokesman*, 1980).

Institutionalization

Persons with epilepsy have most often been confined in facilities with the mentally insane. It was not until 1891 that the first separate institutions for persons with epilepsy were established in the United States, and this was done with the well-being of the insane in mind (Temkin, 1971, p. 256). According to Barrow and Fabing (1956), California, Georgia, Michigan, and New Mexico still permitted a person to be committed to an institution for epilepsy alone if seizure frequency were high and the seizures were not well controlled.

This practice is becoming less problematic, but the historical incarceration of people with epilepsy certainly solidified the connection between epilepsy, insanity, and crime—a connection still made today. Indeed, in 1975 Arangio reported that 17 states still legally allowed the institutionalization of persons with epilepsy.

These legal devaluations support the perceptions that people with epilepsy are undesirable, dangerous, or somehow mentally deficient and capable of passing along that deficiency to their offspring. The reasoning becomes, therefore, that no children should be born to people with epilepsy. So they are forbidden to marry, are sterilized or institutionalized. And certainly no potential adoptive parent would want to adopt a child with epilepsy, at least according to this reasoning. It is quite likely that these laws are not well known and that they are seldom acted upon anymore. Nonetheless, historically they contributed to the legacy of stigmatization, and that some versions of these laws continue to exist is testimony to how hard it is to exterminate old myths.

Public Devaluation

Public Attitudes Toward Epilepsy

Caveness and Gallup (1980) have for the past 30 years been recording trends in the views and feelings people have about persons with epilepsy. Their reports have shown increasing openness and acceptance for people with epilepsy by the general public, especially among the younger, urban, more educated members of society. But other studies contradict the Caveness-Gallup findings.

The Ryan, Kempner, and Emlen (1980) survey of 445 adults with epilepsy and the data of Schneider and Conrad (1983) indicate that there is a certain pressure for people to express socially acceptable attitudes about epilepsy that they may not actually believe or be willing to act on, a conclusion in harmony with Zielinski's (1972) earlier findings.

Evidence to support the conclusions of Ryan et al. (1980), Schneider and Conrad (1983), and Zielinski (1972) comes from many researchers. Remschmidt (1973) found that 30% of 300 questionnaire respondents judged people with epilepsy to have unfavorable personality traits. Harrison and West (1977) interviewed 114 people on the street and found that 50% reported that they had had a negative experience in relating to a person with epilepsy. Vinson (1975) concluded that epilepsy conjures up fear, horror, and superstition in people, and noted that 45% of a sample of 602 adults thought epilepsy to be a mental disorder.

In a 1974 article in *Nursing* magazine, Loy Wiley referred to an unreferenced study that reported that society rejected people with epilepsy at a higher rate than it rejected the mentally ill. There is a great irony here. Society stigmatizes people with epilepsy in part because it perceives them to be mentally ill, and at the same time it is less prejudiced against persons who are mentally ill. An interesting sidelight to this irony was the exchange between the Epilepsy Foundation of America (EFA) and an advocacy organization for mental retardation. The EFA has produced educational information that states that having epilepsy is not the same as being mentally retarded. The other organization has responded by asking how the EFA would feel if the former ran an announcement saying that "most mentally retarded people don't have epilepsy" (Scherer, 1982, p. 5).

Some of the most important research on the issue of prejudice against epilepsy has been conducted by Christopher Bagley (1972), who utilized a questionnaire measuring social attitudes and administered it to three samples of British citizens: 574 high school teenagers, 211 college students, and 104 working-class adults. All three groups objected more to employing people with epilepsy than "spastics." In this same paper, Bagley tested two related hypotheses: (1) People with epilepsy will be rejected as often as immigrants of color; and (2) racial prejudice and prejudice against people with epilepsy will be associated. Using a subset of 230 teens aged 16–18 from the larger sample, Bagley measured their attitudes toward minority groups including people with epilepsy, interracial couples, immigrants of color, Pakistanis, West Indians, and Jews. His findings demonstrate dramatic support for the two hypotheses. Bagley (1972) concludes:

> Prejudice against epilepsy may be akin to racial prejudice (which involves a fear of the unknown and unpredictable). There is a significant correlation between a scale measuring racial prejudice, and one measuring attitudes to the handicapped (this scale being dominated by hostile attitudes to epilepsy). People with epilepsy are seen in hostile terms which are as great as, or greater than, those in which ethnic minorities are viewed. (p. 43)

Another persuasive empirical study documenting the stigma associated with epilepsy comes from Hansson and Duffield (1976). Because it is so important and not widely discussed, it is described in detail here. The authors assembled photographs of 100 female graduating seniors and 100 male graduating seniors from a high school yearbook. Then:

> Using the Thurstone method of equal appearing intervals, 10 female raters rated the 100 male photographs on a 1 to 10 attractiveness continuum, where a score of 10 was least attractive. Similarly, the ten male raters rated the 100 female photographs on the basis of attractiveness. The mean attractiveness score and standard deviation were then calculated for each photograph and used as a basis for selecting 10 target persons for the female lineup and 10 persons for the male lineup. (p. 234)

One hundred college students were then selected and informed that they each would be shown two sets of 10 photos, including one person in each set diagnosed as having grand mal epilepsy. The college students were asked to identify the person in each group of 10 who they thought had epilepsy. Sixty-nine percent of the 100 students selected an "unattractive" female and 83% selected an "unattractive" male as the person with grand mal epilepsy. One conclusion drawn by Hansson and Duffield was this:

> Apparently it was not difficult, in the absence of pertinent cues, to draw upon the stereotype and attribute one further malady (epilepsy) to unattractive persons. Although it has been shown consistently that unattractive persons are judged as possessing less desirable personal traits and as being capable of considerable antisocial behavior, the ease with which Ss [subjects] leaped into relating [un]attractiveness and epilepsy is dramatic. (1976, p. 238)

Physicians' Attitudes Toward Epilepsy

Physicians have not fared much better than the lay public in demonstrating unbiased perceptions of people with epilepsy (Bagley, 1972; Lewin, 1957; Schneider & Conrad, 1983). In a study that sampled 69 Australian doctors on the medical staff of a major Australian teaching hospital, Beran, Jennings, and Read (1981) reported that 91% thought people with epilepsy suffered emotional problems and 54% thought people with epilepsy suffered mood swings—much higher percentages than were attributed to the general population. In addition, 27% of the doctors felt that people with epilepsy were less intelligent, 34% felt people with epilepsy were less productive at work, and 30% felt that people with epilepsy were less reliable at work.

One would expect doctors to possess a more educated and thus enlightened view of epilepsy, but The Commission for the Control of Epilepsy (1978), looking at U.S. data, reports that little attention is given to epilepsy in medical training. This means that the attitudes of physicians may be based more on the prevailing mythology than on scientific information, similar to the situation for the general public.

One especially damaging aspect of this, as many investigators have noted, is that less informed doctors project their limited understandings and negative attitudes about epilepsy onto the rest of society (see especially Bagley, 1972). Through incorrect medical definitions, inaccurate diagnosis, and insensitive labeling and reporting, these less informed doctors substantially influence the direction of the public's view of people with epilepsy just as they influence the public on other sensitive medical maladies in cases where lay knowledge is incomplete, as for example, in cancer, herpes, and AIDS.

The negative attitudes of the legal structure, the public, and the medical establishment constitute serious sanctions against the individual with epilepsy. Schultz (1975) maintains that we have not really removed the deviant label from our perception of epilepsy. We still regard epilepsy as being more than a physical condition. The devaluation of people with epilepsy has been mythologized, collectivized, and internalized until it seems to have become the unquestioned and accepted way of dealing with the malady.

Goffman (1963) states that in order to maintain such a stigma relationship, society must construct a "stigma theory," an ideology that seeks to explain why the stigmatized person deserves to be stigmatized. Or as social psychologist Leigh Marlowe (1975) says, "People know it is not nice to be prejudiced. . . . Therefore, the prejudiced individual must rationalize his attitudes by blaming the victim, i.e. the targets of prejudice are flawed humans" (p. 371).

WHAT ARE THE FACTORS THAT UNDERLIE THE STIGMATIZATION OF EPILEPSY?

This chapter began by noting that there are ancient prejudices toward people with epilepsy that stem from prevailing mythology and ignorance. Vestiges of these age-old perceptions clearly remain, and new factors have emerged to lend additional support to the stigmatization of epilepsy. These include selective misperception of the malady, belief in the relationship between epilepsy and violence, and a belief that epilepsy is related to psychological malfunctioning.

Selective Misperception

In a survey of 114 people, West (1979) found that the public image of epilepsy consisted almost entirely of the grand mal seizure. People tend to associate the outward manifestation of only the grand mal or generalized tonic-clonic seizure (e.g., crying out, falling, foaming at the mouth, rigidity, shaking, loss of bladder or bowel control, turning blue) with their vision of epilepsy. This happens for two reasons. First, the generalized tonic-clonic seizure is more overt, visible, and striking than most other forms of epilepsy. Second, people who have less visible types of seizures (e.g., nocturnal, partial) might choose to keep their epilepsy a secret because of the stigmatization that surrounds the malady. The less overt forms thus dissolve unnoticed into the population at large.

Another group of people who can hide their epilepsy consists of those who are currently seizure free. Zielinski (1976), in his study of epilepsy patients in Warsaw, documents that patients who are seizure free for any length of time are happy to disassociate themselves from any connection to the malady. In a recent article Zielinski (1984) reports, "Many consider themselves 'completely cured' and do not wish to be reminded about their past disorder." People who are either newly seizure free or who have less overt types of seizures may find it possible and preferable to remain more invisible to the public.

This phenomenon is not specific to epilepsy. In a recent editorial in the Archives of Neurology, Herndon and Rudick (1983) note a similar situation in regard to the spectrum of severity for multiple sclerosis, observing that

> those who have MS but have not been diagnosed do not contribute to the image of the disease, nor do those who carry the diagnosis but have few external signs of the disease and function normally in society. (p. 532)

The Commission for the Control of Epilepsy (1978, Vol. 1, p. 21) cites four studies that indicate that generalized epilepsy accounts for about 50% of the epilepsies. And yet generalized epilepsy forms the basis of the public perception of the nature of epilepsy. The work of Crowther (1967), Boshes and Kienast (1970), and Zielinski (1972) all conclude that labeling the most severe cases as "typical" adversely affects the public's feelings and prejudices toward *all* people with epilepsy.

Epilepsy and Violence

It is a common notion that people with epilepsy exhibit violent behavior. In Vinson's (1975) random sample of the perceptions of 602 adults about epilepsy, 50% felt that people with epilepsy were capable of violent crime. When Harrison and West (1977) interviewed 114 respondents on their perceptions about epilepsy, 25% of the sample connected violent behavior and epilepsy. How does this perception arise?

Because many seizures are violent in nature (falling, thrashing about, convulsive motions, odd noises, the loss of control), it might occur to observers that people with epilepsy are purposefully aggressive and violent during the seizure and/or between seizures.

This attitude can be primarily traced to mythology connected to a fear of loss of control (Temkin, 1971). But even in the "enlightened" 1800s, an equation between epilepsy and insanity was widely accepted. This formula was shored up in the work of Cesare Lombroso, a 19th-century Italian physician whose doctrines became the basis for the discipline of criminal anthropology. Lombroso concluded that about 40% of all criminals followed hereditary compulsion and that almost every born criminal suffered from epilepsy to some degree (Lombroso, 1911/1972). This linking of epilepsy and criminal behavior has exerted a dominating influence over common perceptions of people with epilepsy. As Stephen Jay Gould (1981), an evolutionary biologist and historian points out:

> The added burden imposed by Lombroso's theory upon thousands of epileptics cannot be calculated; they became a major target of eugenical schemes in part because Lombroso had explicated their illness as a mark of moral degeneracy. (p. 134)

As Whitman, King, and Cohen discuss in this volume (chap. 13), the Lombrosian theory suggests negative social dynamics that extend far beyond epilepsy.

Epilepsy and Personality Disorders

The relationship between epilepsy and psychological disorder is the subject of a longstanding, intense debate. (In a critical review of the literature of the last 20 years, Hermann and Whitman [1984] analyze 64 studies and provide well over 200 references.) The debate is far from resolved but it is reasonable to argue that the relationship (if any) between epilepsy and psychopathology remains largely undetermined. The debate will not be resolved here. But the alleged relationships will be enumerated. In many important aspects, to pose the question is stigma enough—regardless of what the eventual answer may be.

In the late 1800s, as the equation between epilepsy and insanity began to be set aside, the theory of the "epileptic personality" manifested itself (Temkin, 1971). This theory suggested that (most) people with epilepsy had a similar, global, essentially pathological personality, which has been variously described (see Tizard, 1962).

Soon this theory too gave way to a plethora of nonsupportive evidence—but the basic notion of a link between epilepsy and psychopathology remained (Tizard, 1962). Now, however, it became specific types of psychological disorders (e.g., depression, schizophrenia, sexual dysfunction) that were examined in relationship to epilepsy. More recently, attention has fallen away from "epilepsy" to concentrate on "temporal lobe epilepsy" (Bear & Fedio, 1977; Mungas, 1982; Rodin & Schmaltz, 1983) and most recently to its "laterality," that is, left or right temporal lobe epilepsy (Flor-Henry, 1983). Thus, the "refinements" in this debate have involved not only the shape of the psychopathological characteristics attributed to people with epilepsy, but also the subset of people with epilepsy who are allegedly at high risk. These refinements have not led to significant reductions in the intensity of the debate.

Moreover, it is reasonable to argue that the wider effects of this literature have been damaging. For example, *Omni* magazine interviewed a psychiatrist interested in sexual dysfunction in people with epilepsy (Craig, 1983). Without permission, the magazine accompanied the report of the interview with a photograph of a man biting a woman's foot. The caption under the photograph read, "Some fetishists may not have psychological problems at all but may simply be victims of seizures concentrated in their temporal lobes" (Craig, 1983, p. 37).

In her review of the literature, Janice Stevens (1975) wrote, "The list of psychiatric disabilities attributed to individuals with epilepsy is limited only by one's industry in ferreting out fresh derogations" (p. 85). She then proceeded to list alphabetically 57 alleged negative attributes, ranging from "adhesive" to "willful," used by investigators to describe individuals with epilepsy.

Using the literature on this subject, the following partial list has been assembled of characteristics often ascribed to people with epilepsy: mood fluctuations (Beran et al., 1981; Beran & Read, 1983; Vinson, 1975); emotional problems (Beran et al., 1981; Breger, 1976a, b; Richardson & Friedman, 1974; Vinson, 1975); behavior problems (Richardson & Friedman, 1974); debilitation (Schneider & Conrad, 1981); insecurity (De Haas, 1962; Scambler & Hopkins, 1980); self-centeredness (De Haas, 1962); low self-esteem (Long & Moore, 1979; Matthews, Barabas, & Ferrari, 1982; Ryan et al., 1980; Scambler & Hopkins, 1980); high dependency (Long & Moore, 1979; Matthews et al., 1982); depression, irritability, hostility (Mittan, 1982; Richardson & Friedman, 1974); antisocial behavior (Bagley, 1972; Livingston, 1977; Long & Moore, 1979); deviance and neurotic behavior (Long & Moore, 1979).

The impact of lists like this on the public's perception of people with epilepsy is bound to be confusing, certainly damaging, and conducive to the stigmatization of epilepsy. But, as we have noted, stigma implies a relationship—people with epilepsy not only are reacted to, but also act and react to the reaction. The next section of this chapter will examine some of the social factors that influence the functioning of people with epilepsy.

SOCIAL FACTORS THAT AFFECT THE FUNCTIONING OF PEOPLE WITH EPILEPSY

The actions and reactions of people with epilepsy as they attempt, in Goffman's (1963) words, to "manage a spoiled, threatened identity" have been chronicled over and over. Ryan et al. (1980) found that some persons with epilepsy tend to become preoccupied with feelings of stigmatization and that the devaluation of society becomes so internalized that people with epilepsy feel as if they should not be valued. Bagley (1972) suggests that this internalization of stigma can eventually lead to behavioral anomalies.

The purpose of this section is to discuss some social factors that affect the functioning of people with epilepsy other than the issues of stigma and discrimination that have already been discussed.

Fear

One factor that fits under this category is the fear people with epilepsy experience because of the malady. Mittan, Wasterlain, and Locke (1981) have reported that in a sample of 147 adults with epilepsy, 75% were afraid they might die during their next seizure, and 55% lived in continual fear and dread of attacks. Ryan et al. (1980) call this a sense of vulnerability to physical consequences. Mittan's sample also exhibited fears of what was mistakenly thought to be the typical consequences of epilepsy, for example, significant deterioration of intelligence and loss of mental health. Because of these fears patients often advocate hazardous first aid practices, and the most common (55%) coping response was staying at home, which results in isolation from society at large. These fears, according to Scambler and Hopkins (1980), clearly lead to a self-denial of opportunities that can result in a whole host of problems with employment and personal relations. According to Livingston (1977), these problems can eventually result in antisocial behavior. Mittan (1982) points to the problems caused by medical personnel in their refusal or inability to help patients with epilepsy deal with their fears of death, their depression, thoughts of suicide, loneliness, and fears about leaving home. As this chapter was being written, the correlation between fear of seizures and psychopathology had not been investigated. Mittan's chapter in this book (chap. 4) provides the first documentation of this significant relationship.

One cannot know for sure the impact that harboring these fears has on a person with epilepsy. One can only imagine how it would feel to be confronted, for example, by the daily fear of dying suddenly somewhere from a seizure. It would in the very least seem reasonable to conclude that these social and psychological stresses might affect the individual's ability to function in society.

Parenting Effects

Parental perceptions, expectations, and influences shape the child with epilepsy in fairly intense ways (Bagley, 1972; Ritchie, 1981; Schneider & Conrad, 1980; West, 1979). Beran and Read (1983) suggest that "family members may well represent the single most important aid to patient management" (p. 87).

The literature is clear to point out the effects of both negative and positive parental attitudes on the functioning of persons with epilepsy. Bagley (1972) maintains that negative parental attitudes about epilepsy are the cause, not the result of, disturbed behavior in the child.

Overprotectiveness

Parental overprotectiveness of the child with epilepsy as a coping mechanism is mentioned by several authors as a negative parental response that can be psychologically more dangerous than the physical danger of underprotection (Crowther, 1967; De Haas, 1962; Hauck, 1972; Livingston, 1957, 1977). This overprotection can result from a parent's fears and concerns about seizures, social interaction, mental deterioration, dependence, marital opportunities, other people's reactions, and so on (Ward & Bowen, 1978).

And yet this overprotection, rather than shielding the child from physical or psychological harm, often results in a whole host of other problems. Secrecy and shame about the malady can cause the child to withdraw from social interaction (Kleck, 1968; Long & Moore, 1979; Schneider & Conrad, 1980). The child may perceive an overprotective parent as acting out of guilt and overcompensation (De Haas, 1972; West, 1979; Wiley, 1974). And, of course, overprotection can communicate to a child that she or he is not capable and that the parents have lower expectations in regard to academic achievement, employment opportunities, and healthy emotional well-being.

Unhealthy General Home Environment

The theme of autocratic and domineering parental attitudes is represented well in the literature. Hauck (1972), Ritchie (1981), and Matthews et al. (1982) all assert a connection between autocratic parenting styles and problem behavior in children with epilepsy. In fact, Hauck (1972) suggests that children with epilepsy whose parents are physically abusive and autocratic have more seizures than do children whose parents are not abusive or autocratic. In a 1935 study discussed by Tizard (1962) it is suggested that children with epilepsy who exhibit serious personality disorders have unsatisfactory home environments. Rutter, Graham, and Yule (1970) found that the psychiatric status of the mother was associated with the psychiatric status of the child with epilepsy.

Openness

On the positive side of parental effects, many authors claim that parental openness can encourage a neutral or open view in the child with epilepsy

(Schneider & Conrad, 1980). Hartlage and Green (1972) say that socialization is correlated with parental attitudes, not with seizure type, and that modification of parental attitudes may help children with epilepsy to attain their full potential. De Haas (1961) has hypothesized that the child whose family is the least upset by seizures will have the fewest school problems.

Concealment and Disclosure Issues

Negative and positive parenting effects are directly related to the question each person with epilepsy must ask herself or himself: Do I tell people I have epilepsy or keep it a secret? Because of the stigma surrounding epilepsy, people with the malady, especially including the well controlled and the less noticeable, tend to hide or deny their seizures (Bagley, 1972). To paraphrase Goffman (1963), a person who hides a stigmatizing condition is in effect hiding something that people would devalue if they knew about it (p. 42). The evidence that concealment is the preferred management technique is widely noted, and some authors locate the strategy of concealment firmly in the attitudes and actions of parents (Kleck, 1968; Long & Moore, 1979). West (1984) claims that parents often conceal their child's epilepsy from relatives or friends, even when they are willing to notify the child's school, and Mittan et al. (1981) have reported that concealing epilepsy from one's spouse and children is not uncommon. Schneider and Conrad (1980) call this management technique of concealing from some persons or groups and disclosing to others "selective concealment."

Selective concealment often occurs in relation to employment (Bagley, 1972; Schneider & Conrad, 1980; Zielinski, 1972). Perlman (1977) reports that one fourth of all applicants with epilepsy do not tell employers and that one third lie about their epilepsy on job applications. Scambler and Hopkins (1980) put the percentage closer to 50%, as does Kleck (1968).

But what is the effect of concealment? The literature suggests that concealment may cause problems of its own. Among the effects cited are:

- People who conceal their epilepsy can do deeper emotional damage to themselves (Livingston, 1977).
- Concealing epilepsy to hold a job can generate stress (Crowther, 1967).
- If a person maintains secrecy for many years, the secrecy itself can be a negative influence (Lennox & Markham, 1953).
- A person with concealed epilepsy is still "discreditable" because at any time his or her secret might be revealed (Schneider & Conrad, 1980).
- If a person is hiding something, she or he must monitor all revelations, and this can result in avoidance of social interaction (Kleck, 1968; Schneider & Conrad, 1983).

- Information management becomes the central interpersonal problem in concealment (Schneider & Conrad, 1980); this can lead to less desire for intimacy (Kleck, 1968).
- Parental coaching for concealment results in disability, dependence, and feelings of incompetence (Schneider & Conrad, 1983).

The preceding observations support the conclusion that overprotectiveness and secrecy are in the long term less healthy than openness, and that open disclosure to relatives, friends, employers, and others is a viable management strategy that can be life-giving and positive. Many authors advocate disclosure both for the health of the discloser and for the enlightenment of the public. Some comments on the open style follow:

- Being open about epilepsy to relatives, teachers, and schoolmates can ultimately dispel fallacies (Livingston, 1970).
- If the average person with epilepsy comes out, it helps the average person without epilepsy to understand the malady better (Rodin, Rennick, Dennerll, & Lin, 1972).
- Disclosing can serve a healing, therapeutic function for the teller (Schneider & Conrad, 1983).
- Disclosure broadens public acceptance and lowers stereotypes (West, 1984).
- The sense of stigmatization is broken down with disclosure (Kleck, 1968).
- Maximum disclosure seems to yield the *most* tolerant response (West, 1984).

Another interesting point is raised by Schneider and Conrad (1980), who report that a majority of persons with epilepsy they interviewed did not know another person with epilepsy. If disclosure were the norm instead of the exception, then people with epilepsy could develop networks offering personal, strategic, and political support. Other groups have used this strategy successfully, for example, alcoholics, drug users, gay men and lesbians, and disabled people.

Indeed a substantial epilepsy self-help network is already at work with participating groups across the United States (*Handbook on Self-Help Groups for People with Epilepsy*, 1982; Borman et al., 1980a, b; *Epilepsy Self-Help Newsletter*, 1981; Lieberman & Borman, 1979). This network in its many forms provides the structure in which persons with epilepsy and their families and friends can work and learn together.

Unemployment and Underemployment

Many employers, afraid that people with epilepsy are dangerous, violent, or accident prone, refuse to hire persons they know have epilepsy (Commission for the Control of Epilepsy, 1978; Schneider & Conrad, 1983). Thus people with epilepsy often feel compelled to lie on job applications and risk being terminated if they are discovered. One can understand the statement that knowledge about another's epilepsy can become ammunition in enemy hands (Schneider & Conrad, 1980). This issue has been extensively discussed (Holmes & McWilliams, 1981; Jones, 1965; Livingston, 1977; Richardson & Friedman, 1974; Schneider & Conrad, 1980; Schultz, 1975; West, 1984), and most authors conclude that problems with employment are one of the most significant social difficulties facing people with epilepsy.

Statistics on Employment

Current statistics on unemployment among people with epilepsy show that even those with good seizure control (75%–85% of those with epilepsy) have a 25% unemployment rate (Holmes & McWilliams, 1981). This is about 2½ times the 1983 rate for the whole population of the United States. Fraser (1980) claims that if those persons with epilepsy who have stopped looking for a job are included in the figures, the unemployment rate for all people with epilepsy is 34%. Unemployment causes problems for people with epilepsy as it does for people who do not have epilepsy. Brenner (1973, 1976) has chronicled the personal, emotional, and health problems that result from unemployment in the general population. It seems obvious that being unemployed for whatever cause is reason enough to be depressed and anxious. In fact, that is what Brenner's data show. So why should unemployed people with epilepsy be different? Given that the unemployment rate for people with epilepsy is 2.5 to 4 times higher than the national rate (Fraser, 1980), and given the relationship between unemployment and psychological distress (Brenner, 1973, 1976), one would expect to find people with epilepsy having certain emotional and personal difficulties.

Interviews with Patients

People with epilepsy are quick to document their own difficulties with employment discrimination. Schneider and Conrad (1980) found that 40 out of 80 individuals with epilepsy they interviewed felt that they had serious job problems. Fraser (1980) echoes this percentage. Schultz (1975) quotes an Epilepsy Foundation of America survey that indicates that 40% of adults with epilepsy have experienced job discrimination. This percentage was even noted in an article by Pond and Bidwell (1960). In their survey of 357 people with epilepsy, Hartman, Arntson, Droge, and Norton (1983) found that 60% felt they had trouble getting a job.

Finally, in a 12-year follow-up of 39 persons with epilepsy, Jones (1965) found that two out of three experienced job difficulties related to frequently changing jobs, and to accepting more menial, less lucrative jobs.

Uninsurability

People with epilepsy often have difficulty procuring adequate insurance at a rate they can afford. The Commission for the Control of Epilepsy (1978) notes that 52% of the respondents to a survey experienced problems obtaining life insurance, 40% had problems obtaining medical insurance, 37% accident insurance, and 32% auto insurance.

WHAT NEEDS TO BE DONE?

Stigma is the relationship between the differentness of an individual and the devaluation society places on that particular differentness. Thus stigma is a relationship between the stigmatized and the stigmatizer. And both the individual and the society, the stigmatized and the stigmatizer, need to be accountable for their roles in creating and sustaining stigma. Two strategies for addressing the need for accountability and change will be discussed here: (a) the education of persons and groups about epilepsy; and (b) the political organization of people with epilepsy.

Education of Persons and Groups About Epilepsy

Physicians and Patients

Educating the doctors within our society would seem to be an advantageous place to begin because of their role as interpreters of the disease to their patients and others (West, 1984). Unfortunately, as has been pointed out, doctors are often themselves prejudiced against people with epilepsy (Bagley, 1972; Beran et al., 1981; Lewin, 1957; Schneider & Conrad, 1983). A damaging aspect of this is that physicians' misperceptions are quite easily passed on to the general population. What needs to be passed on instead is a more complete understanding of the malady, both to the public and to persons with the malady.

Does this happen? According to the literature, not often. Many physicians follow a medical model, dealing only with the medical/drug issues of the person with epilepsy to the exclusion of social issues (Richardson & Friedman, 1974). But controlling the frequency of seizures, for example, does not necessarily ameliorate the social consequences for the patient, as noted by Ryan et al. (1980) in their discussion of the "sociopsychological approach." West (1984) reports a "conspiracy of silence" in which doctors appear uninterested, insecure, hurried, and unable to discuss their patients' problems, even the problems related to diagnosis and other more strictly medical issues. Taylor (1982) echoes this perception:

> Many of the sources of human distress manifestly come from difficulties which are beyond medical remedy. . . . But it lies in the hands of all physicians to orient

> themselves and to orient their students towards striving for a form of medical practice which is widely accessible, capable of responding across the wide range of sickness and prepared to influence social policies which are conducive to sickness. (p. 12)

The issues that persons with epilepsy want to discuss, those related to social and psychological factors, are the issues that doctors have the most trouble discussing. Boshes and Kienast (1970) claim that the social condition of the patient affects her or his medical condition as in no other disease and that it might be helpful to pay attention to this issue. Three decades ago Lennox and Markham (1953) challenged doctors to be supportive and comforting and also to be concerned about the social injustices that people with epilepsy face, yet the same problems persist.

The Epilepsy Support Program, a nonprofit organization based in California, trains self-help group leaders and helps develop support groups for parents and children. The August 1983 issue of their newsletter suggests some excellent strategies for "Working with Your Doctor," including a list of questions that patients might need to ask their doctors about medications, the doctor–patient relationship, keeping a journal record of seizure activity, and other treatment issues. This and other efforts like it are a good beginning.

Physicians and the School System

Both Holdsworth and Whitmore (1974) and Crowther (1967) maintain that doctors should seek to communicate about epilepsy to teachers and children in the educational system. This would be a welcome innovation as teachers are rarely trained to deal with the onset of a seizure among the children in their classrooms (Gadow, 1982; Holdsworth & Whitmore, 1974).

Teachers need to understand epilepsy, its causes, treatment, the nature of seizures, how to deal safely with a seizure, and how to convey information and openness to their classes when a child with epilepsy is among them. Examples of persons with epilepsy who have lived in the past and examples of those who are getting along well now are important to share (Rodin et al., 1972). Children pick up cues from adults, and teachers or administrators who see persons with epilepsy as deviant or discreditable may engender these feelings in the children with whom they spend many hours a day.

Educating Society

Educating society about the issues surrounding stigma and epilepsy is an important task (Holmes & McWilliams, 1981) now being done well by many groups including the Epilepsy Foundation of America, an educational and advocacy organization with chapters in every state; the National Epilepsy Self-Help Workshop; and the Epilepsy Support Program. The Epilepsy Task Force of Fort Collins, Colorado, is an active group of persons who either have epilepsy or are related to someone who does. They have initiated a dynamic program that involves going to every elementary school class in the area to present a lecture and discussion session on epilepsy. They see themselves as an advocacy group that seeks to foster acceptance of persons with epilepsy through education and knowledge. They also publish a newsletter designed for laypeople (*Epilepsy Newsletter*, Jo Ann Strader [ed.], Epilepsy Newsletter Service, Ft. Collins, CO) and have initiated a plan for action at the grass-roots level that has as its goal the founding of more local groups across the nation for people with epilepsy. This is one paradigm of the strategy of political organizing that other groups have used to their advantage to obtain just treatment and equal rights. This strategy is discussed more fully in the next section.

Political Organization

One tactic that might address the issue of stigma is the practice by people with epilepsy of full and open disclosure. As was already stated, personal familiarity with someone who has epilepsy fosters greater social acceptance (Breger, 1976b; Schneider & Conrad, 1983; West, 1984). The positive aspects of disclosure and the negative aspects of concealment have already been discussed. But this is a personal strategy only. Another model is needed.

Renée Anspach (1979) offers a model that seeks to build a movement among disabled persons "lodging the sources of disability in an inequitable social structure" (p. 765). Because it directly addresses the relationship between stigma and society, the model could be useful to persons with epilepsy, whether or not they are considered or consider themselves disabled.

Anspach's model calls for the disabled to mobilize their political power and engage in political action centered around forging and presenting an image of strength to the public. Anspach names this "identity politics" and describes its supporters as "politicized deviants, collectively engaged in attempts to reweave the fabric of identity" (1979, p. 767). The goal of identity politics is "to combat the prevailing imagery" (p. 768) and "to alter both the self-concepts and societal conceptions of their participants" (1979, p. 766).

Anspach criticizes the notion conceptualized by sociologists and popularized by the public that assumes the disabled, the mentally ill, and those with epilepsy, etc., are helpless, powerless, and passive. This notion, according to Anspach, has resulted in the belief that the problems of devalued or stigmatized persons are a sort of "personal deviation" (1979, p. 767), rather than a result of the interaction of the stigmatized person and the stigmatizing society. When personal deviation is seen as the cause of helplessness, powerlessness, and passivity, a certain mode of response is offered by the larger society. That mode takes the form of traditional organizations such as volunteer groups, charitable groups, patronization, and telethons. These traditional modes do nothing to empower devalued persons to participate in the mainstream of society.

Identity politics is not a comforting strategy, either for people with epilepsy or the rest of society, because its demands are equality, not friendship; power, not patronage; assertiveness, not adjustment; politicization of life, not individualized despair: The strategy is political rather than therapeutic. Identity politics, as applied to epilepsy, would seek to establish society as the predominant locus of stigma against people with epilepsy. It would demand that the public, when appropriate, view persons with epilepsy as active, viable, strong participants in society who are different because of their seizures but not less than full members of the human race.

Of course, identity politics requires organization and solidarity—two strategies that in and of themselves are power-bestowing. To understand the power and identity possibilities of organization and solidarity, we might look to the union movement of the 1930s, the Black Power movement of the 1960s, the gay rights and women's movements of the 1970s, to name a few. All of these social movements have provided a backdrop and a precedent for a new movement among disabled people, former mental patients, persons with epilepsy, and others who seek to dispel stigma by challenging societal values and forging a strong image of themselves as active participants in society.

SOME CONCLUDING ISSUES

The issue of stigma is important for understanding the relationship of the person with epilepsy to society. Stigma is serious and real; it does limit the quality of life for persons with epilepsy. The problem seems to be in determining how to measure this "limiting of the quality of life." One can measure the percentage of unemployment among people with epilepsy or the number who cannot obtain medical insurance or even how many persons with epilepsy disclose it to their friends and employers.

But it is much more difficult to measure exclusion from the peer group (Breger, 1976a) or lost life opportunities (Breger, 1976a; Rodin et al., 1972) or the sense of vulnerability to physical consequences (Ryan et al., 1980). These configurations are not measurable in the usual etiologic sense. (See chapter 6 in this volume by Paul Arntson and his colleagues, who for the first time document a correlation between stigma and psychosocial consequences of epilepsy.)

One central problem that tends to confound this type of measurement is that research traditionally has been conducted from the perspective of the providers of medical care—doctors and others—rather than from the perspective of the person and her or his experience with epilepsy (Schneider & Conrad, 1983). Thus researchers generate research that reflects their own ideology, which in turn generates more research based on similar ideology. People, even scientists, work out of the particular context of their own histories, social understandings, values, and visions.

This idea is formulated more fully in the work of Stephen Jay Gould (1981), who claims that science has never been, and cannot be, an objective enterprise. He maintains that:

> science, since people must do it, is a socially embedded activity. It progresses by hunch, vision, and intuition. Much of its change through time does not record a closer approach to absolute truth, but the alteration of cultural contexts that influence it so strongly. Facts are not pure and unsullied bits of information; culture also influences what we see and how we see it. Theories, moreover, are not inexorable inductions from facts. The most creative theories are often imaginative visions imposed upon facts; the source of imagination is also strongly cultural. (pp. 21, 22)

Physician-oriented research is thus a problem with several dimensions. Because it is the nature of clinical medicine to understand problems as individual, or as a dualism between mind and body, much research tries to locate the source of people's problems within them individually. Engel (1977) names and explains this phenomenon:

> The biomedical model not only requires that disease be dealt with as an entity independent of social behavior, it also demands that behavioral aberrations be explained on the basis of disordered somatic (biochemical or neuro-physiological) processes. Thus the biomedical model embraces both reductionism, the philosophic view that complex phenomena are ultimately derived from a single primary principle, and mind-body dualism, the doctrine that separates the mental from the somatic. (p. 130)

This concept is especially important when the subject is epilepsy. The main theme of this chapter is that the difficulties, whether mundane or serious, that people with epilepsy must face result from a complex set of relationships involving the whole person and the society of which the person is a part. Reducing psychopathology and even less troublesome problems to biochemical or neurophysiological explanations belies that complexity.

In the field of social science, looking for the source of a relational problem within an individual is called "blaming the victim" (Ryan, 1971):

> As we might expect, the logical outcome of analyzing social problems in terms of the deficiencies of the victim is the development of programs aimed at correcting those deficiencies. The formula for action becomes extraordinarily simple: change the victim. (p. 8)

When the burden of illness is placed solely on the individual who experiences problems with epilepsy and if only the medical establishment's intervention can change the victim, then the role of the larger society in stigmatizing those who have epilepsy is aptly ignored.

Irving Zola (1982), a social psychologist who knows firsthand what it means to be a person stigmatized by a handicapping condition, writes:

> We are experiencing a medicalization of society and with it the growth of medicine as an institution and instrument of social control. And while some have argued that this is a more humane and liberal way to deal with social problems, the notions of health and illness still locate the source of trouble and treatment in individual capacities, not social arrangements. To have a portion of our population declared physically unfit serves an important social function. It is important to recognize that in this country health occupations are the fastest growing category of employment, doctors are in the highest income brackets, and health-related industries are among the ones that make most profits. (p. 245)

We do not know exactly what will work in beginning to eliminate the stigma associated with epilepsy and the damage it causes. But it is clear, as Anspach (1979) maintains, that the battle for humanness is itself health bestowing. For people with epilepsy it is possible that such a battle would be joined by struggling to become fully participating members of society.

REFERENCES

Anspach, R. R. (1979). From stigma to identity politics: Political activism among the physically disabled and former mental patients. *Social Science and Medicine* 13A, 765–73.

Arangio, A. J. (1975). The stigma of epilepsy. *American Rehabilitation* 2, 273.

Bagley, C. (1972). Social prejudice and the adjustment of people with epilepsy. *Epilepsia* 13, 33–45.

Barrow, R. L., & H. D. Fabing. (1956). *Epilepsy and the law*. New York: Harper & Brothers.

Bear, D., & P. Fedio. (1977). Quantitative analysis of interictal behavior in temporal lobe epilepsy. *Archives of Neurology* 34, 454–67.

Becker, H. S. (1963). *The outsiders*. New York: Free Press of Glencoe.

Beran, R. G., & T. Read. (1983). A survey of doctors in Sydney, Australia: Perspectives and practices regarding epilepsy and those affected by it. *Epilepsia* 24, 79–104.

Beran, R. G., V. J. Jennings, & T. Read. (1981). Doctors' perspectives of epilepsy. *Epilepsia* 22, 397–406.

Borman, L., H. Adelstein, P. A. Arntson, B. Bailey, V. Kennan, A. Kopatic, R. Norton, F. L. Pasquale, S. Robinson, & M. Speer. (1980a). *Epilepsy self-help workbook*. Evanston, IL: Northwestern University.

Borman, L., J. Davies, & D. A. Droge. (1980b). Self-help groups for persons with epilepsy. In B. P. Hermann (Ed.), *A multidisciplinary handbook of epilepsy*. Springfield, IL: Thomas.

Boshes, L. D., & H. W. Kienast. (1970). Community aspects of epilepsy. *Illinois Medical Journal* 38, 140–46.

Boshes, L. D., & H. W. Kienast. (1972). Community aspects of epilepsy—a modern re-appraisal. *Epilepsia* 13, 31–32.

Breger, E. (1976a). Attitudinal survey of adolescents towards epileptics of the same age group. Part 1. Awareness and knowledgeability of the epileptic condition. *Maryland State Medical Journal,* January, 61–76.

Breger, E. (1976b). Attitudinal survey of adolescents towards epileptics of the same age group. Part 2. Social acceptance. *Maryland State Medical Journal,* March, 41–46.

Brenner, M. H. (1973). *Mental illness and the economy.* Cambridge, MA: Harvard University Press.

Brenner, M. H. (1976). *Estimating the social costs of national economic policy: Implications for mental and physical health, and criminal aggression* (a study prepared for the use of the Joint Economic Committee, Congress of the U.S.). Washington, DC: U.S. Government Printing Office.

Caveness, W. F., & G. H. Gallup. (1980). A survey of public attitudes toward epilepsy in 1979 with an indication of trends over the past thirty years. *Epilepsia* 21, 509–18.

Chase, A. (1977). *The legacy of Malthus: The social costs of the new scientific racism.* New York: Knopf.

Chorover, S. L. (1979). *From genesis to genocide.* Cambridge, MA: MIT Press.

Commission for the Control of Epilepsy and Its Consequences. (1978). *Plan for nationwide action on epilepsy* (DHEW Publication No. NIH 78-276). Washington, DC: U.S. Government Printing Office.

Committee of the American Neurological Association for the Investigation of Eugenical Sterilization. (1936). *Eugenical sterilization: A reorientation of the problem.* New York: Macmillan.

Craig, C. (1983, January). A temporal kind of love. *Omni,* p. 37.

Crowther, D. L. (1967). Psychosocial aspects of epilepsy. *Pediatric Clinics of North America* 14, 921–32.

De Haas, A. M. L. (1962). Social aspects of epilepsy in childhood. *Epilepsia* 3, 44–55.

Engel, G. L. (1977). The need for a new medical model: A challenge for biomedicine. *Science* 196, 129–36.

Epilepsy newsletter. Epilepsy Newsletter Service, 300 E. Trilby Road., Ft. Collins, CO 80525.

Epilepsy self-help workshop newsletter. (1981). Evanston, IL: The Self-Help Institute, Northwestern University.

Epilepsy support program newsletter. (1983). Vol. 2, no. 1.

Flor-Henry, P. (1983). Determinants of psychosis in epilepsy: Laterality and forced normalization. *Biological Psychiatry* 18, 1045–57.

Fraser, R. T. (1980). Vocational aspects of epilepsy. In B. P. Hermann (Ed.), *A multidisciplinary handbook of epilepsy.* Springfield, IL: Thomas.

Gadow, K. D. (1982). School involvement in the treatment of seizure disorders. *Epilepsia* 23, 215–24.

Goffman, E. (1963). *Stigma: Notes on the management of spoiled identity.* Englewood Cliffs, NJ: Prentice-Hall.

Gould, S. J. (1981). *The mismeasure of man.* New York: Norton.

Handbook on self-help groups for people with epilepsy. (1982). Evanston, IL: Epilepsy in the Urban Environment Project, Center for Urban Affairs and Policy Research, Northwestern University & The Self-Help Center.

Hansson, R. O., & B. J. Duffield. (1976). Physical attractiveness and the attribution of epilepsy. *Journal of Social Psychology* 99, 223–40.

Harrison, R. M., & P. West. (1977). Images of a grand mal. *New Society,* May 12, 282.

Hartlage, L. C., & J. B. Green. (1972). The relation of parental attitudes to academic and social achievement in epileptic children. *Epilepsia* 13, 21–26.

Hartman, E., P. Arntson, D. Droge, & R. Norton. (1983). Initial results from a questionnaire for people who have experienced seizure activity. *Working Papers,* Center for Urban Affairs and Policy Research, Northwestern University, Evanston, IL.

Hauck, G. (1972). Sociological aspects of epilepsy research. *Epilepsia* 13, 79–85.

Hermann, B. P., & S. Whitman. (1984). Behavioral and personality correlates of epilepsy: A review, methodological critique and conceptual model. *Psychological Bulletin* 95, 451–97.

Herndon, R. M., & R. A. Rudick. (1983). Multiple sclerosis: The spectrum of severity. *Archives of Neurology* 40, 531–32.

Holdsworth, L., & K. Whitmore. (1974). A study of children with epilepsy attending ordinary schools. II. Information and attitudes held by their teachers. *Developmental Medicine and Child Neurology* 16, 759–65.

Holmes, D. A., & J. M. McWilliams. (1981). Employer's attitudes toward hiring epileptics. *Journal of Rehabilitation,* April/May/June, 20–21.

Jones, J. G. (1965). Employment of epileptics. *Lancet,* September 4, 486–89.

Kevles, D. J. (1984, October 15). Annals of eugenics. *New Yorker,* pp. 52–125.

Kleck, R. E. (1968). Self-disclosure patterns of the nonobviously stigmatized. *Psychological Reports* 23, 1239–48.

Laughlin, H. H. (1926). *Eugenical sterilization in the United States* (rev. ed.). New Haven, CT: American Eugenics Society. (Originally published 1922, Chicago: Psychopathic Laboratory of the Municipal Court of Chicago).

Lennox, W. G., & C. H. Markham. (1953). The sociopsychological treatment of epilepsy. *Journal of the American Medical Association* 152, 1690–94.

Lewin, G. W. (1957). Some characteristics of the socio-psychological life space of the epileptic patient. *Human Relations* 10, 249–56.

Lieberman, M. A., & L. D. Borman. (Eds.). (1979). *Self-help groups for coping with crisis.* San Francisco: Jossey-Bass.

Livingston, S. (1957). The social management of the epileptic child and his parents. *Journal of Pediatrics* 51, 137–45.

Livingston, S. (1970). The physician's role in guiding the epileptic child and his parents. *American Journal of Diseases of Children* 119, 99–102.

Livingston, S. (1977). Psychosocial aspects of epilepsy. *Journal of Clinical Child Psychology* 6, 6–10.

Lombroso, C. (1972). Introduction. In G. Lombroso-Ferrero, *Criminal man according to the classification of Cesare Lombroso.* Montclair, NJ: Patterson Smith. (Original work published 1911)

Long, C. G., & J. R. Moore. (1979). Parental expectations for their epileptic children. *Journal of Child Psychology and Psychiatry* 20, 299–312.

Ludmerer, K. M. (1972). *Genetics and American Society: A historical appraisal.* Baltimore: Johns Hopkins University Press.

Marlowe, L. (1975). *Social psychology.* Boston: Holbrook Press.

Matthews, W. S., G. Barabas, & M. Ferrari. (1982). Emotional concomitants of childhood epilepsy. *Epilepsia* 23, 671–81.

Mittan, R. J. (1982). *Medical and psychological consequences of inadequate patient education.* Paper presented at the Western Epilepsy Institute, Los Angeles, CA.

Mittan, R. J., C. Wasterlain, & G. Locke. (1981). *Medical misinformation, fears about seizures, and their potential contribution to epileptics' poor psychosocial adjustment.* Paper presented at the Annual Meeting of the American Epilepsy Society, New York City.

Mungas, D. (1982). Interictal behavior abnormality in temporal lobe epilepsy: A specific syndrome or non-specific psychopathology? *Archives of General Psychiatry* 39, 108–11.

National Spokesman (1980). Missouri scuttles marriage law, adoption bill dies. 13, 3.

Perlman, L. G. (1977). *The person with epilepsy: Life style, needs, expecations.* Chicago: National Epilepsy League.

Pond, B. A., & B. H. Bidwell. (1960). A survey of epilepsy in fourteen general practices. *Epilepsia* 1, 285.

Remschmidt, H. (1973). Psychological studies of patients with epilepsy and popular prejudice. *Epilepsia* 14, 347–56.

Richardson, D. W., & S. B. Friedman. (1974). Psychosocial problems of the adolescent patient with epilepsy. *Clinical Pediatrics* 13, 121–26.

Ritchie, K. (1981). Research note: Interaction in the families of epileptic children. *Journal of Child Psychology and Psychiatry* 22, 65–71.

Rodin, E. A., P. Rennick, R. Dennerll, & Y. Lin. (1972). Vocational and educational problems of epileptic patients. *Epilepsia* 13, 149–60.

Rodin, E. A., & S. Schmaltz. (1983). The Bear-Fedio personality inventory and temporal lobe epilepsy. *Epilepsia* 24, 260.

Rutter, M., P. Graham, & W. Yule. (1970). *A neuropsychiatric study in childhood.* Philadelphia: Lippincott.

Ryan, R., K. Kempner, & A. C. Emlen. (1980). The stigma of epilepsy as a self-concept. *Epilepsia* 21, 433–44.

Ryan, W. (1971). *Blaming the victim.* New York: Random House.

Scambler, G., & A. Hopkins. (1980). Social class, epileptic activity, and disadvantage at work. *Journal of Epidemiology and Community Health* 34, 129–33.

Scherer, A. (1982). *Epilepsy and public attitudes: Strategies for change.* Paper presented at the 14th Epilepsy International Symposium, London, England.

Schneider, J. W., & P. Conrad. (1980). In the closet with illness: Epilepsy, stigma potential and information control. *Social Problems* 28, 32–44.

Schneider, J. W., & P. Conrad. (1981). Medical and social typologies: The case of epilepsy. *Social Science and Medicine* 15A, 211–19.

Schneider, J. W., & P. Conrad. (1983). *Having epilepsy: The experience and control of illness.* Philadelphia: Temple University Press.

Schultz, D. (1975). Four million Americans should not have to lie about their health. *Today's Health* 53, 15–20.

Stevens, J. R. (1975). interictal clinical manifestations of complex partial seizures. In J. K. Penry & D. D. Daly (Eds.), *Advances in neurology* (Vol. 11). New York: Raven Press.

Taylor, D. C. (1982). The components of sickness: Diseases, illnesses and predicaments. In J. Apley & C. Ounsted (Eds.), *One child.* London: Heinemann Medical Books.

Temkin, O. (1971). *The falling sickness: A history of epilepsy from the Greeks to the beginnings of modern neurology* (2nd ed.). Baltimore, MD: Johns Hopkins University Press.

Tizard, B. (1962). The personality of epileptics: A discussion of the evidence. *Psychological Bulletin* 59, 196–210.

Vinson, T. (1975). Towards demythologizing epilepsy. *Medical Journal of Australia* 2, 663–66.

Ward, F., & B. D. Bowen. (1978). A study of certain social aspects of epilepsy in childhood. *Developmental Medicine and Child Neurology* 39 (Supp.), 1–50.

West. P. (1979). An investigation into the social construction and consequences of the label epilepsy. *Sociological Review* 27, 719–41.

West, P. (1984). *Becoming disabled: Perspectives on the labelling process.* In U. E. Gerhardt & M. Wadsworth (Eds.), *Stress and stigma: Problems of explanation in the sociology of crime and illness.* Frankfurt: Campus Press.

Wiley, L. (1974). The stigma of epilepsy. *Nursing* 4, 37–45.

Zielinski, J. J. (1972). Social prognosis in epilepsy. *Epilepsia* 13, 133–40.

Zielinski, J. J. (1976). People with epilepsy who do not consult physicians. In D. Janz (Ed.), *Epileptology: Proceedings of the seventh international symposium on epilepsy.* Stuttgart: Thieme.

Zielinski, J. J. (1984). Epidemiological overview of epilepsy: Morbidity, mortality, and clinical implications. In D. Blumer (Ed.), *Psychiatric aspects of epilepsy.* Washington, D.C.: American Psychological Association.

Zola, I. K. (1982). *Missing pieces: A chronicle of living with a disability.* Philadelphia: Temple University Press.

9 / Children with Epilepsy as a Minority Group: Evidence from the National Child Development Study

CHRISTOPHER BAGLEY

MODELS OF EPILEPSY

Despite a century of scientific research, we still have a very incomplete knowledge of the extent and causes of behavioral problems associated with epilepsy (Hermann & Whitman, 1984). In part this has been due to the inefficient application of scientific methods (failure to use control groups, unstandardized or unvalidated measures, failure to measure or control for all relevant variables, premature generalizations, and lack of long-term studies). But in important part too, the failure to understand how people with epilepsy think, feel, and behave in relation to their social world has been due to the application of traditional "scientific" methods that objectify human subjects and ignore gross imbalances of power between the objects of study and other groups in society, including the researchers themselves.

For people with epilepsy (among whom I count myself) the findings of most research and the related statements of professionals (doctors, social workers, and the like) for dealing with "epileptics" are often biased, demeaning, and irrelevant. Reviews of "findings" still treat "epileptics" as deviant, distant objects (e.g., Lewis, Shanok, & Pincus, 1981), and advice for professionals still frequently fails to recognize the subjective aspects of epilepsy, the biases of much research work, and the effects of prejudice (e.g., many of the contributors to Sands [1981], and the work by Freeman [1979] on "the epileptic" in home, school, and society).

We doubt, in fact, whether the categorization of epilepsy that is traditional in neuropsychiatry is of much value for people with epilepsy themselves. Indeed, an English general population survey by Goodridge and Shorvan (1983) suggests that only two thirds of people reporting fits to their general practitioner have an EEG examination, and in at least a quarter of these examinations the EEG was normal. To claim that not all "falling attacks" are epilepsy (Goodridge & Shorvan, 1983; Zander, Graham, Morrell, and Fenwick, 1979) is to assume that diagnosed "epilepsy" rather than having fits is the main area of concern for medical practitioners. This assumption begs the issue of the effect of having a seizure of any kind on an individual, and the reactions of others to these "falling attacks."

The overscholastic, abstract, seemingly scientific but nevertheless biased models of epilepsy have not served people with epilepsy well (Bagley, 1971). They have led to the needless confinement of innocent people in "colonies" (Szasz, 1970); to the exclusion of children from school; and to the overdosing or maldosing of people with drugs and anticonvulsants (Ferrari, Barabas, & Matthews, 1983; Reynolds & Trimble, 1982).

Alternative models of epilepsy have been derived from the sociology of science, in which the implicit meanings and agendas of science are critically analyzed (Pasternak, 1981; Schneider & Conrad, 1981).

Another important model—since it conditions many social responses to epilepsy—involves the ideas of the nature and cause of seizures held by ordinary people (West, 1979). Parents of a child with epilepsy may draw on this folk wisdom (which may actually be extremely negative and stereotyped in its implications) in handling their child (Bagley, 1971; West, 1979). Reactions of the family to a child having seizures are crucial, and negative family reactions may lead to poorer adjustment on the part of the child (Ferrari et al., 1983). However, this finding is by no means universal, and families with a child with epilepsy may react with supportive strength (Bagley, 1971; Karen, 1981). This is particularly likely where a family member already has epilepsy (Schneider & Conrad, 1981). On the other hand, physicians may diagnose and treat "epilepsy" in children when subsequent examinations have shown that diagnosis to be incorrect (Meadow, 1984).

Only one study we can discover (Schneider & Conrad, 1981, 1983) reports data on how people with epilepsy construe their condition. Yet such research on self-conceptions of the label "epilepsy" and of having fits is crucial if we are to understand how children and adolescents react not only to having fits, but also to the reactions of others.

Although there is a large literature in the field of self-concept in handicap (Bowhay & Bagley, 1984) virtually nothing has been written on the self-concept, identity, and self-esteem of children who have fits. Two recent studies suggest, however, that the difficulties parents and teachers have in accepting or understanding epilepsy may be reflected in impaired self-concept in children who have fits (Ferrari et al., 1983; Matthews, Barabas, & Ferrari, 1983). On theoretical grounds at least, it is clear that adequate self-concept is of fundamental importance for the adjustment of the child who has been labeled epileptic (Coulter, 1982). Remschmidt's (1973) social learning hypothesis is consistent with this view: If children who have fits internalize the negative views other people have of them, their self-evaluation will become increasingly negative, in reflection of these views.

THE ADJUSTMENT OF CHILDREN WITH EPILEPSY COMPARED WITH THAT OF ETHNIC MINORITIES

There is an increasing trend for members of some groups of handicapped people to use models derived from the struggle of ethnic minorities in their own claims for an integrated acceptance. This has been particularly true of hearing-handicapped individuals (Bagley & Bowhay, 1982). In the analogy with race relations, people with epilepsy have been forced to "pass" or assimilate, despite a deeply felt but strongly hidden sense of identity as a special group.

People with epilepsy are subject to considerable, but perhaps diminishing, prejudice and rejection on the part of the general population. Indeed, the trends in attitudes to people with epilepsy and toward ethnic minorities show the same curve over time. We showed in fact that racial prejudice and rejection of handicapped people are linked attitudes, and that "epileptics" are the most rejected of all the supposedly handicapped groups (Bagley, 1972; Bagley & Verma, 1979). Moreover, the personality dynamics underlying prejudice toward ethnic minorities and people with handicaps are largely the same (Bagley, Verma, Mallick, & Young, 1979).

Traditionally, self-concept theory has suggested that minority groups will internalize or reflect the stereotyped views others have of them, unless they are able to protect the integrity of their self-image through a strong minority culture (Young & Bagley, 1982). In cultures such as Britain recent immigrants from the Caribbean have had assimilationist aspirations and lacked the social and political organization that could protect children against a variety of stresses (Bagley, 1975a).

It is possible that much of the categorization of black children as behavior disordered in school (with rates far in excess of those of white children) is due to biased perception and labeling by teachers. Such a possibility clearly emerged in a study we carried out in a large population of 10-year-olds in London (Rutter et al., 1974). Teachers completed a questionnaire that measured classroom behavior (Rutter, Tizard, & Whitmore, 1970). This questionnaire was standardized and validated in large general population and clinic samples. According to teacher descriptions of the behavior of black children, 38% of the 354 black children in the study displayed serious behavior disorder, a much higher rate than the 24% in the white children. However, interviews with parents gave a much different picture. The prevalence of parentally described deviant behavior of clinical proportions was 17.5% (62/354) in black children, and 25.0% (422/1,689) in white children. The rate of parentally described behavior is significantly *lower* in black children than in white; yet the rate in black children as described by teachers is significantly *higher*. This could mean either that behavior disorder for the minority children is highly context dependent (perhaps reflecting a rebellious attitude to racist educational systems), or it could reflect biased perception on the part of teachers. Again, this latter suggestion parallels the situation of children with epilepsy, who are often subject to stereotyped perceptions on the part of teachers (Bagley, 1971).

We have reviewed the evidence on teacher prejudice and misconceptions regarding minority children in some detail (Bagley, 1975b; Verma & Bagley, 1979, and 1982). A considerable body of research from both Britain and the United States demonstrates that many (but certainly not all) teachers share commonly held stereotypes and prejudices concerning both ethnic minority and handicapped groups. Such stereotypes may also inform their actions in the classroom in ways that can become self-confirming.

In examining data on ethnic minority children in the National Child Development study of some 15,000 children born in 1 week in 1958, we concluded from the evidence on teachers' descriptions of the behavior and achievement of black children that labeling and misconception had almost certainly taken place. Very early in their school careers black children were seen by many teachers as behavior problems, without learning potential, and suitable for transfer to schools for "subnormal" children. Social background data adequately predicted learning failure and behavioral problems in white children, but most black children whom teachers described as maladapted had no behavior problems at home and came from normal family backgrounds. These findings were quite similar to those obtained by Rutter et al. (1974) in an earlier study.

We argued earlier (Bagley, 1972) that attitudes to people with epilepsy had similar dimensions and dynamics in comparison with attitudes to ethnic minorities. In particular, the crude stereotypes of black people—as dangerous and unpredictable—were similar to the stereotypes held of people with epilepsy, and led to similar types of social exclusion.

In parallel to this argument we contend that prejudiced and stereotyped attitudes (shared by the public and teachers to a significant extent) lead to biased perceptions of minority children of various backgrounds, including children with epilepsy. Moreover, children with epilepsy, like other minority children, may themselves come to accept these negative views. But in any case, we would expect teachers to describe stigmatized groups, such as those with epilepsy, in rather negative terms.

There is little direct evidence of the knowledge and attitudes of teachers toward children with epilepsy, however. An American study by Force (1965) suggested on the basis of a questionnaire completed by teachers that "stereotypes and misconceptions about epilepsy and epileptics exist, knowledge of teachers about epilepsy is often sketchy, and teachers' attitudes toward these children are highly variable and often not based on modern medical or psychological knowledge." In a more recent U.S. study, Gadow (1982) reported of a sample of New York teachers that "teachers were often not informed about the overt features of seizures, side effects of the medication, or seizure management, even in the case of students who experienced seizures and/or side effects in school . . . collectively, these data suggest that in many cases, no one has assumed responsibility for coordinating the delivery of services for psychosocial treatment needs."

No similar studies can be located in the literature although knowledge and attitude studies of this type are not in principle difficult to conduct. We found in a British study (Bagley, 1971) that teachers had little specific knowledge or attitudes concerning children in their classes with epilepsy. However, the teachers frequently underestimated the ability of these children and in a number of cases severely restricted the children's activity. In a few cases children with epilepsy were needlessly excluded from school. An attitudinal study with a mixed population (high school students, teachers in training, university students, and a sample of the general population) indicated that hostility and rejection were the most commonly held attitudes toward people with epilepsy. College students were certainly not immune to these attitudes (Bagley, 1972).

Given the possible biases that teachers have with regard to children with epilepsy, studies such as those by Hackney and Taylor (1976) reporting that children with epilepsy are more disturbed according to teacher descriptions should be treated with caution. Such results could among other reasons be due to:

1. Biased perception by teachers;
2. Situationally specific reactions to negative environments; or
3. An internalization of the negative attitudes of teachers and peers.

In fact, the negative views of teachers can become self-confirming, just as their perceptions of other minority children can become self-confirming (Bagley, 1975b).

METHODS

The British National Child Development Study (NCDS) is a uniquely important long-term study for two reasons. First of all, it has amassed a large amount of perinatal and later data on some 15,000 subjects (Butler & Bonham,

1963; Davie, 1968; Pringle, Butler, & Davie, 1967); second, by taking a complete cohort of all children born in 1 week in 1958 and accessing this group in later follow-ups through the school system, drop-out of subjects has been much lower than if subjects had been followed up by addresses alone (Davie, Butler, & Goldstein, 1972). By using the school system as the source of subjects, the NCDS located some 87% of those studied at birth, by the time they were 16.

This large longitudinal study has been able to identify complete samples of minority populations, including ethnic minorities (Bagley, 1982a), those with special family situations (Bagley, 1985), and groups with special health problems. Children with epilepsy or having seizures in the NCDS cohort have been only briefly described (Ross, Peckham, West, & Butler, 1980). Ross and his colleagues described 64 children with epilepsy (according to strict medical criteria) in the NCDS cohort up to the age of 16. Only 37 of these children were being educated in the normal school system. Most of the remainder had secondary impairments, particularly educational subnormality. Only four children were in special schools for children with epilepsy.

In attempting to analyze data on "epilepsy" from the NCDS cohort, some of the limitations of the data have become apparent. Medical data were collected from teachers and parents, and only atypically by a formal medical examination. Much of the data was gathered in unsupervised settings, and its veracity and validity often have not been established. In all, data on some 2,900 medical, social, educational, and family variables have been collected, which paradoxically has created a number of disadvantages. Computer sorting of such a huge data set is complex and expensive, and still beyond the capacity of many modern computer systems; second, storing this large data set is extremely expensive. Furthermore, the availability of so many variables collected at different points in time makes causal models more, rather than less, difficult to test. For example, in tracing sequelae of maternal smoking during the pregnancy with the NCDS children, we found significant adverse behavioral sequelae in the child at age 16, social class controlled; but it was impossible to test any particular causal model, and the question of whether maternal smoking causes this later behavior has been impossible to answer (Bagley, 1982b).

Our approach to "epilepsy" is that having seizures, both major and minor, is of greater psychological consequence for the individual and his or her parents and peers than the reified medical designation of epilepsy (Bagley, 1972). Because of this theoretical approach, we have defined "epilepsy" as a parental report of the child having at least one seizure after the first year of life, in the absence of other central nervous conditions (including subnormality associated with brain damage, and cerebral palsy). We also excluded from consideration children attending special schools of various kinds, since the main object of this study was to explore the perceptions teachers in the normal school system have of children with seizures. We assume, though we have no direct evidence from the data presented, that teachers can readily identify the majority of children in their classrooms who have had recent seizures. However, previous work suggests that only about 50% of teachers can identify children in their classrooms with a formal diagnosis of epilepsy (Bagley, 1971). In part this may reflect the fact that seizures whose onset was some years earlier may now be controlled by medication. The possibility that some parents may induce or misdescribe seizures in their children also should be borne in mind (Meadow, 1984).

By the time they were 16, 368 children (of the 12,280 on whom reasonably complete data existed) were recorded as having a "seizure" according to parental information on "any form of fit or other turn in which consciousness was lost or any part of the body made abnormal movements." We excluded from these 368, attacks that according to additional medical information appeared to be simple fainting attacks without tonic or clonic involvement (spasms or muscular contractions).

We further excluded any children from the "seizures" category who had a handicap involving some aspect of the central nervous system of such a degree that the child could not be accepted in normal schooling. In this category were 1 child with profound deafness; 6 children who were blind or partially sighted; 4 with cerebral palsy; 23 who were designated educationally subnormal; 12 with other disorders, apparently of CNS origin; and 4 children with chronic, uncontrolled seizures who were in a special colony for people with epilepsy. After these various exclusions we were left with 104 of the original 368 children who had seizures of various kinds past the first year of life and who were not excluded from normal schooling.

Our study group is, then, a selected set of subjects who have seizures of various kinds that resemble those traditionally seen in epilepsy and who have remained in mainstream schooling. The 104 subjects plus the four excluded children in special schools for children with "epilepsy" represent a rate of 9 per 1,000 (108/12,280), which is slightly higher than the range of 4–7 per 1,000 reported in previous studies of children (Ross, 1983). However, the age of our subjects (16) at which prevalence of seizures was assessed should be borne in mind, and the rate of 9 per 1,000 should be compared with a lifetime prevalence of 20 per 1,000 found in a recent British epidemiologic study (Goodridge & Shorvan, 1983). A prevalence rate of 8 per 1,000 in the age group 0–15 has been reported in Swedish work (Blom, Heijbel, & Bergfors, 1978). It is possible that we have included in this study children who, although they have seizures, have not had a formal diagnosis of epilepsy. However, we would argue that having seizures (both major and minor) that can be observed and reacted to by others is the most crucial factor in an individual's adjustment, not the abnormalities (or lack of such abnormality) that underlie those seizures.

Two hundred control subjects were drawn for comparison with the 104 children with a history of seizures. Given the large pool of potential control subjects, we were able to draw controls with the same proportion of children who were male (55%), parents with blue-collar occupation (69%), and of children who experienced perinatal problems including bleeding during pregnancy, difficult birth, and low birth weight (21%), and who had no handicapping conditions requiring attendance at a special school.

The 104 children with seizures were significantly more likely than the children in the cohort who had no seizures of any kind to be male, to have experienced perinatal complications or have low birth weight, and to have a blue-collar background. These are interesting findings in the light of previous research on links between social class, sex, and possible CNS impairment (Bagley, 1971). We will explore these findings elsewhere.

RESULTS

Our basic hypothesis is that children with seizures (who may also be "epileptic" in a formal medical sense) will be viewed (like many ethnic minority children) in more negative or stereotyped ways than children with no history of seizures. We argue further that (as was the case in our previous research with ethnic minorities) parents of these children will see their children more favorably than will teachers in comparison with control subjects for whom parental and teacher perceptions will be more similar.

For purposes of data analysis we have divided subjects into groups according to the most recently reported seizure. The 5-year groupings are unfortunately broad, but were imposed on us by the way the National Children's Bureau had coded the original data. We have assumed that the more recent the seizures, the more likely it is that teachers (for whatever reason) will view the particular students negatively. Further, we assumed that chronic seizures (seizures occurring in more than one 5-year period) would be more likely to be associated with a perceptual bias or labeling set by teachers. It should be acknowledged, however, that alternative psychological or neurological hypotheses could account for such a finding.

Table 9-1 shows that our hypotheses are only partially supported with respect to teacher reports of problems of physical and sensory activity. Overall, children with seizures are described as having significantly more problems than controls. The significant variation of problems within the children with seizures shows that children with the first occurrence of a seizure in the years 11–16 have the highest reported prevalence of sensory and motor problems.

TABLE 9-1. Teacher-Described Problems of Sensory and Motor Activity in Children with Seizures and Controls, at Age 16[a]

Category	*N*	*Some Incapacity of Physical Coordination, Movement, or Hand Control (%)*	*Some Incapacity of Hearing, Speech, or Sight (%)*	*Significance of Chi-squared*
Seizure(s) at age 1–5	22	4.5	9.1	*Motor problems:* within seizure group, $p = .005$; between seizure group and controls, $p = .020$
Seizure(s) at age 6–10	19	10.5	10.5	
Seizure(s) at age 11–16	12	25.0	25.0	*Sensory problems:* within seizure group, $p = .003$; between seizure group and controls, $p = .032$
Seizure(s) at age 1–5 and 6–10	21	9.5	14.3	
Seizure(s) at age 11–16 and 1–5 or 6–10	30	16.7	20.0	
All subjects with seizures	104	12.5	15.4	
Controls	200	5.0	9.0	

[a]All percentages are calculated horizontally, based on the *N* in each category.

However, having had no further seizures past age 5 or age 10 is associated with a lower incidence of these reported problems.

Table 9-2 presents data on teacher-described achievement in English and mathematics. The trend here does support the "chronicity" hypothesis, but only with respect to English achievement. The "selective difficulty with mathematics" that some children with epilepsy have (Bagley, 1971) was replicated in the present population.

Table 9-3 presents data on teachers' perception of the behavior of the children who have seizures. For every category, children with seizures are described more adversely than controls, and in four out of seven comparisons these differences are significant at the 5% level or beyond. The comparisons by age of most recent seizure show that for every behavior described, the

Table 9-2. Assessment by Teachers of Achievement in English and Mathematics in Children with Seizures and Controls, at Age 16[a]

Category	*N*	*"Poor" or "Very Poor" English Achievement (%)*	*"Poor" or "Very Poor" Mathematics Achievement (%)*	*Significance of Chi-squared*
Seizure(s) at age 1–5	22	22.7	40.9	English: within seizure group, p = .024; between seizure group and controls, p = .019
Seizure(s) at age 6–10	19	21.0	36.8	
Seizure(s) at age 11–16	12	33.3	33.3	Mathematics: within seizure group, p = .078; between seizure group and controls, p = .048
Seizure(s) at age 1–5 and 6–10	21	42.8	38.1	
Seizure(s) at age 11–16 and 1–5 or 6–10	30	43.3	40.0	
All subjects with seizures	104	33.6	38.5	
Controls	200	25.0	33.0	

[a]All percentages are calculated horizontally, based on the *N* in each category.

prevalence is higher in those having seizures after age 10. Overall, however, the hypothesis with regard to chronicity is not fully confirmed. It is clear that having no seizures after age 10 is associated with significantly lower rates of problem behavior.

It should be noted that in the English school system most children transfer to their final secondary school at age 11. Seizures occurring before this time might well be "lost" in administrative terms, but seizures occurring in the secondary school period (any time between ages 11 and 16) might well inform the perception teachers in that school have of the child. Alternatively, seizures occurring in the adolescent period could have special psychological or neurological significance for adjustment. The complex interaction of potentially causal variables is likely to give the most complete explanation of behavior problems in children with epilepsy, a hypothesis we have advanced elsewhere (Bagley, 1971), but which we have insufficient data to explore here.

Table 9-4 presents a test of the hypothesis that teachers will view children

TABLE 9-3. Behavioral Descriptions by Teachers of Children with Seizures and Controls, at Age 16 (in%)[a]

Category	*N*	*(a) Very Moody*	*(b) Very Aggressive*	*(c) Very Withdrawn*	*(d) Often or Frequently Steals*	*(e) Very Restless*	*(f) Very Squirmy*	*(g) Very Destructive*
Seizure(s) at age 1–5	22	4.5	0.0	4.5	0.0	13.3	9.1	0.0
Seizure(s) at age 6–10	19	5.3	5.3	0.0	0.0	10.5	0.0	0.0
Seizure(s) at age 11–16	12	16.7	25.0	8.3	16.7	16.7	16.7	8.3
Seizure(s) at age 1–5 and 6–10	21	14.3	9.5	9.5	4.8	19.0	14.3	4.8
Seizure(s) at age 11–16 and 1–5 or 6–10	30	16.7	13.3	10.0	13.3	16.7	13.3	6.7
All subjects with seizures	104	11.5	9.6	6.7	6.7	14.4	10.6	3.8
Controls	200	7.5	3.0	1.0	3.0	7.0	4.0	0.5

Significance:
(a) Moody: within seizure group, $p = .046$; between epilepsy group and controls, $p = .103$
(b) Aggressive: within seizure group, $p = .037$; between epilepsy and controls, $p = .028$
(c) Withdrawn: within seizure group, $p = .081$; between epilepsy and controls, $p = .047$
(d) Steals: within seizure group, $p = .034$; between epilepsy and controls, $p = .081$
(e) Restless: within seizure group, $p = .041$; between epilepsy and controls, $p = .017$
(f) Squirmy: within seizure group, $p = .058$; between epilepsy and controls, $p = .046$
(g) Destructive: within seizure group, $p = .060$; between epilepsy and controls, $p = .105$
[a]All percentages are calculated horizontally, based on the *N* in each category. Significance testing by chi-square.

TABLE 9-4. Teacher's and Parent's Rating of Rutter Scale Items for Children with Seizures and Controls[a]

	Children with Seizures			*Controls*		
Behavior	*Parent's Rating*	*Teacher's Rating*	r *of Two Ratings*	*Parent's Rating*	*Teacher's Rating*	r *of Two Ratings*
Restless "a, c, d"	1.49	1.58	.101	1.45	1.34	.141
Squirmy "a, c, d"	1.67	1.46	.097	1.63	1.18	.134
Destructive "c"	1.07	1.14	.135	1.08	1.06	.095
Fights "c, d"	1.40	1.36	.171	1.42	1.08	.183
Disliked "a, c"	1.14	1.39	.068	1.13	1.14	.082
Worried "a, d"	1.89	1.32	.033	1.82	1.39	.158
Irritable "a, c, d"	1.66	1.40	.043	1.72	1.19	.184
Miserable "a, d"	1.41	1.15	.078	1.35	1.09	.156
Twitches "a, c"	1.09	1.21	.117	1.07	1.01	.063
Sucks thumb	1.04	1.02	.082	1.04	1.01	.145
Bites nails "a, c, d"	1.40	1.20	.088	1.43	1.12	.202
Disobedient "c, d"	1.29	1.36	.035	1.32	1.19	.206
Can't settle "c, d"	1.51	1.57	.179	1.48	1.20	.157
Fearful "a, d"	1.42	1.25	.028	1.43	1.22	.101
Fussy "a, c, d"	1.50	1.24	.091	1.54	1.10	.066
Tells lies "a, c, d"	1.33	1.30	.111	1.30	1.17	.241
Scale total "a, c, d"	22.31	20.95	.107	22.21	18.49	.163
N		100–104			192–200	

Significance: A difference of 0.9 between ratings of parent and teacher for children with seizures is significant at the 5% level or beyond. A difference of 0.8 between ratings for children with seizures and ratings for controls is significant at the 5% level or beyond.
"a" indicates parental rating differs significantly from teacher rating within seizure category.
"b" indicates parental rating for seizure group differs significantly from parental rating in controls.
"c" indicates teacher rating for seizure group differs significantly from teacher rating in controls.
"d" indicates parental ratings for controls differs significantly from teacher rating in controls.
Correlations of .170 and above are significant at the 5% level or beyond in the case of control subjects; correlations of .200 and above are significant in the case of subjects with seizures. Correlations between parent and teacher ratings are smaller in 12 out of 16 cases for children with seizures (p less than .05, using the critical ratio test). Average correlation between parent and teacher ratings for children with seizures is .091, and for controls .145. This difference is significant at the 1% level.
[a]Scores are based on the average of 1 = "doesn't apply", 2 = "applies somewhat"; and 3 = "certainly applies" in response to items in the Rutter Scale (Rutter et al., 1970); e.g., "Very restless. Has difficulty staying seated for long."

with seizures less favorably than they will the comparison subjects and that parental perception of children with seizures will not support teachers' perceptions. In order to test this hypothesis we utilized 16 items from the Rutter Scale for describing behavioral problems in children (Rutter, Tizard, & Whitmore, 1970) that were completed by both parents and teachers. First of all, for 15 out of 16 items, teachers describe children with seizures more adversely than they describe the control subjects. However, parents of the two groups describe children in very similar terms, and both sets of parents describe their children somewhat more adversely than do parents of black children in the NCDS cohort we described earlier (Bagley, 1982).

Correlations between ratings of teachers and parents, although low overall, are more likely to be significant in the case of controls (in five comparisons) than in the case of children with seizures (in none of the comparisons). It appears that in general parents tend to describe their children more adversely than do teachers, but this is less likely to be the case with respect to children with seizures.

DISCUSSION

These findings seem to be compatible with the following competing explanations:

1. Seizures that have not remitted by adolescence imply a more serious neurological dysfunction, and it is this dysfunction that also causes the disturbed behavior. This, it must be admitted, is the most parsimonious explanation of the findings we present.
2. Parents of children with seizures misperceive their children's behavior in overprotective ways: The source of the disturbed behavior children with seizures manifest is an underlying central nervous system pathology, which also causes seizures; or the behavior could also reflect a reaction to anticonvulsant drugs controlling the seizures.
3. The adverse behavior of children with a history of seizures in the classroom is real, but represents a reaction against adverse stereotyping by both teachers and peers. In their homes, children with seizures behave no differently from other children.
4. There is a complex interaction between variables. Dispositions to maladaptive behavior that are neurological in origin, when combined with seizures observable by others, are likely to be exaggerated by the reactions of others. Thus children with seizures come to be observed in a "symbolic" way by some teachers. Teachers' perceptions of many children with seizures are a combination of stereotyping and the reaction of children to the adverse reactions of others. Rejection of a child who has seizures by his or her peer group is likely to be particularly crucial in adolescence in the emergence of classroom-based maladaptation. We acknowledge, in proposing this complex causal model to explain our findings, that we have no direct evidence on biased

> perceptions by teachers of children with seizures; nor do we have information on whether teachers actually knew a child was liable to have seizures.

Probably the fourth model, the theory of complex interaction (which we proposed earlier [Bagley, 1971]), is the most plausible, although it is clear that other explanations are possible. It should be mentioned that analysis of the data on parental and teacher perceptions for the 42 of the 104 children with seizures occurring after age 10 shows larger differences than are shown in Table 9-4, indicating increased support for a labeling hypothesis. However, overall statistical significance is higher (because of the larger *N*) when data on all 104 subjects are utilized.

These data from the British National Child Development Study show that, even in this selected group, children who have seizures but who have not been excluded from normal schooling (a decision that is in itself prejudicial) are more likely to be seen as underachieving, to have behavioral problems, and to have difficulties in sensory and motor areas. Seizures remitting before the age of 10 have the best prognosis in this respect.

The possibility that teacher ratings of children with seizures are biased in ways similar to their biases in perceiving children from ethnic minorities must seriously be considered and is certainly not disproved by our data, although we have no direct measures of such perception. The fullest explanation of the problems children with "epilepsy" experience in school probably comes from a model of the complex interaction of social, psychological, and biological factors, of which the labeling effect is a potentially important part.

We must conclude, however, that whatever the reasons for the often negative reports teachers have of children who have epilepsy (or are seen to have seizures), the long-term prospects for many of these children are not good. The labels and self-conceptions they acquire in school are likely to follow them into the world of work, and any neurological dysfunction causing seizures as well as disturbed behavior may also continue.

CONCLUSIONS

We have been critical of the conceptual and methodological basis of much research on behavioral aspects of epilepsy. Medical models have not served people with epilepsy well in this respect, and many of the "findings" on the nature of behavioral problems in people with epilepsy have been both biased and limited.

A particular gap in the literature concerns the self-esteem and self-conceptions of children and adolescents with epilepsy. Researchers have rarely asked "epileptics" themselves how they feel about having seizures, how they view others' reactions, and the effect those reactions have on them. We have argued that having seizures (both major and minor) that are observable by others is a major factor in adjustment and self-conception, regardless of any medical diagnosis of epilepsy.

We have argued further that the stigmatization people with epilepsy experience is very similar to the stigmatization imposed on certain ethnic minorities. It was hypothesized that results obtained in two studies with black children (Bagley, 1975a, b, 1982b; Rutter et al., 1974) that indicated bias in teachers' perceptions of such children would be replicated in a study of children in the National Child Development Study who have a history of seizures.

The results were generally consistent with this view. More recent seizures were associated with more teacher-described problems of achievement, adjustment, and with more motor and sensory problems. Comparison with parental description for those same children (those with seizures, and controls) suggested that labeling might well be occurring. However, causal models are difficult to test with this data set, and the fullest explanation of the problems of behavior and achievement in these children probably lies in an interaction model, in which various factors (biological, social, and psychological) interact with one another. We would urge, however, that social factors can explain a significant and perhaps a large amount of the variance in the adverse outcomes that affect a significant number of people with epilepsy.

REFERENCES

Bagley, C. (1971). *The social psychology of the child with epilepsy*. London: Routledge & Kegan Paul.

Bagley, C. (1972). Social prejudice and the adjustment of people with epilepsy. *Epilepsia* 13, 33–45.

Bagley, C. (1975a). The background of deviance in black children in London. In G. Verma & C. Bagley (Eds.), *Race and education across cultures*. London: Heinemann.

Bagley, C. (1975b). The teacher expectancy effect. In G. Verma & C. Bagley (Eds.), *Race and education across cultures*. London: Heinemann.

Bagley, C. (1982a). Achievement, behaviour disorder and social circumstances in West Indian children and other ethnic groups. In G. Verma & C. Bagley (Eds.), *Self-concept, achievement and multicultural education*. London: Macmillan.

Bagley, C. (1982b). *Methodological implications of the British National Child Development Study for longitudinal research on children under stress*. Paper given to International Conference on Research Strategies for the Study of Children Under Stress, Concordia University, Montreal.

Bagley, C. (1985). *Child welfare and adoption*. Aldershot, U.K.: Gower Press.

Bagley, C., & C. Bowhay. (1982). *Social and psychological factors in the adjustments of deaf and hearing impaired children.* Calgary: Rehabilitation and Health Monographs.

Bagley, C., & G. Verma. (1979). *Racial prejudice, the individual and society.* Farnborough, U.K.: Saxon House.

Bagley, C., G. Verma, K. Mallick, & L. Young. (1979). *Personality, self-esteem and prejudice.* Farnborough, U.K.: Saxon House.

Blom, S., J. Heijbel, and P. Bergfors. (1978). Incidence of epilepsy in children. *Epilepsia* 19, 343–50.

Bowhay, C., & C. Bagley. (1984). *Self-concept and handicap in children and adolescents.* Calgary: Rehabilitation and Health Monographs.

Butler, N., & D. Bonham. (1963). *Perinatal mortality.* Edinburgh: Livingstone.

Coulter, D. (1982). The psychosocial impact of epilepsy in childhood. *Children's Health Care* 11, 48–53.

Davie, R., (1968). The behaviour and adjustment of seven-year-old children: Some results from the national child development study. *British Journal of Educational Psychology* 38, 1–2.

Davie, R., N. Butler, & H. Goldstein. (1972). *From birth to seven.* London: Longman.

Ferrari, M., G. Barabas, & W. Matthews. (1983). Psychologic and behavioral disturbance among epileptic children treated with barbituate anticonvulsants. *American Journal of Psychiatry* 140, 112–13.

Ferrari, M., W. Matthews, & G. Barabas. (1983). The family and the child with epilepsy. *Family Process* 22, 53–59.

Force, D. (1965). *A descriptive study of the incidence of seizures and teachers' attitudes toward children with epilepsy in the Minneapolis, Minnesota public schools.* St. Paul, MN: Minnesota Epilepsy League.

Freeman, S. (1979); *The epileptic in home, school and society: Coping with the invisible handicap.* Springfield, IL: Thomas.

Gadow, K. (1982). School involvement in the treatment of seizure disorders. *Epilepsia* 23, 215–24.

Goodridge, D., & S. Shorvan. (1983). Epileptic seizures in a population of 6000. *British Medical Journal* (2) 641–47.

Hackney, A., & D. Taylor. (1976). A teacher's questionnaire description of epileptic children. *Epilepsia* 17, 275–82.

Hermann, B., & S. Whitman. (1984). Behavioral and personality correlates of epilepsy: A review, methodological critique and conceptual model. *Psychological Bulletin* 95, 451–97.

Karen, R. (1981). Interaction in the families of epileptic children. *Journal of Child Psychology and Psychiatry* 22, 65–71.

Lewis, D., S. Shanok, & J. Pincus. (1981). Delinquency and seizure disorders: A psychosomatic epileptic symptomatology and violence. In D. Lewis, (Ed.), *Vulnerabilities to delinquency.* New York: SP Medical and Scientific Books.

Matthews, W., G. Barabas, & M. Ferrari. (1983). Achievement and school behavior among children with epilepsy. *Psychology in the Schools* 20, 10–16.

Meadow, R. (1984). Fictitious epilepsy. *Lancet* 2, 25–28.

Pasternak, J. (1981). An analysis of social perceptions of epilepsy: Increasing rationalization as seen through the theories of Comte and Weber. *Social Science and Medicine* 15E, 223–29.

Pringle, M., N. Butler, & R. Davie. (1967). *11,000 Seven-Year-Olds.* London: Longman.

Remschmidt, H. (1973). Psychological studies of patients with epilepsy and popular prejudice. *Epilepsia* 14, 347–56.
Reynolds, E., & M. Trimble. (Eds.). (1982). *Epilepsy and psychiatry*. Edinburgh: Churchill-Livingstone.
Ross, E., C. Peckham, P. West, & N. Butler. (1980). Epilepsy in childhood: Findings from the National Child Development Study. *British Medical Journal* 1, 207–10.
Ross, F. (1983). *Research progress in epilepsy*. London: Pitman.
Rutter, M., J. Tizard, & K. Whitmore. (1970). *Education, health and behaviour*. London: Longman.
Rutter, M., B. Yule, M. Berger, N. Yule, J. Morton, & C. Bagley. (1974). Children of West Indian immigrants. *Journal of Child Psychology and Psychiatry* 15, 241–62.
Sands, H. (Ed.). (1981). *Epilepsy: A handbook for the mental health professional*. New York: Brunner/Mazel.
Schneider, J., & P. Conrad. (1981). Medical and sociological typologies: The case of epilepsy. *Social Science and Medicine* 15A, 211–19.
Schneider, J., & P. Conrad. (1983). *Having epilepsy*. Philadelphia: Temple University Press.
Szasz, T. (1970). *The manufacture of madness*. New York: Harper.
Verma, G., & C. Bagley. (1979). The labelling effect in education. In G. Verma and C. Bagley (Eds.), *Race, education and identity*. London: Macmillan.
Verma, G., & C. Bagley. (1982). Prejudice in teachers? In G. Verma & C. Bagley (Eds.), *Self-concept, achievement and multicultural education*. London: Macmillan.
West, P. (1979). Making sense of epilepsy. In D. Osborne (Ed.), *Research in psychology and medicine* (Vol. II). London: Academic Press.
Young, L., & C. Bagley. (1982). Self-esteem, self-concept and the development of black identity: A theoretical overview. In G. Verma and C. Bagley (Eds.), *Self-concept, achievement and multicultural education*. London: Macmillan.
Zander, L., H. Graham, D. Morrell, & P. Fenwick. (1979). Audit of care for epileptics in a general practice. *British Medical Journal* 2, 1035–37.

10 / Sources of Stigma Following Early-Life Epilepsy: Evidence from a National Birth Cohort Study

NICKY BRITTEN,
MICHAEL E. J. WADSWORTH, and
PETER B. C. FENWICK

The child with epilepsy has more problems to contend with than do children who suffer from less stigmatizing illnesses. In addition to the seizures themselves, the child has to cope with the attitudes and prejudices of parents, teachers, doctors, and society at large. Bagley (1972) attributes behavior disorders of people with epilepsy to their widespread social rejection and demonstrates, in the case of aggressive behavior, that environmental factors have importance over and above that of neurological factors. The Office of Health Economics (1971) suggests that many psychiatric and social consequences of epilepsy would be eliminated by changes in the attitudes of society as a whole, in the same way that reduction of birth trauma, brain infections, and accidents would prevent many cases of epilepsy from developing at all.

But where do such stigmatizing ideas originate? Generally speaking they come from perceived and visible differences in appearance and/or behavior or, by repute, from expected differences. Therefore, if we are to tackle the problem of the stigmatizing nature of a particular illness we have to discover the sources of stigma and endeavor to understand how it is maintained.

Goffman (1963) characterizes the stigmatized individual as someone disqualified from full social acceptance, someone reduced in the minds of others from a whole and normal person to a tainted and discounted being. He uses the term *stigma* to refer to an attitude that is deeply discrediting and points out that the attribute in question is neither creditable nor discreditable in itself. He describes various forms of discrimination by which the life chances of the stigmatized individual are reduced and shows that a wide range of imperfections are imputed on the basis of the original one. Such stigmatization is demonstrated by the literature on the "epileptic personality" in the early part of this century, reviewed by Bagley (1971). Clark (1925) even stated that "the epileptic makeup has its roots in a narcism [sic] which is based upon a repressed or illy-repressed homosexuality." This literature has since been discredited on the grounds of poor methodology (inadequate definitions, unspecified populations, false inferences, and so on), but it demonstrates that stigmatization may well be reinforced, even if not initiated, by professionals as well as laypeople. Bagley (1971) suggests that such prejudice against epilepsy is based on a common fear of sudden loss of control of the movements of the body, so that people liable to this loss are subjected to rejection and hostility; he also likens it to racial prejudice (Bagley, 1972).

It is arguable that from such poor research the notion of an "epileptic personality" took root in everyday clinical thinking and language, and there is some evidence to suggest that this is so. Books of advice on how to rear children are a valuable source of health care professionals' ideas, and although it can be objected that they are generally read only by a minority of middle-class parents, they nevertheless will repeat the ideas that are in common circulation among professionals and that are put forward to patients from all kinds of social backgrounds. Changes in such sources are likely to be forerunners of changes in public views, just as they continue to be in other topics in health education. In Truby King's widely distributed book *Feeding and Care of Baby* (1937) mothers are advised that

> convulsions are not only dangerous to life but they tend to do permanent damage to the nervous system. Many cases of epilepsy come on in people who have had convulsions during infancy, and the seeds of many other grave nervous affections are sown in the same way. (p. 191)

As this passage makes clear, getting things right in childhood carries with it the implication of guilt for those who apparently get things wrong. So, for example, mothers were ambiguously advised, under the heading *epilepsy,* that "many nervous disorders are brought on by wrong habits in childhood" (Liddiard, 1944, p. 156).

It is reassuring that today's mothers can read readily accessible explanations of epilepsy and especially of its effects.

> A tendency to epileptic fits does not in itself affect a child's personality. It is now realised that many of the behavioural and emotional problems suffered by people with epilepsy and previously ascribed to the disease were the result of other people's reactions to the condition and the way patients were treated. They used to

> be ostracised by society, especially if they were put together in an "epileptic" colony. Children with epilepsy should never be referred to as "epileptics." (Jolly, 1980, p. 585)

Current authors also reflect present-day clinicians' much increased awareness of the need to explain what to expect of childhood illness in day-to-day life (Illingworth & Illingworth, 1984), and in particular of epilepsy.

Stigmatizing ideas about epilepsy have thus been sustained partly by professional concepts of this illness and its effects, which are inevitably passed on to patients with epilepsy. However, health care professionals' notions of the stigmatizing nature of epilepsy are gained not only from published work, but also through contact with patients. These latter views of epilepsy are patients' self-concepts of what it is to have this illness, and they may be assumed to be built up from patients' own interpretations of their experiences, and from their feelings about what others expect of someone with epilepsy. Many researchers into stigma in this illness and in other areas have also relied on patients' self-concepts of stigma for information about how far epilepsy is in fact, as well as in the sufferers' perceptions, an impediment in everyday life and in personal achievements (Schneider & Conrad, 1980). And although inferences about the effects of stigma made on the basis of data collected from sufferers are important in knowing what it is like to have epilepsy, it is not appropriate to assume that this information may be treated as objective data about personal achievement. Assessments of personal achievements of individuals with epilepsy should be based on comparisons of their achievements with those of others from similar social backgrounds.

Three different and quite separate strands of data about the stigmatizing nature of epilepsy may therefore be identified: first, the views of other people about the expected and likely social and personal consequences of epilepsy; second, the actual consequences of epilepsy in terms of such things as education, occupational achievement, and marriage; and third, the perceptions of sufferers from epilepsy about what life is like for them.

The aim of this chapter is to describe these different strands of data that may reflect different aspects of the stigmatizing effects of epilepsy, and to do so using information from a 36-year developmental follow-up study of a large national birth cohort. Cohort children who developed epilepsy in childhood and adolescence are compared with healthy cohort children from similar social backgrounds using data on teachers' views of their behavior at school and with others, on their educational, occupational, and marital histories, and on their own self-conceptions of life achievements. Because we believe that potentially stigmatizing experiences are likely to be very different for those with idiopathic as compared with symptomatic epilepsy, we have divided children with epilepsy into these two groups in our comparisons.

METHODS

The Medical Research Council's National Survey of Health and Development is a longitudinal study of a national sample of children born in 1 week in March 1946 in England, Wales, and Scotland. The sample comprises all legitimate single births to wives of nonmanual workers and to wives of agricultural workers, and one in four births to wives of other manual workers, a total of 5,362 children. These children have been studied at intervals of 2 years or less throughout childhood and adolescence, and at somewhat longer intervals in adult life, so far up to age 36. Information has been collected on a wide range of medical, sociological, psychological, and educational topics, and a full description of the study and a summary of work is given in Atkins, Cherry, Douglas, Kiernan, and Wadsworth (1981). Information on the cohort's health and illnesses was collected at school medical examinations carried out specifically for the study, and from hospital records followed up after reports of hospital admissions. Losses from the birth cohort have occurred through death and emigration, leaving 3,875 people as of 1982. When those still resident in England, Wales, or Scotland were last visited at home, 86% (n = 3,322) were contacted.

Cases were included in the study if they had experienced two or more seizures, at least one of which occurred after the age of 5, and if they had no evidence of acute illness accompanying the second or subsequent seizure(s). Prevalence of epilepsy thus identified in the cohort up to age 26 years was 46 cases; of these, 42 had been confirmed by a hospital specialist and four by reports from a school doctor or general practitioner (Britten, Morgan, Fenwick, & Britten, in preparation). Contact with the cohort at age 36 suggests that a maximum of 3 cases may have been missed, but at the time of writing these have not been confirmed. All of the 46 children with epilepsy had taken anticonvulsants continuously over long periods of time. Cases in which there was no evident cause for the seizures, and no evidence of other central nervous system pathology, were graded as idiopathic (30 cases), and the remaining 16 were graded as symptomatic. This follows the classification of Graham and Rutter (1968), in which we have used the term *idiopathic* where they used *uncomplicated*, and *symptomatic* for their term *complicated*. By the age of 26 (in 1972), 9 of the 46 cases had died, 2 had refused to cooperate with the survey, and 5 were not contacted, leaving 30 cases with complete information.

Two matched controls were obtained from within the study population for each child with epilepsy, and cases were matched on the basis of sex, father's social class, and area of residence when the child was 4 years old. Controls were chosen at random from among the remaining survey members who had not experienced any major illness and who had no mental or physical handicaps. Two kinds of comparison were made: The cohort members with epilepsy were compared with the whole of the rest of the cohort and also with their matched controls.

Teachers' ratings for each cohort child were used to construct an index of social visibility of children at school at 15 years, in other words, a measure of their conspicuousness in the eyes of other people. Teachers were asked to rate each child's behavior by choosing, for 19 different aspects of behavior, one of three possible statements that described that child best (Douglas, Ross, & Simpson, 1968). In most cases the teacher who made the ratings was the teacher who knew the child best. Pupils were rated regardless of type of school attended, and so the nine children with epilepsy who attended special schools for educationally subnormal children of all kinds (seven of the symptomatic and two of the idiopathic cases) are also included in the following discussion. The 19 aspects were roughness, attention seeking, daring, competitiveness, happiness, aggression, ability to make friends, physical energy, anxiety, reaction to criticism, truancy, disobedience, reaction to discipline, tendency to daydream, cribbing, lying, ability to work hard, concentration, and neatness in class work. Any behavior pattern teachers perceived as being uncommon (in the sense that fewer than about 20% of children were so described) was given a score of 1, and the common behaviors were given a score of zero. These scores were then summed to produce the index of visibility, values of which ranged from zero (no conspicuous behavior patterns) to 18 (visible on all but one of these aspects of behavior).

FINDINGS

Prevalence, Incidence, and Mortality from Epilepsy

Table 10-1 shows the incidence of epilepsy by age of onset. The figures given are population estimates, obtained by statistical weighting to compensate for

Table 10-1. Incidence of Epilepsy by Age of Onset[a]

Age of Onset in Years	*Idiopathic*	*Symptomatic*	*All*	*Rate per 1,000*[b] *Idiopathic*	*Symptomatic*	*All*
0–4	34 (10)	16 (7)	50 (17)	2.8	1.3	4.1
5–9	6 (3)	14 (5)	20 (8)	0.5	1.2	1.7
10–14	16 (7)	4 (1)	20 (8)	1.4	0.3	1.7
15–19	17 (8)	2 (2)	19 (10)	1.4	0.2	1.6
20–26	5 (2)	1 (1)	6 (3)	0.4	0.1	0.5
0–26	78 (30)	37 (16)	115 (46)	6.4	3.1	9.5

[a]Figures are population estimates, and the unweighted numbers are in parentheses.
[b]Apparent discrepancies are due to rounding errors.

the sampling procedure. The incidence for the first 26 years of life is 9.5 per 1,000. Overall, highest incidence occurred during the first 5 years, but whereas most symptomatic cases had arisen in childhood (0–9 years), most idiopathic cases had arisen after the age of 10. Ten years later in 1982, 12 of the 46 cases with epilepsy had died, 5 had refused to participate, 4 were abroad, and 4 were not traced in time to be included, leaving 21 who were successfully contacted. Thus the cumulative mortality of the group with epilepsy was 261 per 1,000 by age 36, compared with 58 per 1,000 for the rest of the cohort. In addition, a maximum of 12 cases of late onset (after 26 years) have yet to be confirmed. If all the possible new cases were to be confirmed, this would correspond to a prevalence of 11.8 per 1,000 at 36 years.

Since the cases have been identified at onset and subsequently followed up regardless of their current state, this study includes those in remission as well as those still having seizures. It also includes those with age of onset ranging from the earliest years to the mid-twenties, and this must be taken into account in the interpretation of findings about the effects of stigma.

Others' Views and Assessments

Many aspects of the debate about the role of stigma in the lives of children with epilepsy depend on the notion that children with this illness are recognizably different in various ways. If any such differentiation has occurred in this study it is likely to be reflected in teachers' reports on children's behavior and attitudes to school work. No information is available about whether teachers knew of children's illnesses when these reports were made, but we guess that in many cases teachers must have been aware; and as Wolff (1969) noted, "Once a handicap is recognised allowances are generally made for a child's failures."

The validity of the measure of social visibility (described earlier) for the cohort as a whole was assessed in an attempt to discover whether visibility as defined here made any difference to the final educational qualifications of children of comparable attainment and social background. Educational qualifications refer to the highest level of academic or vocational examinations passed by the individual concerned. Those survey members with high visibility scores were more likely to have no qualifications and less likely to have high qualifications, and this result is statistically significant at the 1% level. Social visibility is also associated with lower attainment test scores, described later, at 16 and 26 years. A multivariate log linear analysis (using the method of Nelder & Wedderburn, 1972), which took account of fathers' social class and the child's measured reading attainment at age 15, showed that not only was visibility associated with attainment at age 15, but it was even more strongly associated with final educational qualifications. Thus visibility as measured here certainly has some bearing on the progress of the whole cohort.

Having established the importance of the visibility score, is it associated with the poorer educational qualifications of the whole group with epilepsy? To assess the importance of the visibility score for the children with epilepsy, another multivariate log linear analysis was performed that also included the distinction between children with idiopathic epilepsy and those without epilepsy, but no significant associations were found either between idiopathic epilepsy and visibility or between idiopathic epilepsy and qualifications. It may be concluded that for the idiopathic group social visibility at school was not a problem either because they were not affected by visibility or because visibility was not associated with attainment for this group. Conclusions concerning the symptomatic group are less easy to draw because of the smaller numbers.

On the individual ratings, children with epilepsy were more likely to be rated as extreme in aggressiveness (being either unduly timid or aggressive) and in attention seeking (either showing off or avoiding attention) than the rest of the cohort children (for aggressiveness $\chi^2 = 5.92$ with 1 d.f., $p < 0.05$; for attention seeking, $\chi^2 = 4.37$ with 1 d.f., $p < 0.05$). On none of the other individual ratings were the differences between children with and without epilepsy (shown in Table 10-2) statistically significant.

Behavior Measures

Previous studies have shown that some children with epilepsy may experience behavior problems (e.g., Stores, 1975, 1978). They may also experience psy-

TABLE 10-2. Individual Behavior Ratings for Children With and Without Epilepsy (in %)

		Children with Epilepsy	*Rest of Cohort*
1. Roughness	Liable to get unduly rough during playtime	6.1[a]	4.3
	Rather frightened of rough games	27.3	19.5
2. Attention seeking[b]	Avoids attention, hates being in the limelight	18.2	15.0
	Shows off, seeks attention	21.2	7.6
3. Daring	A daredevil	6.1	4.5
	Extremely fearful	9.1	2.1
4. Competitiveness	Overcompetitive with other children	6.1	1.0
	Diffident about competing with other children	27.3	20.5
5. Happiness	Usually gloomy and sad	8.8	5.1

TABLE 10-2. Individual Behavior Ratings for Children With and Without Epilepsy (in %) (continued)

		Children with Epilepsy	*Rest of Cohort*
6. Aggressiveness[b]	A quarrelsome and aggressive child	2.9	1.7
	A timid child	23.5	9.9
7. Ability to make friends	Makes friends extremely easily	12.1	16.8
	Does not seem able to make friends	15.2	3.7
8. Energy	Extremely energetic, never tired	6.1	6.3
	Always tired and "washed out"	9.1	7.2
9. Anxiety	Very anxious, apprehensive, or fearful	6.1	1.2
10. Reaction to criticism or punishment	Tends to become unduly resentful	6.1	7.3
	Tends to become unduly miserable or worried	12.1	4.5
11. Truancy	Occasionally	5.9	3.5
	Frequently	0.0	0.7
12. Disobedience	Sometimes disobedient	29.4	21.2
	Frequently disobedient	0.0	1.7
13. Discipline	Sometimes difficult to discipline	14.7	10.8
	Frequently difficult to discipline	2.9	1.0
14. Daydreaming	Frequently daydreams in class	12.5	6.8
15. Cheating	Sometimes cheats	17.6	17.1
	Frequently cheats	0.0	1.6
16. Lying	Sometimes evades the truth to keep out of trouble	20.6	15.7
	Frequently evades the truth to keep out of trouble	0.0	1.6
17. Work	A poor worker or lazy	14.7	10.9
18. Concentration	One with high power of concentration	5.9	10.7
	Little or no power of sustained concentration	29.4	15.1
19. Neatness	Very untidy in class work	14.7	7.7

[a]I.e., 6.1% of children with epilepsy were rated as unduly rough and 27.3% were rated as rather frightened. Both groups were given a score of 1 when computing the visibility index.
[b]$p < .05$

chiatric problems (see Rutter, Graham, & Yule [1970] and Bagley [1971] for reviews of the literature). In the present study, although children with epilepsy tended to be rated as aggressive and attention seeking by their teachers, it is possible that these reports were biased by the teachers' knowledge of the child's illness. It was therefore important to see whether more objective indicators taken from the later years, when cohort members had left school, would reveal other signs of behavior difficulties.

Two indicators of behavior difficulties were used to compare children with epilepsy with others. First, data on delinquency in males up to age 21 were investigated using official reports of offending (Wadsworth, 1979). Of 21 boys with epilepsy, 5 (24%) were found to have been delinquent and all 5 had early onset of the illness. Though a higher proportion of those with epilepsy were reported as delinquent when compared with other boys (15% of whom were delinquent), the difference did not reach statistical significance. Delinquency in girls was too rare to permit a similar comparison for females.

Indicators of emotional disturbance were also examined. Reports of hospital admissions and of outpatient and general practitioner treatment for emotional disturbance, as well as self-assessments of stress collected while cohort members were aged 15–26, were assessed by a psychiatrist and made into a scale of disturbance that reflected treatment seeking. On this scale, 7 (18%) of 39 sufferers from epilepsy had had some medical treatment for emotional disturbance that had lasted a year or more, or had been admitted to a hospital for psychiatric care, as compared with 6.8% of the 4,572 men and women who had not had epilepsy ($\chi^2 = 5.85$ with Yates' correction and 1 d.f., $p < .05$).

Although there has been very little discussion of the "epileptic personality" in recent years, there is evidence that different types of personality may be associated with different types of epilepsy (Nuffield, 1961). Nuffield concluded that although environmental factors may determine the presence or absence of behavior disorders, it is the underlying physiology that determines the type and quality of the reaction. In the present study the short version of the Maudsley Personality Inventory (Eysenck, 1958) was used to assess two dimensions of personality, namely, neuroticism and extraversion, at ages 15 and 26. The personality scores of the cohort members with epilepsy were not significantly different from those of their matched controls at age 15, but this was not the case 11 years later. At age 26, idiopathic epilepsy was associated with increased neuroticism ($p < .025$). This is consistent with the view that neuroticism is a consequence of having epilepsy, whether or not it is largely a neurological consequence, a psychological consequence, or perhaps a result of the stigmatizing effects of other people's attitudes.

When we looked for associations of neuroticism with teachers' reports of behavior at school it was clear that high social visibility at school was associated with increased neuroticism at ages 15 and 26. However, in a log linear analysis the association between epilepsy and neuroticism remained significant even after the effect of social visibility at school had been taken into account, suggesting that it may not have been the attitudes of others that brought about the increased neuroticism of those with epilepsy.

From the information available to us in this cohort study we are unable to discern whether epilepsy as an illness is directly associated with the atypical signs of behavior described here, or whether it is rather more indirectly associated with individuals' reactions to having the illness, and possibly also to others' treatment of them; but it is evident that those with epilepsy were more inclined to emotional disorder than others. Hoare (1984) found that children with newly diagnosed epilepsy and those with chronic epilepsy had psychiatric disturbance, whereas children with newly diagnosed diabetes were less disturbed than those with chronic diabetes. He concluded that the simplest explanation was that the neurological dysfunction responsible for epilepsy also predisposed individuals to psychiatric disorder.

Education, Occupation, and Marital Status

We already have evidence that in this cohort children with chronic illness of all kinds were inclined to significant educational underachievement in comparison with healthy children from similar social circumstances (Wadsworth, 1985). This seems, in general, not so much the result of disruption of their school work as an effect of their emotional reaction to their illness; as Pless (1968) observed of the chronically ill cohort children in general, "Some become depressed, dependent and neurotic, while others show signs of aggression and assume an air of defiance and independence in an attempt to deny themselves and others the fact that they are in some respects disabled." Given that children with idiopathic epilepsy seem not to have been assessed as especially disruptive at school, apart from an increase in aggressive and attention-seeking behavior, it seemed particularly important in this longitudinal study to see whether their generally inconspicuous classroom behavior was associated with good educational achievement, and in due course with relatively stable job histories.

At the age of 15 cohort members took tests of both verbal and nonverbal attainment; the Watts-Vernon test assesses reading ability and the Group Ability Test (AH4) has separate verbal and nonverbal sections (Pidgeon, 1968). The tests were administered to the study children by their own class teachers, and the testing was carried out in conjunction with the National Foundation for Educational Research in England and Wales and the Scottish Council for Research in Education.

It was to be expected that some children with epilepsy would have learning problems (Stores & Hart, 1976). However, the only evidence of learning difficulties in this study was shown by the group with symptomatic epilepsy whose nonverbal test scores at age 15 were significantly lower than those of their matched controls.

We also compared the final achieved educational levels of children with epilepsy with those of their controls. To do this we used as scores the highest educational qualification achieved by the age of 26. Educational qualifications of the symptomatic and idiopathic cases, taken together, were significantly lower than those of their controls (Wilcoxon matched pairs test $p < .05$), but this lower performance was accounted for by the scores of those with symptomatic epilepsy, and those with idiopathic epilepsy were not significantly lower.

There was no evidence of poorer occupational achievement as measured by socioeconomic position (Office of Population Censuses and Surveys, 1970) at age 26 for the idiopathic group when compared with matched healthy controls. There seemed to be a link between socioeconomic achievement and teachers' assessments during the school years, in that those with high visibility scores were more likely to have manual jobs than those who had been less socially visible. It may be, however, that these measures of socioeconomic status based on occupation are not sufficiently sensitive to detect lack of achievement by, or discrimination against, survey members with epilepsy.

A log linear analysis was carried out to examine the associations between verbal attainment at age 15, the experience of epilepsy, father's social class, social visibility at the school, and occupational achievement at age 26. There was no association between social class in adulthood and either epilepsy or social visibility, suggesting (for the idiopathic group at least) that visibility, if it may be seen as an indicator of stigma, was not a serious problem.

When cohort members were 36 years old, seven of the nine male idiopathic cases were in paid employment, compared with all nine controls; three of the seven female idiopathic cases were in paid employment, compared with five controls. Too few of the symptomatic cases remained for comparisons of their occupational achievements by this age, partly as a result of a high death rate (20% of them had died by this age) and also because of the relatively high failure-to-contact rate (26.7% of the 30 were not contacted).

There is some evidence in the literature that the sexuality of men with epilepsy may be affected (Lindsay, Ounsted, & Richards, 1979) and that the fertility of women with epilepsy may be lower than that of women in the general population (Dansky, Andermann, & Andermann, 1980). However, there is no evidence of any differences in marital status or fertility between survey members with and without epilepsy at the age of 26.

Thus, there is a suggestion of change in the fortunes of those who had suffered childhood idiopathic epilepsy. In terms of educational qualifications they seemed to differ very little from controls, nor did they differ in respect to their socioeconomic circumstances achieved by the age of 26. But 10 years later, at 36, their socioeconomic circumstances were worse than those of the controls, though differential loss makes it difficult to conclude with certainty that the economic circumstances of the whole group had deteriorated. For the symptomatic cases there was evidence of poorer educational qualifications, but not of poorer occupational attainment.

Self-perceptions

So far, our findings reveal very little that is different when comparing the early adult social lives of children who had idiopathic epilepsy with those of controls, and these findings are not in accord with what the literature led us to expect. We imagined that the effect of the stigma of epilepsy would have been revealed in some aspects of the sufferers' school and work lives, but we have found very little to support this expectation. However, we have not yet looked at possible effects of stigmatization in the self-concepts of those who had idiopathic epilepsy and it is here that we should also expect to find evidence of a difference between sufferers and controls.

Our data on self-concept were collected when cohort members were 36 years old and derive from questions that asked the study population to review their lives, particularly in respect to their education, work, and family lives. When compared with controls, significantly more of those who had had idiopathic epilepsy felt that life had, in general, not been good to them, and more felt discontented with their working lives, but not with education or family life. This particular difference in discontent accords with the evidence of falling socioeconomic fortunes by this age of those who had had childhood idiopathic epilepsy.

It is not clear from these differences in self-perception whether cohort members actively felt stigmatized by their epilepsy, although we do know that they tended to attribute their difficulties to bad luck rather than to some fault of their own, but these replies are nevertheless not inconsistent with a stigmatizing effect.

The differences between subjects with epilepsy and their matched controls are summarized in Table 10-3.

CONCLUSIONS

It is clear that the number of individuals with epilepsy who were contacted by age 36 years was considerably lower than the number originally identified. Of the 46 cases identified by age 26, half were not contacted 10 years later

TABLE 10-3. Summary of Differences Between Subjects with Epilepsy and Their Matched Controls[a]

	Subjects with Symptomatic Epilepsy	*Subjects with Idiopathic Epilepsy*
Reading test at 15 years	n.s. ($p > .025$)	n.s.($p > .025$)
Nonverbal ability at 15 years	$0.01 < p < .025$	n.s.($p > .025$)
Neuroticism at 15 years	*	n.s.($p > .025$)
Extraversion at 15 years	*	n.s.($p > .025$)
Reading test at 26 years	n.s. ($p > .025$)	n.s.($p > .025$)
Neuroticism at 26 years	*	$p < .005$
Extraversion at 26 years	*	n.s.($p > .025$)
Level of educational and vocational qualifications achieved at 26 years	*	n.s.($p > .05$)
Social class at 26 years	*	n.s.($p > .05$)
+Marital status at 26 years	n.s. ($p > .1$)	n.s.($p > .8$)
+Children at 26 years	n.s. ($p > .5$)	n.s.($p > .5$)
Paid work at 36 years	*	*
Self-perception at 36 years	*	$p < .05$

[a]*Indicates that there were too few cases with nonmissing data to perform the test. +Statistical significance was assessed by means of the Wilcoxon matched pairs test (which distinguishes only three levels of significance for a one tailed test: .025, .01 and .005), except for dichotomized variables, marked +, which were tested using the Pike-Morrow test (Pike & Morrow, 1970). This latter test produces a test statistic that is distributed approximately as chi-square on one degree of freedom. n.s. = not significant.

but the most prominent reason for this was death (12 had died). At 36 years five people refused to be interviewed, a considerably higher rate of refusal than among controls, and this may reflect a desire for concealment among those with epilepsy; it is also possible that the four we could not trace wanted to conceal their illness.

However, the importance of this study lies not so much in the numbers of cohort members with epilepsy as in the unusual opportunity it provides both to look at the problems of childhood and early adult epilepsy across time, and to look at stigma associated with this illness in several different ways.

Adolescence is a sensitive time, when children are especially anxious to conform with their age peers. Children who are different in some way usually react by trying particularly hard to be liked, either by their age peers, or by their teachers, and they are therefore likely to be more visible in a social sense than others as a result of their behavior. Adolescence is also a time when teachers' and parents' expectations of children's behavior and achievements are strongly associated with later educational success (Douglas, 1964; Douglas et al., 1968). Such expectations and assessments by self and others are the basis for stigma (Schneider & Conrad, 1980; West, 1976, 1983), and therefore adolescence is a good time to look for evidence of stigma associated with epilepsy. It is also, in this study, a time when 34 of the 46 children with epilepsy were already diagnosed, and therefore data on teachers' views of cohort children's behavior and educational chances collected at 15 years were examined. It is arguable that the teachers' opinions will have a strong influence on the children's educational achievements and that they are therefore potentially damaging sources of stigma.

From the evidence of this birth cohort study we suggest that it may be helpful to move away from assumptions that stigmatizing effects of epilepsy can be seen as unidimensional and static in time. We propose that, contrary to common research practice, it is important to examine possible stigmatizing processes and effects separately from several different points of view. For example, it is valuable to separate evidence of self-perceptions of stigma from more objective evidence about possible effects of the process of stigma, and to do so taking into account the severity of the illness.

On the more objective measures available in this study, such as the childrens' test scores, their teachers' assessments, and their occupational and educational achievements, there was little evidence of either poorer abilities or discrimination among those with epilepsy. It is therefore difficult to conclude that active discrimination or "enacted" stigma (Scambler, 1982) from these sources was a critical factor for children with epilepsy. It is true that there is some suggestion of poorer occupational achievement at age 36, but this may be due to differential loss of the more successful of this group, or a reflection of either economic circumstances or the tendency of discriminating attitudes to gain force with the passage of time. But the bulk of our results do not support the view that objective manifestations of stigma were a potent discriminating factor.

However, the more subjective measures used in this study do support the notion of "felt" stigma (Scambler, 1982). Children with epilepsy were more prone to emotional and psychiatric disturbance, and were markedly more neurotic than their peers from similar backgrounds. As adults, their self-concepts were significantly poorer than those of these same peers.

The disparity between these objective and subjective measures requires some explanation, which cannot be given using the existing data in this study. Our results suggest that stigma may have been felt by those with epilepsy, and it would be surprising if none was experienced. We must conclude from our findings that these people have managed to overcome or to accommodate the prejudice they feel from others, that prejudice is not as strong as they think, or that they have deliberately chosen concealment as a method of coping with the attitudes of others.

We also found that stigma seemed to vary with age. Our concept, described here, of the changing views of health care professionals about what causes epilepsy and about its effects on the lives of sufferers shows a cohort effect in this aspect of stigma, but we had not anticipated changes within the lives of our cohort members. We were therefore surprised at the suggestion that although those who had had idiopathic epilepsy in childhood were apparently little different from controls in their socioeconomic achievements at the age of 26, at age 36 there was some indication that in comparison they might have slid into relatively worse socioeconomic circumstances. If this has, in fact, occurred we suspect that it may be the result of changing self-perceptions. Whereas in their school years the children with epilepsy seemed to have reacted to their illness with some form of aggression and attention seeking, it may be that later in life coping takes a more withdrawn form, anticipated in this study by the greater neuroticism and, later, worse self-perceptions of those who had epilepsy in childhood. At work, this might take the form of an uncomfortable awareness of the need to conceal their illness or its history (Rodin, Lennick, Dendrill, & Lin, 1972), and in due course being obliged to take work of a lower social status.

Although we do not have all the necessary data to confirm these notions of a change in the process of stigma in epilepsy, it seems evident from our data that changes occur, and that in order to detect them and search for their causes, it is necessary to examine stigma from several points of view.

REFERENCES

Atkins, E., N. Cherry, J. W. B. Douglas, K. E. Kiernan, & M. E. J. Wadsworth. (1981). The 1946 British birth cohort: An account of the origins, progress and results of the National Survey of Health and Development. In S. A. Mednick and A. E. Baert (Eds.), *Prospective longitudinal research: An empirical basis for the primary prevention of psychosocial disorders. Oxford: Oxford University Press.*

Bagley, C. (1971). *The social psychology of the child with epilepsy.* London: Routledge & Kegan Paul.

Bagley, C. (1972). Social prejudice and the adjustment of people with epilepsy. *Epilepsia* 13, 33–45.

Britten, N., K. Morgan, P. B. C. Fenwick, & H. Britten. Incidence of epilepsy in the first 36 years of life. In preparation.

Clark, L. P. (1925). Some psychological data regarding the interpretation of essential epilepsy. *Journal of Nervous and Mental Disease* 61, 51–59.

Dansky, L. V., E. Andermann, & F. Andermann. (1980). Marriage and fertility in epileptic patients. *Epilepsia* 21, 261–71.

Douglas, J. W. B. (1964). *The home and the school.* London: MacGibbon & Kee.

Douglas, J. W. B., J. M. Ross, & H. R. Simpson. (1968). *All our future.* London: Peter Davies.

Eysenck, J. H. (1958). A short questionnaire for the measurement of two dimensions of personality. *Journal of Applied Psychology* 42, 14–17.

Goffman, E. (1963). *Stigma.* Harmondsworth: Penguin Books.
Graham, P., & M. Rutter. (1968). Organic brain dysfunction and child psychiatric disorder. *British Medical Journal* 3, 695–700.
Hoare, P. (1984). The development of psychiatric disorder among schoolchildren with epilepsy. *Developmental Medicine and Child Neurology* 26, 3–13.
Illingworth, C. M., & R. S. Illingworth. (1984). Mothers are easily worried. *Archives of Disease in Childhood* 59, 380–84.
Jolly, H. (1980). *Book of child care.* London: Sphere Books.
Liddiard, M. (1944). *The mothercraft manual.* London: Churchill.
Lindsay, J., C. Ounsted, & P. Richards. (1979). Long-term outcome in children with temporal lobe seizures. II. Marriage, parenthood and sexual indifference. *Developmental Medicine and Child Neurology* 21, 433–40.
Nelder, J. A., & R. W. M. Wedderburn. (1972). Generalised linear models. *Journal of the Royal Statistical Society* 135A, 370–84.
Nuffield, E. J. A. (1961). Neuro-physiology and behaviour disorders in epileptic children. *Journal of Mental Science,* 107, 438–58.
Office of Health Economics (1971). *Epilepsy in society.* London: Office of Health Economics.
Office of Population Censuses and Surveys. (1970). *Classification of occupations 1970.* London: Her Majesty's Stationery Office.
Pidgeon, D. (1968). Appendix I: Details of the fifteen year tests. In J. W. B. Douglas, J. M. Ross, & H. R. Simpson, *All our future.* London: Peter Davies.
Pike, M. C., & R. H. Morrow. (1970). Statistical analysis of patient-control studies in epidemiology. *British Journal of Preventive and Social Medicine* 24, 42–44.
Pless, I. B. (1968). A heavy load of illness. In J. W. B. Douglas, J. M. Ross, & H. R. Simpson (Eds.), *All our future.* London: Peter Davies.
Rodin, E. P., P. Rennick, Y. Dennerell, & Y. Lin. (1972). Vocational and education problems of epileptic patients. *Epilepsia* 13, 149–60.
Rutter, M., P. Graham, & W. Yule. (1970). *A neuropsychiatric study in childhood.* London: Spastics International Medical Publications.
Scambler, G. (1982). Deviance, labelling and stigma. In D. L. Patrick & G. Scambler (Eds.), *Sociology as applied to medicine.* London: Bailliere Tindall.
Schneider, J. W., & P. Conrad. (1980). In the closet with illness: Epilepsy, stigma potential and information control. *Social Problems* 28, 32–44.
Stores, G. (1975). Behavioural effects of anti-epileptic drugs. *Developmental Medicine and Child Neurology* 17, 647–58.
Stores, G. (1978). School-children with epilepsy at risk for learning and behavioural problems. *Developmental Medicine and Child Neurology* 20, 502–508.
Stores, G., & J. Hart. (1976). Reading skills of children with generalised or focal epilepsy attending ordinary school. *Developmental Medicine and Child Neurology* 18, 705–16.
Truby King, F. (1937). *Feeding and care of baby.* Auckland: Whitcombe & Tombs.
Wadsworth, M. E. J. (1979). *Roots of delinquency.* New York: Barnes & Noble.
Wadsworth, M. E. J. (1985). Intergenerational differences in child health. In Office of Population Censuses and Surveys, *Measuring Socio-Demographic Change.* Occasional paper No. 34. London: Office of Population Census Surveys
West, P. B. (1976). The physician and the management of childhood epilepsy. In M. Wadsworth & D. Robinson (Eds.), *Studies in everyday medical life.* London: Martin Robertson.

West, P. B. (1983). Acknowledging epilepsy: Improving professional management of stigma and its consequences. In M. Parsonage, R. H. E. Grant, A. G. Craig, & A. A. Ward (Eds.), *Advances in epileptology: XIVth Epilepsy International Symposium.* New York: Raven Press.
Wolff, S. (1969). *Children under stress.* London: Allen Lane.

11 / The Social Meaning of Epilepsy: Stigma as a Potential Explanation for Psychopathology in Children

PATRICK WEST

> It's all connected with a disease of the mind and that's a dirty word. Anybody who's had something wrong with their mind is looked down upon by other people . . . Because you lose control of your senses same as a silly person does, there seems to be some stigma there which everybody—even doctors—tries to keep under cover.

> I don't think it's anything like being completely deaf or completely blind. I don't think of it as being a really serious handicap. I'd put it just a bit worse than being shortsighted.

These contrasting views about the social meaning of epilepsy were expressed by two parents, each of whom had a child with epilepsy. Clinically, the children presented with rather similar characteristics. Both had a normal perinatal history, an onset around 2 years of age, and a diagnosis corresponding to the classification "primary generalised epilepsies" (Commission on Classification and Terminology of the International League against Epilepsy, 1981). The first, a girl, had several intermittent seizures until the age of 8 and thereafter some ill-documented "vacant attacks"; the second, a boy, commenced with numerous absences and by age 15 had developed tonic-clonic seizures.

The differences in gender and seizure pattern apart, on clinical criteria alone the two cases are as near equivalent as is likely to be found in most studies of epilepsy. In terms of the "effects" of biological variables such as seizure type or onset age on personality or behavior, it might be expected the children would display similar profiles. According to their parents, they did not. The girl was depicted as "backward, lazy, immature, defiant, and terribly bad-tempered"; the boy as "intelligent, good-natured, and extroverted."

If biological variables do not in these two cases explain differences in personality, there are other factors of a social nature that might. With regard to the meaning of epilepsy and ensuing consequences for parents and children, the cases could hardly be more different. The girl's parents, acutely conscious of the "stigma" of epilepsy, were committed to a policy of concealing the child's disorder and, to minimize the risk of exposure, restricted her participation in activities outside the home. Inasmuch as she had not had a seizure in public, the strategy had proven effective. The boy's parents, in contrast, expressed a belief in the tolerance and understanding of others and were committed to a policy of maximum disclosure and maximum participation in activities. The strategy had been reinforced by the sympathetic reactions experienced on the occasions his seizures had been witnessed.

For both sets of parents, the adoption of these diverse strategies was intended to achieve the same goal—to "keep their child as normal as possible." The first may have been outwardly successful but had failed in their attempts to secure a normal identity for the child, perhaps in part because of the very strategy pursued to achieve that end. In their eyes, she had become "epileptic." Their "explanation" of her identity was in terms of defects attributable to her epileptic condition; it was not something within their control. In the second case, the combination of a policy of disclosure and participation in activities had resulted in the achievement of normality both inside and outside the family. The boy remained a "normal child with seizures," and as a consequence there was simply less to account for. His parents perceived the maintenance of normal identity as being within their own and the boy's control.

The focus on these contrasting cases, both drawn from a study of 24 families, sets the scene for this chapter. For the most part, scientific explanations of the relationship between epilepsy and psychopathology have concentrated heavily on biological variables (Hermann & Whitman, 1984). As the two cases illustrate, such an exclusive orientation seriously underestimates the potential significance of social factors. Yet when such factors have been included in research, they typically fail to address the issue of what epilepsy means to families, the type and effectiveness of strategies adopted, and the ensuing consequences for the child. Even the best studies that show the importance of parental attitudes and behavior treat those variables as if they existed in a social vacuum. The study reported here, although not directly designed to investigate the relationship between epilepsy and psychopathology, is intended to draw attention to the potential importance of the meaning of epilepsy as a factor in its genesis. In particular, it suggests the need to reformulate social factors in terms of stigma and its consequences for the identity of children with epilepsy.

EXPLANATIONS FOR PSYCHOPATHOLOGY

Nuffield (1961) observed more than 20 years ago that explanations of the relationship between epilepsy and psychopathology sharply divided the "organicists" from the "environmentalists." That observation seems to be as true now as it was then. Indeed, with the refinement of variables of both an organic and environmental nature, the addition of treatment variables and the emphasis on multifactorial etiology, the situation seems ever more complex. What, though, are the essential features of organicist and environmental explanations, and how might some of the problems of interpretation associated with them be clarified by a focus on the social meaning of epilepsy?

Organicist Explanations

Organicist explanations rest on the proposition that there is some inherent defect in the person, or some persons, with epilepsy that is causally linked to the genesis of psychopathology. In that respect, it stems from the now universally rejected concept of the "epileptic personality" (Tizard, 1962; Williams, 1967). With the demise of constitutional explanations, attention switched to an examination of the effects of brain damage, of which seizures were only one manifestation. Bradley's (1951) distinction between "primary behavior disturbances," attributable to "disordered cerebral function," and "secondary" disturbance arising as a consequence of reactions to the disorder provided a conceptual framework that distinguished between epilepsies associated with structural brain damage and those that were not. Recent work has formulated the issue in much more sophisticated terms, focusing in particular on seizure type and electroencephalographic categories. Of particular interest is the relationship between a temporal lobe focus and psychopathology.

Research in the organicist tradition has by and large failed to produce a consistent pattern of findings. Some investigators (Bridge, 1949; Grunberg & Pond, 1957) found no correlation between brain damage in epilepsy and "personality" or "conduct disorder"; others, like Rutter, Graham, and Yule (1970), did. Similar contradictions are apparent in what has become known as the temporal lobe controversy. Nuffield (1961) found children with a temporal lobe focus to be more aggressive than those with a "3/sec spike and wave" pattern; others, like Wilson and Harris (1966), did not. Stores (1978) found the presence of a left temporal focus to be related to "behavioural disorder." Whitman, Hermann, Black, and Chhabria (1982) found neither a seizure type nor laterality effect, though some relationship existed between a focus in the anterior temporal lobe and higher scores on an aggresssion scale. These investigators, however, placed this finding in the context that the vast majority of neurological and biological variables included in their study showed no relationship at all with aggression or other measures of psychopathology.

Although the one certain conclusion of research in this tradition is that the scope of possible etiologic significance attributable to biological factors appears to have gradually narrowed from all sufferers to those with brain damage and subsequently to those with temporal lobe epilepsy, this does not explain why recent broadly comparable studies produce such diverse findings. One major reason why this might be so resides in the problematic assumption that in the identification of subjects with similar characteristics such as onset age, seizure type, or EEG focus equivalence of effect has been achieved. The assumption is true only if it is held that such variables are uncontaminated by environmental or social factors. As the two cases in the introduction show, quite diverse meanings can be associated with similar clinical profiles. The implication, of course, is that without controlling for social variables, it is not possible to assess the true etiologic significance of organic factors that might paradoxically turn out to be more important than current research suggests is the case.

Environmental Explanations

The potential significance of environmental variables in the genesis of psychopathology is suggested by the continual references made by investigators and other commentators to the problem of prejudice and discrimination epilepsy sufferers are believed to encounter in society. This prejudice and discrimination would seem to be at the heart of environmental explanations of psychopathology, yet the environmentalists have not approached the problem from this perspective but have focused instead on the pathogenic consequences of particular environments to which children are exposed. The approach, therefore, fails to address in a direct way the social meaning of epilepsy either as it underpins the reactions of others or as it shapes the experience of having a child with epilepsy in the family.

One of the earlier studies in this tradition (Grunberg & Pond, 1957) found that children with epilepsy who displayed "conduct disorder" were distinguished from another group who did not by an excess of environmental problems that included disturbed parental attitudes, sibling rivalry, restrictions, and changes in environment. Later work by Bagley (1971) confirmed these findings and drew attention in particular to parental attitudes such as maternal overprotectiveness in the development of aggressive "behavior disorder." Further evidence of the importance of parents' attitudes was provided by Hartlage and Green (1972) and Long and Moore (1979). The latter found parents had lower expectations and were stricter and more dominant with their child with epilepsy than they were with a nonepileptic sibling. The possible significance of the "overprotective" mother, alluded to by several investigators, was further highlighted in another pilot study conducted by Mulder and Suurmeijer (1977).

One of these investigators (Suurmeijer, 1980) provides the best example of research in the environmentalist tradition to date. The sample consisted of 109 matched pairs of children with epilepsy and healthy controls whose parents provided information on a range of issues including their emotional and "pedagogic" relationship to the child, restrictions imposed, reactions of peers, and behavioral characteristics and academic achievements of the child. Both mothers and fathers of the epilepsy group were found to be more worried and frustrated, more overprotective, and more likely to impose restrictions than those in the control group. Correspondingly, the children with epilepsy were reported to have experienced more negative peer reaction, more isolation, and to have more behavioral problems and lower educational achievement. In contrast to organic variables, which had little effect on the functioning of the child with epilepsy, the environmental variables were correlated in rather complex ways. Suurmeijer concluded that negative reactions were both a cause and effect of restrictions that, in turn, promoted withdrawal, further restrictions, and lowered expectations for the child.

If it is admitted that much greater consistency of findings characterizes the environmentalist than the organicist tradition, it is by no means self-evident what the variables of etiologic significance are meant to represent and what position in a chain of cause-effect relations they occupy. For example, the oft-cited overprotective mother could be a descriptor of a personality trait possessed by some individuals and not others just as well as it could indicate a particular style of coping developed as a reaction to a child's epilepsy. Similarly, protectiveness or restrictiveness may be conceptualized simply as styles of reacting to the child, or they may be seen, however implicitly, as components of a broader strategy of averting perceived negative consequences of epilepsy. The parents of the girl featured in the introduction are undoubtedly overprotective and extremely restricting, but to label them as such singularly fails to recognize that for them these behaviors are logical corollaries of a commitment to concealing at almost all costs.

The problem, in short, is that although research into environmental factors has produced significant advances in our knowledge, the independent variables (parental attitudes and behavior) are conceptualized as fixed properties of individuals that somehow exist in a social vacuum. We know how these attitudes are distributed and the effects on the child but we do not know very much about why they are held. Without examining the broader context in which such attitudes and behaviors develop, there is a danger that we investigate only part of the whole issue and misrepresent the reality of what it means to have a child with epilepsy. Nevertheless, the cumulative evidence of research into environmental factors does suggest that the interrelationship among negative reaction, parental worries, restrictiveness, and the child's identity might themselves be components of an overarching orientation adopted by families toward epilepsy. A reformulation of the environmental factor in terms of social meaning rather than sociopathy may go some way to resolving the problem.

Potential Stigma Explanations

To date, no study has specifically addressed the way in which the subjective meaning of epilepsy might be related to psychopathology. There is, however, an increasing body of research, principally focusing on adult sufferers, which endeavors to document what epilepsy means to people, particularly in terms of stigma and its management. For persons with epilepsy, whose situation is generically "discreditable" rather than "discredited" (Goffman, 1963), a central possibility is that normal identity may be achieved by concealing potentially discrediting information. The evidence so far suggests there is greater variation than the generic situation implies.

Scambler and Hopkins (1980; Scambler, 1982, pp. 184–92) have proposed that the situation of epilepsy sufferers is characterized less by "enacted stigma," overt prejudice and discrimination by others than by "felt stigma," a deep sense of shame about "being epileptic," and an oppressive and largely erroneous belief that others are ever poised to stigmatize. In their study of 94 adults with epilepsy, Scambler and Hopkins found that only a minority recalled any instances of stigmatization at all, a pattern contrasting markedly with the pervasive sense of shame and fear of negative reaction that made up their sense of felt stigma. Typically, the sense of felt stigma preceded episodes of stigmatization and predisposed these individuals to concealment. Typically, too, felt stigma constituted a major source of unhappiness exceeding that attributable to enacted stigma.

A less all-embracing view of the situation of adult sufferers emerges from Schneider and Conrad's (1980) study. They found in their sample that a sense of the shamefulness of epilepsy was not invariably experienced. Despite the potential for concealment, the majority adopted a selective strategy of managing information, concealing from some audiences, disclosing to others. To a large extent, which strategy was adopted in which circumstances depended on what others as "stigma coaches" encouraged them to do. Parents were especially important in this respect, because the more they had conveyed an attitude of shame the greater the commitment to concealing. Paralleling the earlier findings of Kleck (1968), when sufferers did risk disclosure, however, they often found that the reactions of others were not as hostile as they had supposed. For these persons, "testing" societal reaction reinforced a belief that having epilepsy was compatible with normal identity.

Further evidence that epilepsy does not invariably involve a stigma was found in another study of 445 adults with epilepsy (Ryan, Kempner, & Emlen, 1980). Using a measure of perceived stigma, these investigators found considerable variation in the extent to which it was experienced. Furthermore, it was only very moderately related to an index of seizure severity derived from data on seizure type and frequency, the effect of which was further mediated by other social and psychological characteristics of respondents. Although the authors did not comment on the relative importance of felt and enacted stigma, it is clear that inasmuch as seizure severity denotes visibility and, therefore, differential likelihood of stigmatization, that perceived stigma was largely independent of the negative reactions of others.

To the author's knowledge, there has been no research into families with a child with epilepsy that directly addresses the issue of stigma. Its potential importance must be inferred from a small number of studies in which some data were collected on disclosure patterns. Ward and Bower (1978) in a study of 81 families found that the great majority of parents had informed the school and that, although there was more evidence of concealing from other family members and friends, in general most had adopted an open policy with, it seems, a broadly sympathetic reaction from others. A similar picture of general assent to disclosure was documented in another study (Goldin, Perry, Margolin, Stotsky, & Foster, 1971). The authors found that only 21% of parents believed it was in the child's interests to conceal epilepsy. More evidence of concealing is implied by Hodgman, McAnarney, Myers, Iker, McKinney, et al. (1979), who, although not reporting disclosure rates, found in a group of adolescents that those with better seizure control were less likely to be open about their epilepsy. Long and Moore (1979), too, noted that one third of the parents in their sample were unwilling to discuss epilepsy with the child, which suggests a tendency to concealment. It also suggests, of course, that for some parents their commitment to concealing may extend to the children themselves.

The cumulative evidence from these studies suggests that the situation of epilepsy sufferers is characterized more by felt stigma than episodes of actual stigmatization, that it is not universally experienced, that it is largely unrelated to seizure type and frequency, and that while predisposing to concealment this is not invariably practiced. The attitude of parents appears to be crucially related to the extent of felt stigma and the strategy adopted to manage it. The importance of parents as stigma coaches also suggests that their advocated management styles are not only adopted on behalf of the child, but may reflect what they themselves feel about having a child with epilepsy. In that respect, they can be generically depicted as having a "courtesy stigma" (Birenbaum,

1970). That they may themselves experience shame suggests their problem is not confined to the management of information alone but to securing a normal identity for the child that does not threaten their claim to normality.

These observations point to a way in which the potentially stigmatized situation of families with a child with epilepsy might be linked to the findings of environmentalists that parental attitudes are of etiologic significance for the development of psychopathology. It suggests that those attitudes are at least in part a consequence of the degree to which parents experience felt stigma, the strategies adopted to manage it, and their effectiveness in achieving normal identity. In terms of the effects on the child's identity, what epilepsy means to parents and the way they cope with it could have consequences in at least three ways: first, by affirming or ameliorating the sense of shame experienced by the child; second, by limiting or facilitating the child's participation in activities; and third, by decreasing or increasing the likelihood of stigmatization. In view of the documented effects of negative peer reaction, the effectiveness of stigma strategies in making this reaction more or less likely would seem crucial.

One further aspect of the hypothesized interplay between stigma, strategies, and the reactions of others merits consideration, and this relates to parents' own knowledge and interpretations of the child's identity. Parents, like anybody else, are not without knowledge at the outset of their child's epilepsy; they have certain ideas and images that might be expected to resemble those found in a number of studies of public knowledge (Remschmidt, 1973; Vinson, 1975; West, 1981, pp. 3–12). Such knowledge often contains a stereotyped image of "epileptic" identity and is likely not only to comprise a component of felt stigma, but also to constitute a framework within which the parents may judge their own child. It may generate expectations, represent what the child might become, or provide an "explanation" of identity. The question arises, then, as to how parents interpret those images and what the consequences of their interpretations are.

We now turn to the interrelationship among these hypothesized features of the experience of having a child with epilepsy. The investigation reported cannot prove a link between these factors and psychopathology, but it does suggest ways in which diverse meanings associated with epilepsy might be related to different identity profiles in children.

PERSPECTIVE AND METHODS

The starting point of the study was precisely that which the environmentalists might have adopted: to treat the meaning of epilepsy as the central focus of investigation. In contrast to the prevalent model of research into the relationship between epilepsy and psychopathology, which seeks to establish statistical relationships between variables, the approach taken in this study was essentially qualitative. The key distinguishing feature of this perspective is that instead of defining the subject's reality in terms of the investigator's concepts, an attempt is made to understand and reproduce the way that people themselves experience and interpret their world (Schwartz & Jacobs, 1979). It may complement existing quantitative research in the sense that it provides fuller interpretations for observed statistical regularities, but in its focus on subjective experience it offers a means of attending to the complexity of social processes not easily captured in survey methodology.

Twenty-four families containing 26 children with a confirmed or suspected diagnosis of epilepsy were selected from the EEG department and outpatient clinics in a children's hospital. As far as possible they were consecutive attenders, the only criteria for inclusion being (a) that the children should not have associated disabilities contingent on structural brain damage, and (b) that they were of secondary school age or thereabouts. The former was adopted to minimize the likelihood that parents' definitions of the disorder were complicated by other medical conditions; the latter because it was thought older children would be better informants in a proposed complementary child-based study. For largely practical reasons (West, 1979), it proved impossible to accomplish this latter goal in a consistent manner. What data there are on the child's perspective, though often illuminating, are essentially anecdotal.

Three of the 26 children were cases of suspected epilepsy that was subsequently rejected as a diagnosis. These children are excluded from the analysis along with one other whose parental data were very incomplete. The remaining group was slightly biased toward females (12 girls, 10 boys) but comparable in social class to community-based samples. Clinically, they displayed a variety of seizure types; 13 children had a history of tonic–clonic seizures, 2 experienced absences, and 7 had a mixed pattern, 4 of whom had attacks suggestive of temporal lobe epilepsy. They had later onset ages (mean: 7 years 3 months) and more severe seizure disorders than would be expected in an unselected sample. Given the central focus of the investigation, however, it was essential to maximize the probability that epilepsy was perceived as a current problem for families. Although the sample is clearly not representative of the population of children with epilepsy of comparable age, the observed patterns may be quite typical of the situation many families experience at some more critical stages in their child's career.

In order to elicit and comprehend the meanings associated with epilepsy, a tactic of getting as close to the families as possible was adopted, a strategy corresponding to what Lofland (1976) termed the development of "intimate familiarity." Accordingly, interviews of a loosely structured conversational type, usually lasting between 2 and 4 hours, were conducted with one or both parents in their own home. In addition, every opportunity was taken to maintain informal contact, which varied from casual conversation in outpatient clinics to participation in family activities. Most of the parents were contacted on at least two occasions over the course of about 1 year, the most extensively researched case comprising 10 major interviews and numerous informal contacts. With the exception of one family, all interviews were taped and transcribed.

The interviews were designed to cover a range of topics organized around the child's biography, including onset of seizures, initial definition of the event, contact with medical agencies, and any salient events up to the time of interview. In addition, much broader topics were addressed relating to parents' previous experience and knowledge of epilepsy, their perception of societal views of epilepsy, evaluations of doctors, strategies for managing the child's problem, descriptions of the child and why they thought he or she was like that, aspects of family life, the reactions of others, and their own "theories" of epilepsy. From the mass of data collected, the focus here is on the nature and extent of parents' felt stigma; the range of strategies they, as stigma coaches, practiced; the effectiveness of those strategies in securing normality; and their interpretations of the child's identity.

FINDINGS

Felt Stigma

Data relating to parents' feelings of stigma are available from several sources in the interview transcripts. Of particular importance are the stories they told about people with epilepsy they encountered prior to the onset of their child's seizures.

For five of them, the characters they recalled were essentially "ordinary" persons, living normal lives in a context of sympathetic tolerance. For example:

> A lad who used to play cricket with us and used occasionally to have a fit. It was almost part of the game. Any new player of course would be somewhat taken aback at first but the rest of the lads used to accept it, and because the rest accepted it they'd accept it in the same manner.

For another seven, the characters were portrayed quite differently:

> A pure outcast. Nobody used to say very much to her . . . Daren't talk to her, you know, she's not right in the head. I'll never forget her.

Or:

> Now years ago there was a lad on our estate. He was mental with it, and I can remember him going down the street and our mum says to me, "Keep away from Billy Eye," and course we did. When we saw him, we ran.

Stories such as these are the best evidence of the kind of knowledge parents had at the outset of their child's career as seizure sufferer. They typically contained an image of identity and referred to the reactions of others; thus negative stories featured "backward," "mad," "violent" characters who were "shunned," "avoided," or "feared." Their significance appears to reside in the way they symbolized how others were likely to perceive and judge their child and the reactions to expect. They constituted one source of influence on parental perceptions of their situation that preceded experience of others' reactions, and along with other stories they told about sufferers they provided an ever-present source of reference for checking the identity of the child.

Fueled or not by images conveyed in stories, the more general accounts parents gave about the social meaning of having a child with epilepsy were like those provided by the two parents who opened this chapter. These accounts represent a combination of the imagined and actual reactions of others. In 15 of the 20 cases, parents' views indicated a perception of their situation as one infused to varying degrees by felt stigma. For them, having a child with epilepsy meant a disvalued identity with potential or actual consequences for stigmatization ranging from rejection, being "put away," to more moderately phrased problems such as losing friends.

That the disvalued status not merely attached to the child but implicated other family members was also indicated by a number of parents. This is more difficult to demonstrate because their accounts tended to focus on the implications for the child rather than the family as a whole. Its importance, therefore, must largely be inferred, though some parents expressed a feeling of courtesy stigma with particular clarity. For example:

> People shy away, and they immediately think there's something wrong with the rest of the family because you've got one like that.

A sense of shame that having a child with epilepsy damages the reputation of the whole family is rather more important than might at first appear. There is a widespread lay belief that epilepsy "runs in families" (West, 1981); it is a view that without exception the parents at one time held. Typically they said they couldn't understand why their child had seizures because "there was nobody else in the family." In the course of making sense of what had happened, however, over half of these parents uncovered a suspect relative, information that had usually been hidden from them. That in itself is confirmation of the shamefulness of the disorder, but it also conveys a sense of blame—the child's epilepsy might have been avoided—and implicates others in the family as potential sufferers.

It is not suggested that all or even most parents experienced this sense of courtesy stigma, but it does mean that for some, felt stigma is likely to have more profound connotations of blame and shame than is at first apparent. It might explain why parents as stigma coaches appear so especially prone to the maintenance of secrecy.

Strategies for Managing Information

The extent to which parents experienced stigma underpinned the strategies adopted to manage information about their child. There were a variety of ways of attempting to do this, one of which involved the presentation of the child's seizure disorder as something other than epilepsy. Almost all parents at some time or for some audiences practiced this strategy. Typically, it involved the use of terms like *dizzy spells, funny turns, faints,* or *blackouts.* In at least three cases, it meant that the children themselves did not know they had epilepsy. Its particular relevance appeared to derive from the importance in the home context of trying to ensure that all children, including the sufferer, did not deliberately or unwittingly talk about epilepsy outside the home except in terms that suggested a relatively normal problem. This strategy aside, the major way of managing their situation resided in the potential afforded by epilepsy to conceal the condition from others.

For parents of a child with epilepsy, the strategy of concealing involves a major dilemma. To conceal is to risk involuntary disclosure and possible misadventure; to reveal is to risk stigmatization. The dilemma appears to explain why among this group the predominant pattern was one of selective disclosure. There were certainly those committed to concealing at almost any cost, and there were others who believed in a policy of disclosing the child's epilepsy to as many people as possible. There was no child, however, whose epilepsy was entirely concealed from people outside the family, school authorities being the most frequently informed nonfamily audience. Only three parents failed to reveal any information to the school authorities, and in each case the strategy failed when the child had a seizure.

Much greater evidence of concealing was apparent in other contexts, a pattern that characterized or had previously characterized the situation of most of the families. For some, it was strictly adhered to:

> We never discuss it with people outside the family, even relations really. Lots of relations don't know anything about it, and that's how we'll keep it.

Like the girl referred to in the introduction, the strategy had proven effective. In another case, a boy with absences, the policy was even more extreme.

His sister had not been informed, the problem posed by attendance at hospital clinics being passed off as "dental appointments." All of these families, of which there were six, may be depicted as successful concealers in that the child had not been witnessed outside the family having a seizure.

For another group of six, the strategy of concealing failed. Each of the children had seizures in a variety of situations outside the family and without exception experienced stigmatization by others. Despite the fact that the strategy had not proved effective, in the wake of often hostile reaction parents seemed to redouble their efforts to conceal the child's disorder and encouraged the child to do the same. As one mother put it:

> You try to avoid anybody sort of knowing . . . as long as you can.

In this group, parents' felt stigma had, through involuntary disclosure, been put to the test. It had been amply confirmed.

The remaining parents may be described as displaying a pattern of selective disclosure. Typically, they picked the people who were informed often in the expectation of a positive response, concealing from others about whom they were less sure. One parent summarized the situation rather well:

> There is sort of people around I suppose who are really illiterate, and it's no good telling [them], but to the average intelligent person I think yes, they should [be told].

These parents adopted this selective strategy often in the wake of the failure of earlier attempts at concealment that on occasions resulted in stigmatization. In general, however, they expressed surprise that the reactions of others when informed of the child's epilepsy were not as unsympathetic and intolerant as they had supposed. In consequence, felt stigma was much less apparent among these parents than among either the successful or failed concealers.

The extreme of this pattern was indicated by two families committed to a policy of disclosure, one of which is the family of the boy featured in the introduction. Both made it their business to inform as many people as possible, a decision made in the light of the additional benefits of minimizing the risk of misadventure and maximizing participation in activities outside the home. Neither recounted any instance of stigmatization despite the fact that both children had seizures in public on several occasions. Both sets of parents displayed less evidence of felt stigma than any others in the study.

The pattern of strategies adopted in this group indicates that concealing is a major, but not invariable, feature of the lives of families with a child who has epilepsy in which parents play a particularly important role. What data there are from the children themselves strongly suggest that they echoed the practices advocated by their parents. What is also apparent is that a two-way relationship existed between felt stigma and the effectiveness of strategies adopted to manage potentially damaging information. Not surprisingly perhaps, those parents who experienced stigma most strongly were most likely to practice concealment. When successful, felt stigma remained high. When concealing failed by virtue of involuntary disclosure, it was confirmed, which in turn predisposed to further concealing. When parents risked disclosure, it appeared on balance to reduce felt stigma and correspondingly to encourage more openness. Finally, though some forms of epilepsy like absences lend themselves to concealing, in this group both felt stigma and related strategies were largely unrelated to seizure type or frequency, an observation according with Ryan et al.'s (1980) findings.

Keeping the Child "Normal"

In terms of the effectiveness of information management, normal identity is secured when either the child's epilepsy is successfully concealed or, when revealed, it does not have the consequence of tarnishing either the child's or the family's reputation. Whichever strategy is adopted, though, is not just concerned with the management of information but with creating the conditions in which children can remain as normal as possible. In that respect, the various strategies practiced by parents were designed to achieve the same goal. The possibility is, though, that the associated consequences of those practices may not produce a normal child, with the additional risk that a deviant identity will undermine the whole family's precarious claim to normality.

One of the more obvious consequences of stigma strategies is that they may fail and result in stigmatization. In this study, instances of enacted stigma were much fewer than the rather pervasive sense of felt stigma would suggest. Of the eight parents who recalled episodes of stigmatization, six reported that it followed involuntary disclosure. When stigmatization did occur, it typically took the form of naming. Thus, various children were known as "mental," "nutter," "noddy," "peelegs," or "Dracula." In a few cases it took an extreme form and involved hostile reactions. For example, a family friend commented on what happened to one girl at school following a seizure:

> They wouldn't go near her . . . [they thought she was] going mad. Ought to be shot because she looks like a dog when she's foaming at the mouth.

This and similar episodes resulted in the parents' condoning avoidance of situations outside the home. As a result, the girl remained confined indoors for lengthy periods. Similar instances occurred in other cases where children were stigmatized though none involved such total isolation.

This pattern was not merely a reaction to the experience of stigmatization;

it was an associated consequence of the practice of concealing even when it was outwardly effective. To maximize the chances of success, parents minimized the extent of participation in outside activities. Typically, this took the form of restrictions on going out or staying overnight with friends or relatives, and involved chaperoning the child in public settings. The case featured in the introduction is an extreme example of this practice. In addition to restrictions on swimming and cycling, the parents forbade their daughter to go on school trips or participate in a range of activities with her schoolmates. The mother avoided traveling by bus on the occasions they had to attend clinic. Neither did the family go on vacation because of the increased risk of exposure. The parents, in consequence, went to extreme lengths to compensate:

> A lot of children will go down the playing fields and climb things and slides and do things over there. Well, we try to provide that sort of thing here . . . She's got it on hand. She hasn't had to go out and look for anything.

Concealing and restrictiveness, then, are closely associated. It is not the only way this pattern can develop—some restrictions may emanate from the clinic or result from a parental conception of the child as "fragile" (West, 1984)—but it does appear to be a major corollary of this particular style of managing stigma. The association is highlighted by the situation of other families who adopted a policy of disclosure. In these cases, particularly those committed to openness, informing others about their child's epilepsy was closely linked with the parental aim of maximizing participation in outside activities. It was perceived as a means of reducing the risk of misadventure and creating conditions for keeping the child normal.

This points to a central dilemma for those parents whose strategy of concealing involves restrictions on the child's activities, for while their goal is the same the extent to which it is achievable is problematic. Quite apart from the effects of stigmatization, to be isolated, protected, and restricted is not typically thought of as conducive to normal development. It is a real possibility, therefore, that the effects on the child will be such as to produce deviant identity and undermine the very strategy designed to secure normality.

Identity and Interpretations

Although no standard tests of personality or behavioral ratings were used in this study, parents provided a great deal of data about their child's identity, often comparing them with siblings and other people with epilepsy they had encountered. This information provides a basis for evaluating the possible role of stigma and related strategies in the development of psychopathology. In their interpretations of the child's identity, it is also possible to assess the extent to which they perceived the production of normality to be within their control.

Almost all parents described their child as normal prior to the onset of seizures, a claim substantiated by the earliest entries in their medical records. The profiles they gave of their children showed wide variation in the extent to which their goal of keeping the child normal had been achieved. Among successful concealers, there is evidence that some children were not perceived as deviant. Two of them were described as normal, intelligent, and doing well at school. Four others, however, were felt to be either shy, nervous, and highly strung or disturbed, moody, bad tempered, and defiant. Among the failed concealers, though, there is more evidence of deviant identity. Here, five of the six children were described in extremely negative terms, as aggressive, maladjusted, the sort to cause trouble, to give just three examples. There is also an indication that some of the children whose parents rather belatedly adopted a policy of selective disclosure were similarly depicted, but overall negative attributions were much less common. Of the two cases committed to disclosure, one was described as emotional and moody, the other as normal.

It is obviously the case that there is no neat association between the strategies parents adopted to manage stigma and the child's identity as indicated in parental profiles. Nevertheless, it seems clear that the combination of concealing and stigmatization is associated with greatest deviation and that concealing by itself is more likely to be associated with deviant identity than disclosure. These findings, tentative though they must be, do correspond to those of other studies where negative peer reaction and restrictiveness have been linked to psychopathology.

Finally, we may ask what it meant to parents when they perceived their child to deviate from normal and how they interpreted his or her identity. Its importance resides in the extent to which the production of normal identity remained within their control.

Most parents had an image of the typical "epileptic," most vividly portrayed in the stories they told, which at one and the same time constituted a component of their felt stigma and provided an ever-present means of checking the identity of their own child. It was to the production of normality and avoidance of any correspondence between the child's identity and the stereotyped image that their efforts were directed. When their child was perceived to retain normal identity, they could rest assured that he or she was not a typical "epileptic." When the child's behavior or personality was perceived as deviant, a major problem was raised for parents in explaining why this was so.

The mechanism by which parents came to see their child as "epileptic" has been described in some detail elsewhere (West, 1979, 1984). Essentially, it rested on the attribution of likeness between the child's identity and that of one or more characters they knew who represented the typical "epileptic." In this process was revealed an interpretation of identity that predominantly explained the child's deviant behavior or personality in terms of defects attributable to epilepsy. It was, in short, a lay equivalent of the outmoded concept of the "epileptic personality" that allowed them to interpret almost any aspect of the child's identity as evidence of an inherent defect.

The use of this "theory" has one very important implication: It carries with it the idea that how the child is, or appears to be, is unavoidable. It means that parents, other children in the family, or others outside are not implicated as responsible through their conduct for producing the child's deviant identity. As such, it may be used to justify stigmatization or serve to sustain patterns of conduct, like restrictiveness, which make it more likely the child will confirm their "theory." It means above all else that parents no longer have control over the production of normal identity; it could not have been otherwise.

In this study, interpretations of identity in terms of epileptic defect were most common among those families whose strategy of concealing failed by virtue of involuntary disclosure. It was also employed in at least two cases in the group of successful concealers. What this suggests is that through a combination of the effects of concealing and its associated practices, coupled with the experience of stigmatization, are created the conditions of a self-fulfilling prophecy. The child becomes "epileptic" as a consequence of effects that parents by virtue of their use of "defect" explanations largely do not see. In contrast, among those who disclosed voluntarily, there was the least evidence of interpretations of this sort. That this was the case would seem to have resulted from the fact that in the combination of disclosure and participation in activities was a policy that made the achievement of normality more likely. These parents believed so and in that respect they retained control over the production of normal identity. When successful and the child remained a normal child with seizures, there was simply less to account for.

CONCLUSION

In an attempt to advance our understanding of the complex processes that underlie the relationship between epilepsy and psychopathology, this chapter has been concerned to place the social meaning of epilepsy on the research agenda. It is an issue constantly alluded to, but, except rather implicitly, it is constantly ignored as a variable in research in the environmentalist tradition. Without taking account of what epilepsy means to people in terms of stigma, stigma strategies, stigmatization, and consequences for identity, we are investigating only part of the problem and are in danger of conceptualizing what is a dynamic process as fixed properties of sociopathogenic environments.

The study reported here represents an exploration of the diverse meanings associated with epilepsy and their ultimate consequences for children who suffer from seizures. As such, it may go some way toward a reformulation of the environmentalist perspective.

Because of the small sample, conclusions must be tentative. Nevertheless, the findings do broadly concur with those of the increasing number of investigators studying stigma among adult sufferers and—with some reinterpretation—those who have identified parental attitudes as an important factor in the genesis of psychopathology. It seems clear that the link resides in the association between stigma strategies and other practices designed to create conditions in which children may preserve a normal rather than deviant identity. Of particular importance is the association between concealing and the condoned avoidance of activities that finds expression as a pattern of restrictiveness and overprotection and that, in turn, may have deleterious consequences for the child. At the very least, concealing, even when outwardly effective, perpetuates the shame associated with epilepsy. In complete contrast is the association between disclosure and maximum participation in activities that on available evidence is more likely to result in normal identity.

It is also the case that these diverse strategies are, for reasons that are not entirely clear, differentially linked to the likelihood of stigmatization. One explanation is that when people are informed, they are more likely to judge the child as normal: Children whose epilepsy is first revealed through seizures may already have a deviant identity, perhaps as a direct consequence of the practices associated with concealing. At any rate, the evidence from this and other studies strongly suggests that voluntary disclosure is more likely than is often supposed to result in a judgment that epilepsy is compatible with normal identity.

Reconceptualizing environmental factors in terms of a process rather than fixed properties of individuals also means that the achievement of normal identity is to an extent at least within the control of families who have a child with epilepsy. That this was perceived by some parents but not by others was in no small measure due to the kind of knowledge they had about epilepsy and the interpretations they made about the child's identity. Explanations that invoked the idea of "epileptic" defect parallel those of organicists and mean that the achievement of normal identity is limited by biological factors. Obviously in some children this is a real enough constraint, but in this study parents employed this "theory" much more pervasively than the biological facts would allow. When that occurred, it signaled they were no longer in control of the production of normal identity and promoted conditions with further deleterious consequences for the child.

A focus on the dynamics of families who have a child with epilepsy directs attention to what might be done to avert some of the consequences of certain ways of coping with the problem. What was striking in this group of families was the way many of the parents were attempting to make sense of their situation in an "official vacuum." They simply lacked information. The one situation in which they might have obtained it, the medical consultation, was with few exceptions felt to be of little or no help (West, 1976, pp. 13–31; 1983, pp. 41–50). In consequence, they predominantly depended on lay knowledge and their own immediate experience to understand, cope with, and "explain" the problem. It is precisely such knowledge that sustains felt stigma and promotes practices and interpretations that can damage the child. It is the author's contention that with more comprehensive and positive professional input, some of the environmental problems associated with psychopathology are entirely avoidable. That professionals themselves are prone to secrecy means that it is not enough to urge a more open policy with greater transfer of information. People with epilepsy and their parents should know that normal identity is at least in part within their control.

REFERENCES

Bagley, C. (1971). *The social psychology of the child with epilepsy.* London: Routledge & Kegan Paul.

Birenbaum, A. (1970). On managing a courtesy stigma. *Journal of Health and Social Behaviour* 11, 196–206.

Bradley, C. (1951). Behavior disturbances in epileptic children. *Journal of the American Medical Association* 146, 436–41.

Bridge, E. (1949). *Epilepsy and convulsive disorders in children.* New York: McGraw-Hill.

Commission on Classification and Terminology of the International League Against Epilepsy. Proposal for revised clinical and electroencephalographic classification of epileptic seizures. (1981). *Epilepsia* 22, 489–501.

Goffman, E. (1963). *Stigma: Notes on the management of spoiled identity.* Harmondsworth: Penguin Books.

Goldin, G. J., S. L. Perry, R. J. Margolin, B. A. Stotsky, & T. C. Foster. *The rehabilitation of the young epileptic.* Lexington: Lexington Books.

Grunberg, F., & D. A. Pond. (1957). Conduct disorders in epileptic children. *Journal of Neurology, Neurosurgery and Psychiatry* 20, 65–68.

Hartlage, L. C., & J. B. Green. (1972). The relation of parental attitudes to academic and social achievement in epileptic children. *Epilepsia* 13, 21–26.

Hermann, B. P., & S. Whitman. (1984). Behavioral and personality correlates of epilepsy: A review, methodological critique and conceptual model. *Psychological Bulletin* 95, 451–97.

Hodgman, C. H., E. R. McAnarney, G. J. Myers, H. Iker, R. McKinney, D. Parmelee, B. Schuster, & M. Tutihasi. (1979). Emotional complications of adolescent grand mal epilepsy. *Journal of Paediatrics* 95, 309–12.

Kleck, R. E. (1968). Self-disclosure patterns of the non-obviously stigmatised. *Psychological Reports* 23, 1239–48.

Lofland, J. (1976). *Doing social life: The qualitative study of human interaction in natural settings.* New York: Wiley.

Long, C. G., & J. R. Moore. (1979). Parental expectations for their epileptic children. *Journal of Child Psychology and Psychiatry* 20, 299–312.

Mulder, H. C., & T. B. P. M. Suurmeijer. (1977). Families with a child with epilepsy: A sociological contribution. *Journal of Biosocial Science* 9, 13–24.

Nuffield, E. J. A. (1961). Neuro-physiology and behaviour disorders in epileptic children. *Journal of Mental Science* 107, 438–58.

Remschmidt, H. (1973). Psychological studies of patients with epilepsy and popular prejudice. *Epilepsia* 14, 347–56.

Rutter, M., P. Graham, & W. Yule. (1970). *A neuropsychiatric study in childhood.* London: Spastics International Medical Publications.

Ryan, R., K. Kempner, & A. C. Emlen. (1980). The stigma of epilepsy as a self-concept. *Epilepsia* 21, 433–44.

Scambler, G. (1982). Deviance, labelling and stigma. In D. L. Patrick & G. Scambler (Eds.). *Sociology as applied to medicine.* London: Balliere Tindall.

Scambler, G., & A. Hopkins. (1980). Social class, epileptic activity and disadvantage at work. *Journal of Epidemiology and Community Health* 34, 129–33.

Schneider, J. W., & P. Conrad. (1980). In the closet with illness: Epilepsy, stigma potential and information control. *Social Problems* 28, 32–44.

Schwartz, H., & J. Jacobs. (1979). *Qualitative sociology: A method to the madness.* New York: Free Press.

Stores, G. (1978). School-children with epilepsy at risk for learning and behaviour problems. *Developmental Medicine and Child Neurology* 20, 502–508.

Stores, G., & N. Piran. (1978). Dependency of different types in schoolchildren with epilepsy. *Psychological Medicine* 8, 441–45.

Suurmeijer, T. B. P. M. (1980). *Kinderen met epilepsie: Een onderzoek naar de invloed van een ziekte op kino en gezin.* Doctoral dissertation, University of Groningen.

Tizard, B. (1962). The personality of epileptics: A discussion of the evidence. *Psychological Bulletin* 59, 196–210.

Vinson, T. (1975). Towards demythologising epilepsy: An appraisal of public attitudes. *Medical Journal of Australia* 2, 663–66.

Ward, B., & B. D. Bower. (1978). A study of certain social aspects of epilepsy in childhood. *Developmental Medicine and Child Neurology* 20 (Supp. 39), 1.

West, P. (1976). The physician and the management of childhood epilepsy. In M. Wadsworth and D. Robinson (Eds.), *Studies in everyday medical life.* London: Martin Robertson.

West, P. (1979). An investigation into the social construction and consequences of the label epilepsy. *Sociological Review* 27, 719–41.

West, P. (1981). From bad to worse: People's experience and stereotypes of epilepsy. In S. McGovern (Ed.), *Epilepsy 1980–81.* Crowthorne: British Epilepsy Association.

West, P. (1983). Acknowledging epilepsy: Improving professional management of stigma and its consequences. In M. Parsonage, R. H. E. Grant, A. G. Craig, & A. A. Ward (Eds.), *Advances in epileptology: XIVth Epilepsy International Symposium.* New York: Raven Press.

West, P. (1984). Becoming disabled: Perspectives on the labelling process. In U. E.

Gerhardt & M. Wadsworth (Eds.), *Stress and stigma: Problems of explanation in the sociology of crime and illness.* Frankfurt: Campus Press.
Whitman, S., B. P. Hermann, R. B. Black, & S. Chhabria. (1982). Psychopathology and seizure type in children with epilepsy. *Psychological Medicine* 12, 843–53.
Williams, D. (1967). Epilepsy. *Royal Institute of Public Health and Hygiene Journal* 30, 38–41.
Wilson, D. P., & B. S. H. Harris. Psychiatric problems in children with frontal, central and temporal lobe epilepsy. *Southern Medical Journal* 59, 49–53.

IV / *Psychosis and Violence in Epilepsy: Two Social Analyses*

Part IV contains chapters about two behavioral disorders that are particularly controversial in the epilepsy/psychopathology literature—psychosis and violence.

For quite some time investigators have hoped that the study of individuals suffering from both epilepsy and psychosis would yield clues as to the biological determinants of that psychopathology. Several methodological aspects of this research are problematic, leaving many basic issues unresolved. For instance, debates still exist as to whether there is an overrepresentation of psychosis in epilepsy (the affinity hypothesis), whether epilepsy protects against psychosis (the antagonism hypothesis), or whether there is no special relationship between the two (the coincidence hypothesis).

The one issue most investigators in this area seem to agree on is that, whatever the prevalence of psychosis in epilepsy, its causes are most likely biological. This of course corresponds to a large extent to one of the theories about the etiology of psychosis in the general population. Despite this agreement, the evidence that the causes of psychosis are likely to be biological, in both the general population and in people with epilepsy, remains inconclusive.

Peter Wolf, Rupprecht Thorbecke, and Werner Even from the Free University of Berlin take a unique approach to this problem in chapter 12. They define their terms carefully and then empirically test several social factors to determine if they are significantly related to psychosis in people with epilepsy. Several are, and these findings suggest new areas of research and new approaches to this important question.

In chapter 13, Steven Whitman, Lambert King, and Robert Cohen examine the relationship between epilepsy and violence. These authors have in the past written two reviews of what is known about epilepsy in prison and have carried out two major empirical investigations of this issue. Moreover, as directors of medical services in two of the largest jails in the United States, King and Cohen have encountered many prisoners with epilepsy on a clinical and personal basis. All of this evidence has suggested to these authors that there is no special relationship between epilepsy and violence. Furthermore, the vast majority of the literature suggests the same. Nonetheless, the belief in this relationship remains prominent and the use of epilepsy as a defense against criminal charges actually seems to be increasing.

Rather than review the evidence in detail yet again, Whitman and his colleagues briefly discuss the more prominent studies in this area and then present opposing social and biological explanations of three scenarios in which epilepsy was used as an explanation for violent behavior. Their chapter goes beyond the data, which is always a risky and potentially controversial endeavor. We hope, however, that this will be an illuminating and stimulating conclusion to the book.

12 / Social Aspects of Psychosis in Patients with Epilepsy

PETER WOLF, RUPPRECHT THORBECKE,
and WERNER EVEN

Psychiatrists' discussions about the significance of social factors in the pathogenesis of "functional" or "endogenous" psychoses such as schizophrenia often end up in ideological arguments, sometimes restricted to dogmatic statements of beliefts that are as dear to their defenders as they are difficult to prove. Is schizophrenia a brain disease with still undetected causes, or is it no disease at all but rather the indicator of the corruptness of our society, becoming manifest in the experiences of unfortunates doomed to the role of the scapegoat?

In the recent literature, there is a strong but ill-founded (Wolf, 1980) tendency to baptize some psychotic disorders of epilepsy as "schizophrenialike," and to subsequently use them as a paradigm of true schizophrenia. This approach has been adopted mostly by advocates of biological psychiatry who hope to gain insight into the pathogenesis of schizophrenia by studying a supposedly related disorder of known organic background. Social psychiatrists have not followed a parallel path, and one wonders why. Is the field of psychoses with organic background a priori left to biological psychiatrists because it seems hopeless to gain a social footing there? Or is a possible constraint felt, and then avoided, to accept multifactorial pathogenesis where social factors, as all other factors, would be of limited significance?

Sarcastic considerations of this kind are difficult to avoid. The longer a clinician works with patients in a neurological epilepsy clinic, the more puzzled he or she becomes by the psychiatric complications these patients experience; nor can the clinician help noticing the contribution of social factors to these complications. Further, trying to read and learn more about the issue, the clinician becomes aware of having come across something of a blind spot in social psychiatry.

In the literature on psychoses of epilepsy, the possible influence of social factors has been mentioned occasionally (Herrington, 1969; Landolt, 1972; Pond, 1971), and there are some illustrative case reports (Kury & Cobb, 1964; Müller-Suur, 1942; Trethowan, 1952). Little systematic research, however, seems to have been undertaken in this field (Bruens, 1980).

CONDITIONS OF EPISODIC PSYCHOSES WITH EPILEPSY

The psychoses of patients with epilepsy attending an outpatient seizure clinic within a neurology department are predominantly episodic. They may or may not require admission to a hospital ward; in our department, we prefer admission to the neurology ward, where the patients remain in the care of doctors with whom they are already familiar. Some of our patients were primary neurological admissions, mainly for status epilepticus.

The causes of the psychotic episodes that can be observed in such a clinical setting are by no means uniform. An attempt to categorize the various pathogenic conditions led to the delineation of nine classes (Table 12-1):

1. *Ictal episodes.* The psychotic condition is identical with a (prolonged) seizure event. Typical examples of this are stuporous and twilight states with continuous spike-wave discharge in generalized epilepsies, and various forms of acute organic psychoses *(akute exogene Reaktionstypen)* caused by focal minor status epilepticus (see note).
2. *Postictal episodes.* Their most common cause is grand mal status but they may follow single grand mal seizures as well as, occasionally, complex focal seizures. They last from some days to a few weeks. These are, again, psychotic states of an organic type. Delirious states and hallucinoses are more common than simple twilight states. Not infrequently, the psychotic content is of a religious or erotic kind or both, and the mood is typically ecstatic or nihilistic.
3. *Parictal episodes.* This term is suggested for episodes occurring in a period of distinctly increased seizure activity without, however,

TABLE 12-1. Pathogenetic Classification of Psychotic Episodes in Epilepsy

1. Ictal episodes
2. Postictal episodes
3. Parictal episodes
4. Alternative syndromes ("forced normalization")
5. Toxic psychoses
6. Withdrawal psychoses
7. Paranoid reactions
8. Psychoses unrelated to the epilepsy
9. Psychotic episodes of multifactorial pathogenesis

apparent relation to any individual seizure event. Presumably, this category is not fundamentally separated from the two previous ones. The clinical syndromes are, again, of an organic-psychotic type.
4. *Alternative syndromes ("forced normalization").* The most extraordinary relation of epilepsy and psychiatric disorder is that of alternative episodes or of forced normalization. The history and definition of these concepts have been dealt with in detail by Wolf and Trimble (1985), and the various clinical syndromes of forced normalization by Wolf (1984). The essence is that, in some patients, seizure control does not result in well-being but in some kind of psychiatric symptomatology, mostly paranoid episodic psychoses in clear consciousness. The condition has been reported in temporal lobe epilepsy but seems to be more common in adolescents and adults with absences who receive intense antiabsence treatments with succinimides. Of these patients, as many as 7.8% seem to be at risk (Wolf, Inoue, Röder-Wanner, & Tsai, 1984).
5. *Toxic psychoses.* These may be observed with an overdose of various antiepileptic drugs; however, there has never been a study comparing the drugs in this respect. In our own experience, toxic psychoses were caused by phenytoin at serum levels above 32 μg/ml or carbamazepine at serum levels above 13 μg/ml. The symptomatology was paranoid without organic signs.
6. *Withdrawal psychoses.* They have been observed with the withdrawal of barbiturates, clonazepam, and pheneturide. The psychoses are paranoid in type, mostly with vivid hallucinations and increased psychomotor activity. If associated with withdrawal seizures, distinction from Classes 1–3 may be difficult or impossible.
7. *Reactive psychotic episodes.* Paranoid reactions to relevant life events *(sensitiver Beziehungswahn)* may be observed in occasional patients. There is nothing to indicate that patients with epilepsy are at a higher risk than the average population although the precipitating event may be connected with the epileptic disorder.
8. *Psychoses of various pathogeneses unrelated to the epilepsy.* An example of this would be periodic dysphoric states and dyscontrol syndromes that occasionally may include paranoid delusions.
9. *Multifactorial pathogenesis.* This is rather common as various factors of pathogenic importance often interact in ways that may be too intricate to determine the weight of individual causes.

Of these nine categories, 7 and 8 will not be considered further as they are not directly related to epilepsy whereas all others are connected either with epilepsy or its treatment.

EPISODIC PSYCHIATRIC DISORDERS AND THE LAW OF IDENTITY

There has never been a comparative study of patients with different kinds of psychotic episodes although, for many reasons, it would be of high interest. It seems questionable, however, that such a study is feasible because it appears that the manifestation of any kind of psychotic episode increases the risk of further psychotic complications of whatever pathogenesis (unpublished data). Consequently many patients cannot be assigned to one category or the other as they have experienced several types over time. Two examples may illustrate this:

Ursula R. suffered, since age 19, from sleep grand mal with an aura of fear, and left versive seizures probably due to perinatal damage. At age 23, she had a series of grand mal seizures on one day that was followed by a confused state with severe anxiety and delusions of persecution lasting 6 weeks. When she was 25, having left her hometown and living by herself, she had some difficulties with her colleagues and superiors with which she seemed unable to cope, and developed a psychotic state that lasted, with some fluctuations, about 1 year. She had visual and auditory hallucinations, cenesthetic sensations in her sexual organs, and erotic delusions. Two years later, a delusion of persecution of 2 weeks' duration was the consequence of an elevation of antiepileptic drug dose (1.5 g primidone plus 300 mg phenytoin, drug levels not known). In the following 7 years, there were three short exacerbations of her sexual delusions and haptic hallucinations that seemed to be caused by social stress and overfatigue. Thus, she had postictal, reactive, and toxic episodes, all with similar symptomatology.

Another patient, Anneliese E., with absences since age 6 and grand mal on awakening since age 18, had grand mal status followed by a simple twilight state of 1 week's duration at age 34. At 39, another status epilepticus was followed by a delirious state with paranoid fears and visual hallucinations indicating that death was impending. At 43, intensive therapy with phenytoin and ethosuximide that led to complete seizure control caused a lucid stuporous psychosis with auditory hallucinations, and cosmic and nihilistic delusions that repeated some of the themes of her previous psychoses (serum level: 17 μg/ml phenytoin, 70–80 μg/ml ethosuximide). The condition could be controlled by additional administration of 30 mg clobazam. Three years later, at an unchanged medication and slightly lower drug levels, still seizure free, there was a short paranoid burst with delusions of persecution following a disappointing love affair. Three pathogenic types of psychotic episodes—postictal, alternative, and psychoreactive—were thus observed over time in this patient, but important parts of their contents were identical.

In other patients, different sequences were observed.

Although the literature on psychoses associated with epilepsy contains many case reports, this multietiologic aspect has received remarkably little attention, and psychotic episodes have always been looked at as isolated acute events. This is obviously inadequate for a more comprehensive understanding of psychosis in epilepsy. A psychotic episode, even if not experienced in full consciousness, and apparently remitting without residue, seems not to become extinguished but to remain part of a patient's history and identity. Remarkably, longitudinal observations of the kind just reported indicate that such experiences may be reactivated both by physical and psychosocial pathogenic factors. Delusions once experienced seem to become part of a person's disposable pattern of behavior and may serve as a response to various extreme conditions.

Delusions substitute an imaginary world for reality. Most often this includes imaginary social relations, positive or negative. It has been noted (Wolf, 1980) that psychotic delusions of patients with epilepsy often express, unusually directly, their actual life problems as they seem to represent the imaginary repair of the patients' most bitter frustrations in love, social standing, or attempts at leading independent lives.

Tellenbach (1965) reported that, in the majority of patients with alternative epileptic psychoses, the relation to their parents became a motive of their psychotic symptomatology, often as a delusion of being an adopted child. He believed that this reflected these patients' experiences of a high degree of dependency on their parents.

It was, again, with patients with alternative psychiatric complications that we found indications of social pathogenic factors. It is to this topic that we now turn.

FORCED NORMALIZATION: PSYCHOSIS, PREPSYCHOSIS, AND SOCIAL STATUS

The clinical manifestation of forced normalization is not uniform (Wolf, 1984), but the most common condition is a paranoid psychosis. This is often precipitated by a dysphoric state with insomnia, and feelings of oppression or fear (Tellenbach, 1965). Its most characteristic feature is the patient's withdrawal from his or her surroundings and usual activities (Wolf 1976a). The importance of this is that, if this "prepsychotic dysphoria" is recognized in time, the development to a psychotic state can often be prevented (Wolf, 1976a). If this succeeds, the "prepsychotic dysphoria" will have been the isolated manifestation of forced normalization.

Wolf (1976b) looked at possible differences between patients with paranoid psychoses and patients with alternative prepsychotic dysphorias. He found only one significant difference: The majority of patients who developed psychotic episodes were vocationally disintegrated, having no job or professional training. This was not true for dysphoric patients. This unpredicted finding became the motivation for further studies conducted by our group and reported in the next section.

At present, our material comprises 9 patients with prepsychotic dysphorias, 7 of whom were employed and two of whom were in training at the time of forced normalization. Of the 19 patients with alternative psychoses only 6 were employed, 8 were in training, and 4 were unemployed ($p < .05$ comparing employed patients with the others). Two hypotheses can be formed to explain the differences:

1. Social integration is a stabilizing factor in a psychically critical situation.
2. Better social integration is an indicator of a more stable primary personality that is more able to cope with a critical situation.

CONTROLLED STUDIES

Two retrospective studies were performed by our group with the objective to develop more detailed hypotheses about these conditions.

Family Development of Patients with Epilepsy and Psychosis: A Pilot Study

Are there peculiarities in psychosocial development that may help to explain why some patients in the course of their illness become psychotic? In our first study we started with the assumption that the family's reaction to the manifestation of epilepsy could be crucial in the further development of children with epilepsy. Do the parents believe, as a consequence of the seizures, that their child needs intensive care during all his or her life? Are the seizures frequent and embarrassing? Do they have a menacing appearance, for example, in a patient with running seizures who tramples over any obstacle? Or do they seem to be a matter of little consequence, causing only short interruptions of the child's activity, or, in the case of auras, do they enable the patient to avoid dangerous situations? Does the disorder influence the parents' expectations for the intellectual, professional, and social development of their child?

As a result of such factors, the family can be expected to develop a specific role structure as an adaptation to the presence of epilepsy in one of its members. This structure may remain stable even if the clinical condition changes, e.g., if the individual's seizure frequency decreases or side effects disappear.

As a consequence, improved possibilities for the child's development may be neglected.

The scheme of Figure 12-1 may help to describe some typical role patterns that may appear as a reaction to the child's epilepsy (Dreitzel, 1972).

There are two dimensions: (1) the variety of roles a child is allowed to adopt (many or all activities outside the home such as football, dancing, and meeting friends may be excluded); and (2) the control of the child's activities (e.g., time restrictions, control of how activities are performed).

We conducted extensive, unstructured, open-ended interviews with 10 patients with epilepsy with a history of paranoid episodic psychoses, and used as controls 13 adolescents with epilepsy, most of whom had been sent to us because of difficulties concerning vocational training and employment. The main areas of questioning centered on:

- The meaning of the child's epilepsy for the family
- Typical role patterns in the family

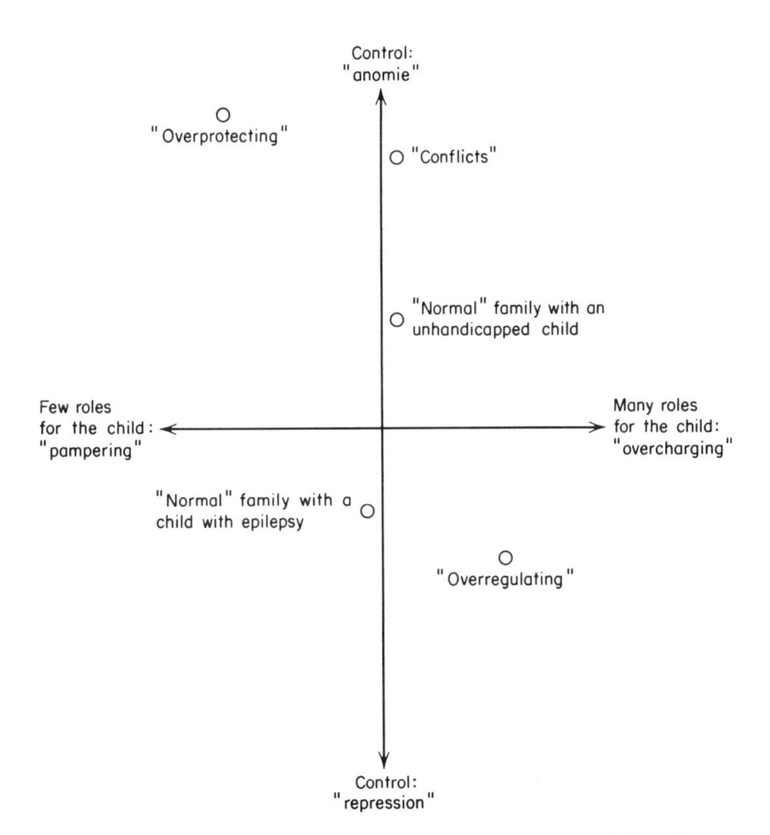

Figure 12-1. Typical role patterns as a reaction to the child's epilepsy

- Contacts with persons outside the family
- Schooling and professional education
- Sexual relations and marriage
- The religious orientation of the parent and patient
- The family and professional situation before the psychotic episode.

When evaluating our data, we tried to differentiate the families according to the scheme presented in Figure 12-1, and tried to determine peculiarities in the families of the patients who had experienced a psychotic state.

The main results were as follows (Thorbecke, 1980): Both psychotic patients (Group P) and controls (Group C) came from families rated as "normal" or "overprotective". In both family types, however, there had been, in the P patients, a higher tendency to regulate their activities. For example, they were not allowed to meet a friend during the weekend or to choose a certain profession. In the 4 overprotective families of Group C, this overprotective behavior could be explained by the parents' feeling of guilt whereas in the 4 families of Group P, it seemed to be caused by the perception of the child with epilepsy as defective and dangerous.

The 4 families (of 23) rated as "overregulating" all belong to Group P. The peculiarities concerning the "normal" and "overprotective" families of Group P were rediscovered here in much more pronounced form: Everyday life was strictly regulated even by use of physical force; the patients were charged and overcharged with household tasks (cooking, cleaning, babysitting, etc.) to a degree that left them no time for hobbies and their own interests. In addition, sexual prudishness prevailed; for example, adolescent patients were not informed about sexual matters and were not allowed to be out in the evening or to visit friends of the same or opposite sex. In three families the parents' exaggerated religiosity did not help to cope with the child's disability but fulfilled the function of legitimating the parents' claims of control and conformity.

On the other hand, the patients belonging to the three families that were characterized by open conflicts between parents and patients were all control patients.

We concluded from this study that the family structure as a whole seems less important as a risk factor for psychosis than the presence of the specific traits just described.

As a consequence we constructed a questionnaire of 167 items to be used in a more systematic study.

Social Risk Factors in Psychosis with Epilepsy: A Controlled Study

The study comprised 32 patients with a history of paranoid psychosis (Group P) and 32 matched controls (Group C). The matching criteria are given in

TABLE 12-2. Matching Criteria for Controlled Study

Kind of Epilepsy	*Group P*	*Group C*
Generalized	10	11
Generalized and focal	6	3
Focal-temporal	12	13
Focal-cortical	4	5

Sex: 18 F 14 M (P)
18 F 14 M (C)

Age of onset of epilepsy
14.0 years (P)
14.1 years (C)

Duration of epilepsy at onset of first psychotic episode was matched with duration of epilepsy at first consultation in our epilepsy clinic in C patients

15.3 years (P)
17.4 years (C)

Table 12-2. It was difficult to find adequate matched controls using the four criteria listed in the table, and medication as an additional control criterion could not be introduced as we originally desired. As a consequence, it was found that ethosuximide was given more often and in higher doses to patients of Group P ($p < .01$) whereas for valproic acid the reverse was found ($p < .03$).

Comparison of both groups revealed the following conditions.

Socioeconomic Characteristics

Regarding the social class indicators for the parents (schooling and professional education), we could not find any substantial difference between the two groups. Fathers and mothers of P patients are about 2 years older at the birth of the child with epilepsy than parents of controls (not significant). In seven families of Group C and six families of Group P, the child with epilepsy is the only child. There was no difference in the age rank of patients among the siblings. Patients did not significantly differ in schooling and professional education from the nearest sibling. In the families of Group C more often than in Group P, a second child was handicapped ($p < .08$).

The Meaning of the Child's Epilepsy for the Family

The patients of Group P significantly more often reported a feeling that their parents were uneasy about having a child with epilepsy ($p < .02$). Patients of Group P much more rarely than controls reported that they had a friend with whom they talked about the epilepsy ($p < .01$). The P patients more often than C patients reported that their parents believed that a child with epilepsy must be saved from strain ($p < .13$) or that they forbade things for reasons related to the child's epilepsy ($p < .01$).

The Family's Inner Structure and Control of the Child's Activities at Home and Out

Whereas almost all patients from Group P grew up with both parents, one third of those in Group C grew up with relatives or shifted between the care of relatives and parents ($p < .05$). In both P and C groups, a traditional role pattern prevailed: The main part of the family's income was earned by the father, the mother being the most important person for the children when they needed help with the solution of everyday problems and homework. P patients reported more often that one parent alone made all important decisions, whereas in Group C both parents seem more often to have been involved ($p < .06$). There were clear differences in the methods used to control the children's behavior: Patients of Group P reported more often to have been punished by their parents ($p < .03$). In the same group a greater variety of punishment was used, and physical punishment prevailed ($p < .03$). In Group C, on the other hand, punishments such as not talking to the child or denying the fulfillment of certain wishes predominated ($p < .02$). It is worth noting that four patients who reported always to have agreed with their parents' orders all belong to Group P ($p < .05$).

Patients in Group P were less independent than those of Group C. They were subject to more prohibitions created in reaction to their epilepsy. As long as the patients lived with their parents, intake of antiepileptic drugs was more rarely and at a higher age controlled by themselves ($p < .01$). If drug intake was the patient's own responsibility, there was more supervision by parents in Group P than in Group C ($p < .07$). Patients of Group P less frequently reported to have had friends in the neighborhood or in the school, to have participated in a youth club or to have been out in the evening ($p < .07$). Finally, the four patients who were not allowed to participate in a dancing course all belonged to Group P ($p < .03$).

Sexuality

The patients of Group P more often felt they did not know their parents' attitudes concerning sexuality ($p < .001$). They were more rarely and at a higher age informed about sexual life. Also, they seem to have had the first friendship with a partner of the opposite sex at a higher age than controls ($p < .08$). More often than in Group C, parents were opposed to such friendships or these were kept secret from the parents.

In both Groups P and C women were more often married than men ($p < .05$). Loose relationships with members of the opposite sex before marriage were less frequent in Group P patients ($p < .03$). Patients who still lived with their parents at the time of our interview were more often observed to have no experiences with partners of the opposite sex ($p < .09$). Further, nearly all patients who still lived with their parents were not married; patients who had left their parents' home late had a higher rate of divorce ($p < .01$).

Religious Orientation

In both groups the majority of parents are members of the Protestant church. In Group P, however, a higher proportion of the parents belong to the Roman Catholic church or religious minority groups such as Jehovah's Witnesses or Baptists ($p < .03$ if comparing mothers). Members of minority groups all belong to Group P. Patients of Group P more often than controls described their parents as highly engaged in religious affairs ($p < .01$ if fathers are compared).

When patients' religious interests in childhood and adulthood were compared, most P patients reported a constant or increasing occupation with religious issues whereas in most controls such interest decreased from childhood to adulthood or they had little religious interest at all age levels ($p < .01$).

Several relationships between high religious interest of the parents and other variables could be demonstrated. Families with religious interests more often had discussions about who was guilty for having an epileptic child ($p < .01$). Patients from these families were, as adolescents, rarely out to see friends in the evening ($p < .08$) and usually were not allowed to participate in a dancing course ($p < .01$). Sexual matters were discussed more rarely in these families ($p < .12$).

To sum up, this retrospective study (Even, 1983) indicated some substantial differences in patterns of everyday life between the families of the patients with epilepsy and psychoses and matched controls. The adolescents of Group P were less often or at a later age allowed to adopt certain roles and perform them according to their own interests. This restrictive practice is supported by the prevailing pattern of physical punishment. No relationship between these family characteristics and indexes of social class could be found. The families of Group P comparatively often adhered to religious minority groups. Further studies should look more closely at the significance of this factor for the everyday life of the families. In the families of patients with psychoses, there is a higher uncertainty about issues such as sexuality and the meaning of the member's epilepsy for the family. This may result in uncertainty with regard to the adoption of social roles in general and could be linked to the indexes of social instability in adulthood that were apparent in patients with psychotic episodes as reported in the previous section.

Our findings, however, must be taken with the reserve appropriate for retrospective studies. Particularly, the psychotic experience may have influenced the patients' recall of their own history. Another drawback is that, in retrospect, no differentiation is possible between the family situation before and after the onset of epilepsy. Studies aimed at this are difficult but more desirable.

SOCIAL FACTORS IN THE PATHOGENESIS OF PSYCHOSIS WITH EPILEPSY: POSSIBLE MODES OF ACTION

In the previous sections we have reviewed findings indicating that social factors may contribute to the pathogenesis of psychoses in epilepsy. It seemed that social influences contributing to the development of personality may be involved in the formation of a person's fitness to cope with difficult and critical life situations. Another possibility is that primary personality insufficiency contributes to social adjustment problems that would have to thus be considered as mere indicators of risks. These hypotheses that do not necessarily exclude each other are difficult to assess in retrospective studies, and the problem, at present, remains open.

It might be asked, however, if any modes of action of such factors are apparent from the case histories. For this, it should be kept in mind that the pathogenesis of psychotic episodes in epilepsy is not homogeneous. The different pathogenetic groups should, therefore, be considered separately.

Ictal Episodes

Little is known about the causes and conditions of ictal episodes, and apart from anecdotal experiences, there is at present nothing that indicates the influence of social factors.

Psychotic Episodes Related to Increased Seizure Activity (Postictal and Parictal Psychoses)

With our present therapeutic means the seizures of many patients still cannot be completely controlled but, apart from exceptional cases, seizure frequencies of the scale that may precipitate a psychotic state have become unusual. If they occur, the most common cause is status epilepticus as a consequence of drug withdrawal. But also the parictal psychoses related to increased seizure frequency are often related to situations of relative withdrawal due to noncompliance. Thus, all factors that influence compliance seem to be indirectly involved.

Forced Normalization

The most common pathogenesis is seizure control by some antiepileptic drug, and the first clinical symptom is insomnia. The condition seems particularly common in patients with absences who are treated with ethosuximide (Wolf et al., 1984). In these patients at least, the background of the insomnia seems organic and caused by the drug in question. An additional factor could be that the alteration of sleep structure by ethosuximide might facilitate intrusion of dream material into wakeful consciousness (Röder & Wolf, 1981). At present, however, it is uncertain whether the drug does anything more specific than to get somebody with absences into a critical state of mind as a consequence of a sleep deficit. The influence of a drug like ethosuximide on sleep is ubiquitous, but only a minority of patients experience a critical state of mind and, again, only part of these develop psychosis. It is not known what factors predispose to the "critical" response, and the quality of this response could in turn be influenced by several factors. Social status seems to represent one of these factors.

It could be active in a most simple way: The most important means of prevention of alternative psychosis seems to be early control of insomnia (usually by transitory administration of some tranquilizer). This is only possible if the patient quickly reports the onset of insomnia or other prepsychotic symptoms. To wait until the next routine appointment at the clinic may mean to wait too long. Several of our nonpsychotic patients with forced normalization did indeed see us urgently because they did not feel well whereas others presented at the routine appointment with psychotic symptoms that had long been preceded by warning signs of a similar order.

Patients of inadequate social adjustment may be more reluctant to leave the routine. To take an extra step and ask for an urgent appointment requires a minimum of social versatility that some patients seem not to possess. This may prove deleterious in such a situation.

Toxic and Withdrawal Psychoses

These are closely related to the course of therapy and are thus mainly iatrogenic. The patients of our own observation (eight toxic and one withdrawal psychosis) all had important social problems but it would be difficult to connect these with the development of the psychosis.

Reactive Psychoses

The stressful events that seem responsible for the development of these psychoses are, as usual in this kind of psychosis, mainly of a social order.

Multifactorial Psychoses

Multifactorial psychoses form quite a heterogeneous group with individual differences too important to allow for any general conclusion. However, the most common known or possible factors appear to be increased seizure frequency, recent seizure control, and reaction to stressful life events. The social relations of these factors have been discussed here.

CONCLUSIONS

Clinical observations and results of methodical studies indicate that some of the pathogenetically inhomogeneous forms of psychotic episodes in epilepsy have a multifactorial etiology and that social disabilities may belong to the factors involved. Should they not be factors, they are at least indicators of risk. It seems that such disabilities emerge from the development of the personality of patients with epilepsy in the family. The respective roles, however, of possible primary personality insufficiency, restrictions imposed by the disease, primary family setting, and the family's reactions to the disease are difficult to assess and remain to be elucidated.

NOTE

The authors are aware that some readers, especially of American background, will be unfamiliar with the concept of organic psychoses that is in common use in most European countries. This is not the place for a detailed discussion of this point. The interested reader is referred to European textbooks of psychiatry such as Bleuler (1983).

REFERENCES

Bleuler, E. (1983). *Lehrbuch der Psychiatrie (15th ed.). Berlin: Springer-Verlag.*

Bruens, J. H. (1980). Psychosoziale Bedingungskonstellationen von Psychosen bei Epilepsie. In P. Wolf & G.-K. Köhler (Eds.), *Psychopathologische und pathogenetische Probleme psychotischer Syndrome bei Epilepsie.* Bern: Huber.

Dreitzel, H. P. (1972). *Das gesellschaftliche Leiden und das Leiden an der Gesellschaft.* Stuttgart: Enke.

Even, W. (1983). *Zur psychologischen und sozialen Entwicklung von Patienten mit Epilepsie und Psychosen in Familie, Schule, Beruf und Partnerschaft—Eine kontrollierte Studie.* Thesis, West Berlin.

Herrington, R. N. (1969). The personality in temporal lobe epilepsy. In R. N. Herrington (Ed.), *Current problems in neuropsychiatry: Schizophrenia, epilepsy, and the temporal lobe.* Ashford (U.K.): Headley.

Kury, G., & S. Cobb (1964). Epileptic dementia resembling schizophrenia: Clinicopathological report of a case. *Journal of Nervous and Mental Disease* 138, 340–47.

Landolt, H. (1972). Epilepsie und Psychose. In *Psychiatrie der Gegenwart (2nd ed., Vol. II). Berlin: Springer-Verlag.*

Müller-Suur, H. (1942). Beitrag zur Kenntnis der epileptischen Psychosen. *Psychiat.-neurol. Wschr.* 44, 185–89.

Pond, D. A. (1971). The psychological disorders of epileptic patients. *Psychiatria, Neurologia, Neurochirurgia.* 74, 159–62.

Röder, U. U., & P. Wolf. (1981). Effects of treatment with dipropyl-acetate and ethosuximide on sleep organisation in epileptic patients. In M. Dam, L. Gram, J. K. Penry (Eds.), *Advances in epileptology, XIIth Epilepsy International Symposium.* New York: Raven.

Stevens, J. R. (1975). Interictal clinical manifestations of complex partial seizures. In J. K. Penry & D. D. Daly (Eds.), *Advances in Neurology: Vol. 11. Complex partial seizures and their treatment.* New York: Raven.

Tellenbach, H. (1965). Epilepsie als Anfallsleiden und als Psychose. Ueber alternative Psychosen paranoider Prägung bei "forcierter Normalisierung" (Landolt) des Elektroencephalogramms Epileptischer. *Nervenarzt* 36, 190–202.

Thorbecke, R. (1980). Gibt es soziale Faktoren, die das Risiko, im Verlauf einer Epilepsie eine Psychoses zu erleiden, erhöhen? *In* P. Wolf & G.-K. Köhler (Eds.), *Psychopathologische und pathogenetische Probleme psychotischer Syndrome bei Epilepsie.* Bern: Huber.

Trethowan, W. H. (1952). Diagnostic and therapeutic problems in a patient with epilepsy, psychosis and temporal lobe abnormality. *American Journal of Medicine* 12, 338–43.

Wolf, P. (1976a). The prevention of alternative epileptic psychosis in outpatients. In D. Janz (Ed.), *Epileptology.* Stuttgart: Thieme.

Wolf, P. (1976b). *Psychosen bei Epilepsie, ihre Bedingungen und Wechselbeziehungen zu Anfällen.* Thesis, West Berlin.

Wolf, P. (1980). Zur Kritik des Begriffs schizophrenie-ähnliche Psychose bei Epilepsie. In P. Wolf & G.-K Köhler (Eds.), *Psychopathologische und pathogenetische Probleme psychotischer Syndrome bei Epilepsie.* Bern: Huber.

Wolf, P. (1984). The clinical syndromes of forced normalization. *Fol. psychiat. neurol. Japon.* 38, 187–92.

Wolf, P., Y. Inoue, U. U. Röder-Wanner, & J. J. Tsai. (1984). Psychiatric complications of absence therapy and their relation to alteration of sleep. *Epilepsia* 25, S56–S59.

Wolf, P., & M. Trimble. (1985). Biological antagonism and epileptic psychosis. *British Journal of Psychiatry* 146, 272–76.

13 / Epilepsy and Violence: A Scientific and Social Analysis

STEVEN WHITMAN, LAMBERT N. KING,
and ROBERT L. COHEN

An important part of the epilepsy/psychopathology controversy concerns the relationship between epilepsy and violence. This relationship may be the most dramatic aspect of this controversy because epilepsy is not infrequently used as a defense in criminal trials, often in the most spectacular cases. For example, epilepsy has been implicated in the cases of Jack Ruby, who killed President Kennedy's assassin; Robert Torsney, a white New York City police officer who killed Randolph Evans, a black teenager; and Mehmet Ali Agca, who shot Pope John Paul II. An important social consequence grows out of these cases since an "epilepsy defense" of an individual who allegedly committed a violent act serves to stigmatize people with epilepsy by correlating epilepsy with violence.

Another indicator of the importance of the epilepsy/violence hypothesis is the central role Cesare Lombroso gave epilepsy during the 1870s in his formulation of the "criminal man"—one of the first systematic attempts to demonstrate that violent behavior is biologically determined. Efforts to demonstrate biological roots of social behavior generally rise and fall as a function of changing social and political conditions and are once more becoming prominent under the name of "sociobiology."

Delineating the relationship between epilepsy and violence would therefore be valuable for several reasons. It would provide insight into the relationship between the brain and social behavior, it would allow us to deal more appropriately with the stigma that accrues to people with epilepsy as a result of its alleged relationship to violence, and it would facilitate an examination of the axes of debate around the more general but related issue of sociobiology.

We proceed in the following manner: First, we define the issues that must be addressed if there is to be clarity in this area. Too often, separate issues are confused and discussions crisscross in an unhelpful manner. Second, we briefly summarize relevant parts of the literature, including our own work.

This is done not for detail, but to provide a sense of how research in this area proceeds. Next, we discuss the work of Lombroso, his notion of "criminal man," and the school of criminal anthropology that he helped found and that is still active today. Fourth, we describe three purported examples of the relationship between epilepsy and violence. We present opposing social and biological (epilepsy) explanations and note the policy and political implications of each. Finally, we generalize this issue beyond the epilepsy/psychopathology debate and suggest a framework for policymaking in the area.

THE ISSUES

Is there a relationship between epilepsy and violence? Before summarizing the pertinent available data, we first must establish several definitions. By *epilepsy* we will mean the manifestation of at least two seizures that occur without acute metabolic or structural cause such as head trauma, high fever, or alcohol withdrawal. If a person has had two or more such seizures but has not had a seizure in at least 5 years, and has not been on antiepilepsy medication during this time, that person no longer has epilepsy (or has "inactive epilepsy"). These are established definitions (Hauser & Kurland, 1975) although there are, of course, variations. For example, some investigators require a minimum of three seizures, whereas some require only one; inactive cases are often not excluded; seizures from acute metabolic causes are often included; and electroencephalographic (EEG) confirmation is sometimes required and sometimes not required.

Other diagnoses, which range from selected abnormal but nonepileptiform EEG patterns to "subclinical epilepsy," can be and have been seen as precursors or conditions associated with epilepsy, and efforts also have been made to correlate these conditions with violence. However one evaluates these diagnoses, they do not constitute "epilepsy" as it is generally defined. (See Rodin's [1982] excellent survey of the literature about these pseudoepilepsy conditions.)

Another important section of the literature that will not be reviewed here involves physiological data that may have some relationship to epilepsy. Such data stem in large part from brain stimulation experiments in animals (Goldstein, 1974) and studies of humans involving brain lesions, neurochemistry, and pharmacology (Eichelman, 1983). These data are certainly intriguing but their relationship to epilepsy is, at this moment, totally speculative. The interested reader should consult the comprehensive government report that provides an in-depth review of all of these issues (Goldstein, 1974).

Once epilepsy is defined, further considerations remain. When we discuss the relationship between epilepsy and violence, we must specify whether we are discussing violence that occurs during or in close temporal proximity to a seizure (often referred to as "ictal violence") or violence that occurs when a seizure does not occur (often referred to as "interictal violence"). This is a distinction with important legal, empirical, and theoretical implications.

It is also important to understand the meaning of the terms *violence* and *aggression.* Most authors seem to act implicitly as if they were the same, or at least part of the same continuum, but it would appear that important differences exist (Nelson, 1974). For example, shouting at someone is not the same as hitting someone and hitting someone is not the same as killing someone. Additionally, the social context of such acts is always crucial: Who is more violent, parading Ku Klux Klan members or people who attack the parade? Finally, measuring all these concepts is very difficult. Such "technical" problems have no easy resolutions but they are essential and need to be kept in mind when evaluating the "epilepsy/violence" literature.

To summarize, in this chapter we discuss only "epilepsy" as defined here and not the relationship of violence to nonepileptiform EEG patterns, "subclinical epilepsy," and so on. Furthermore, we treat violence as either ictal or interictal and maintain this distinction throughout. Additionally, we regard violence and aggression as distinct phenomena, and name and define them as they are utilized in the reviewed studies. Finally, we do not discuss the literature involving aggression in children with epilepsy. Differing dependent measures and the effects of maturation on both epilepsy and aggression make the childhood literature a topic for separate analysis.

THE DATA

As noted, there have been many instances of the use of epilepsy as a defense in criminal trials. In such cases it is maintained that the crime was committed during a seizure, or immediately after one, while the defendant was in a state of postictal confusion. It is relevant to note that almost every research project that investigates this area fails to find even one case of ictal violence. Rodin notes that the "personal, extensive experience" of Hughlings-Jackson, the father of modern studies of epilepsy, "did not include a single case of directed, aggravated assault upon another person" (1982, p. 187). Rodin also summarizes his own very substantial experience with this matter: "Over the mentioned time span of 21 years, we have observed somewhat more than 10,000 epileptic seizures with automatic components." Although seizures with automatisms are the only kind capable of generating ictal violence, Rodin did not, he continues, "have a single case" that could be regarded as involving "directed exertion of physical force so as to injure, abuse or destroy" (p. 197). This same author has also provided an empirical investigation of this topic

(Rodin, 1973) as have Ramani and Gumnit (1981) and Delgado-Escueta et al. (1977, 1982). Not one case of ictal violence was located in any of these studies.

In an effort to provide the definitive study about the issue of ictal violence, the Epilepsy Foundation of America and the National Institute of Neurological and Communicative Disorders and Stroke appointed an international panel of 18 epileptologists to examine this matter (Delgado-Escueta et al., 1981). The panel solicited simultaneous video-EEG recordings from 16 epilepsy programs in the United States, Canada, Germany, Italy, and Japan that might have observed ictal violence. They were sent recordings of 19 patients (from a pool of approximately 5,400) and rated the aggression involved from a low of 1 ("non-directed aggressive motion") to a high of 6 ("severe violence to a person"). In 6 of the 19 patients the diagnosis of epilepsy was unsubstantiated. In the remaining 13 subjects, 1 received an aggression rating of 4 (she tried to scratch her psychologist's face during a seizure) and none received ratings of 5 or 6. The panel's conclusion was that *directed* ictal violence was unlikely, a conclusion consistent with that of another major government report (Goldstein, 1974).

In opposition to these studies, only the group of researchers associated with Jonathan Pincus and Dorothy Lewis have consistently generated data that support the existence of ictal violence (Pincus, 1980, 1981). Their research, however, has been based on highly selected samples of incarcerated delinquent boys (Lewis, Pincus, Shanok, & Glaser, 1982; Lewis, Shanok, Pincus, & Glaser, 1979) and children referred to a juvenile court (Lewis, 1976). Further, they have employed unusual EEG definitions (Lewis et al., 1982) and concepts like "psychomotor epileptic symptoms" (Lewis, 1976; Lewis et al., 1982). Underlying all these differences have been these researchers' determined prevalence rates of psychomotor epilepsy of 6% (Lewis, 1976) and 18% (Lewis et al., 1982). These may be contrasted with the results from the definitive epidemiologic study of epilepsy in the United States that found the prevalence of epilepsy to be 0.6% in a middle-class community (Hauser & Kurland, 1975), and another study that found the prevalence to be between 2.4% and 4.7% in a poor urban community (Hauser, Tabaddor, Factor, & Finer, 1984). Since only about half of all cases of epilepsy are psychomotor, we can see that the studies of Lewis et al. are generating prevalence rates of epilepsy that are 3–15 times higher than those established for poor people and 20–60 times higher than those for middle-class communities. All of these methodological peculiarities make it difficult to set their research in a proper perspective.

In summary, although the research of Lewis and Pincus and their colleagues suggests that ictal violence is not rare, and a few other reports, anecdotal in nature, suggest that ictal violence is not nonexistent (e.g., Mark & Ervin,

1970; Saint-Hilaire, Gilbert, Bouvier, & Barbeau, 1980), the vast majority of research in this area argues against these findings. Treiman and Delgado-Escueta (1983), for example, review this literature in great detail and locate many studies that we have not discussed that also support our conclusion. Understanding the balance of this evidence is crucial since these are the data relevant to criminal defense claims. This is because if a person commits a crime during a seizure, then presumably he or she cannot be held responsible for the act.

What about interictal violence or aggression? The hypothesis in such research is that although it might be impossible to effect directed ictal violence while the seizing person is suffering from unconsciousness or altered consciousness, interictal violence may be more likely and thus easier to detect. Furthermore, since interictal violence could occur in people with generalized epilepsy (GE) as well as in those with temporal lobe epilepsy (TLE), the TLE specificity can be tested against an appropriate control group—similar people with GE. Thus, a specificity effect could be shown either by demonstrating that violence was more common in people with TLE than in people with GE or was more common in people with epilepsy than in some control group such as people with another chronic malady like diabetes or asthma or in healthy people. These two types of comparisons (TLE vs. GE, epilepsy vs. nonepilepsy) would answer different questions and stimulate different hypotheses—but both would indeed indicate if there was a relationship between epilepsy and violence. What has previous research demonstrated?

First let us consider data about incarcerated people. Several studies of epilepsy among prisoners have revealed an elevated prevalence and for a while this was viewed as support for the hypothesized relationship between epilepsy and violence. Now, however, it is apparent that this elevated prevalence results from the fact that poor people have more epilepsy than wealthier people (Hauser et al., 1984; Shamansky & Glaser, 1979; Whitman, Coleman, Berg, King, & Desai, 1980) and that it is mostly poor people who go to prison (Sourcebook of Criminal Justice Statistics, 1981). As Treiman and Delgado-Escueta (1983) write:

> A relationship between socio-economic status or racial factors and epilepsy would explain the higher incidence of epilepsy amongst criminals and prisoners. It is possible, then, that the presence of epilepsy has no immediate relationship to violence or crimes. Epilepsy simply occurs more frequently in these populations as do other neurological disorders and a variety of psychiatric syndromes. In other words, coexistence of an increased prevalence of epilepsy and of violent behavior is not evidence of a causal relationship. (p. 185)

In addition to the reports of Lewis and her colleagues, there have been two major studies of epilepsy among prisoners—one in the United Kingdom (Gunn, 1977) and one in the United States (Whitman et al., 1984). Both have gone beyond the noncausal observation of elevated prevalence and performed controlled investigations of crime and violence, comparing prisoners with epilepsy to prisoners without epilepsy.

In the U.S. study, we screened all male prisoners (more than 5,000 men) entering the Illinois prison system through its main intake center over a 12-month period. Those who indicated any history of "epilepsy," "seizures," "convulsions," or "fits," or who had experienced seizurelike phenomena (e.g., episodes of lip smacking or strange feelings), were identified by the screen and entered into our diagnostic process. The screen located 162 men who were then administered an hour-long seizure history questionnaire, an hour-long general medical and social history questionnaire, and a half-hour physical exam. The project internist, who had examined the patient, and the project neurologist, who had never seen the patient, then made independent diagnoses based upon the information gathered. The diagnoses involved conclusions about whether the subjects had epilepsy and, if they did, about seizure type and etiology. The independent diagnoses were in agreement in 95% of the cases. When there were divergent diagnoses the two physicians met and reconciled their differences.

Eventually, 132 of the 162 men were diagnosed as having epilepsy. Then a control group of 132 men without epilepsy, individually matched on race and age, was selected and the two groups were compared on the seriousness of the crime for which they were incarcerated (as determined by the five-category Illinois Felony Classification System); whether or not violence (as indicated by 13 kinds of crimes) was involved; and whether or not "major violence" (defined as murder, attempted murder, rape, attempted rape, and armed violence) was involved. In all three comparisons there were no statistically significant differences between the epilepsy group and the control group. Those prisoners with TLE were then compared to those with GE. These two seizure groups also did not differ on any of the foregoing three measures. Finally, "none of the 132 men attributed any directed criminal act to an ictal event or to post-ictal confusion" (Whitman et al., 1984, p. 780).

Gunn's findings (1977) in the United Kingdom were very similar to these. He found no differences in criminal behavior or violence involvement between prisoners with epilepsy and prisoners without epilepsy, no differences in seizure type for violence associated with crime of conviction, and no ictal involvement. This last point had been previously reported in even greater detail (Gunn & Fenton, 1971).

Thus, independent replications in two very large prison systems on two separate continents have failed to discern a specificity of crime or violence to either epilepsy in general or TLE in particular.

What do available data say about this relationship in nonincarcerated individuals? In a recent review of the last 20 years of literature concerning psychopathology in adults with epilepsy, we located seven studies that made seizure-type comparisons (e.g., TLE vs. GE). We noted:

> The measures of aggression included MMPI indices, interview-based rating scales, specialized measures of hostility and aggression, standardized psychiatric rating scales, and clinical evaluations by psychiatrists. The populations were selected from general out-patient clinics, neurology departments, special epilepsy centers, and psychiatric facilities. All of the seven investigations failed to document increased aggression in TLE. (Hermann & Whitman, 1984, p. 470)

In addition, we know of only two studies comparing aggression in patients with epilepsy and patients with other chronic maladies. One found that patients with epilepsy were more aggressive (Guerrant et al., 1962), but the other found no significant difference between the two groups (Standage & Fenton, 1975). There have also been two comparisons with normal controls (Cairns, 1974; Mungas, 1983). Both found that epilepsy patients were more aggressive. However, it is not clear if these findings were due to epilepsy, sampling artifact, or a nonspecific chronic illness effect (Mungas, 1983).

In brief, the empirical evidence overwhelmingly suggests that there is no relationship between epilepsy and violence. This does not mean that people with epilepsy can never be violent or aggressive. It simply means that, as of now, a dozen major studies have all failed to detect either *directed* ictal violence or disproportionate interictal violence. A more detailed analysis of the studies discussed here may be found in recent review articles (Hermann & Whitman, 1984; Stevens & Hermann, 1981). An excellent review of the entire epilepsy/violence literature is provided by Treiman and Delgado-Escueta (1983).

LOMBROSO AND "THE CRIMINAL MAN"

In the next section we illustrate some of the social implications of inaccurately linking epilepsy with violence. But before we do this it will be helpful to understand the roots of this link.

Rodin (1982) cites the earliest known connection between epilepsy and violence as occurring between 529 and 522 B.C. when Cambyses, King of Persia, alleged to have epilepsy, impulsively killed the son of one of his servants. This was neither the beginning nor the end of linking epilepsy to unusual behavior. For example, Temkin (1971) describes the centuries of debates over whether epilepsy had a physical cause or a metaphysical cause. He also notes how those with the malady were often ostracized: "To the ancients the epileptic was an object of horror and disgust and not a saint or prophet as has sometimes been contended" (p. 9). In addition there was a pervasive conjoining of the word *epilepsy* with words like *insanity, easy mor-*

als, and so on. All these formulations, however, were apparently ad hoc or unsystematic. That is, there was not yet a concerted, theoretically directed effort to link epilepsy with violence. Such a task awaited modern medicine, social science, and a man named Cesare Lombroso.

Many events combined to make Lombroso's work possible. First, the 19th century brought with it the intensifying industrialization of Europe, which gave rise to cities and new forms of poverty, crime, and disease. Intense dialogue ensued to examine how these factors were interrelated and how society should respond to these new social dimensions of life (Rosenberg, 1976). Second, data collection and quantitative analysis were becoming established scientific processes. For example, researchers in France led by Quetelet and Guerry collected and published the first set of national criminal data between 1825 and 1833 (Lindesmith & Levin, 1937); the Registration Act of 1836 in England facilitated the processing of medical statistics (Chase, 1977); and quantitative data on brain size, shape, and weight were being surveyed in an effort to gain insight into the location of individuals in the social hierarchies of emerging industrial societies (Gould, 1981). Third, the two previous centuries had lifted the supernatural stigma from epilepsy and pronounced it a disease, thus turning it over to medicine and science (Temkin, 1971).

Lombroso was born in 1835 and worked, among other jobs, as a professor of psychiatry and as a prison physician (Wolfgang, 1961). He thus reached his professional maturity in the wake of the work of Darwin, Maudsley, Broca, and Galton, writing his major works between 1870 and 1880 (Wolfgang, 1961). He no doubt thought of himself as a rationalist seeking to bring science to the study of crime, a researcher seeking to professionalize the study of this growing social problem (Jeffery, 1959).

Lombroso, in an introduction to his daughter's summary volume of his work, traces the evolution of his thinking from an amorphous feeling to a scientific theory of the biologically determined nature of the criminal.

> I began dimly to realize that the a priori studies on crime in the abstract, hitherto pursued by jurists, especially in Italy, with singular acumen, should be superseded by the direct analytical study of the criminal, compared with normal individuals and the insane. (Lombroso, 1911/1972, p. xxiv)

The "dim realization" grew no longer slowly but now by leaps and bounds. The first "insight" occurred when Lombroso participated in the autopsy of "the famous brigand Vilella."

> This was not merely an idea, but a relevation. At the sight of that skull, I seemed to see all of a sudden, lighted up as a vast plain under a flaming sky, the problem of the nature of the criminal—an atavistic being who reproduces in his person the ferocious instincts of primitive humanity and the inferior animals. (Lombroso, 1911/1972, pp. xxiv–xxv)

One final quote brings us to the end of Lombroso's formulations as far as the purpose of this chapter is concerned.

> The various parts of the extremely complex problem of criminality were, however, not all solved hereby. The final key was given by another case, that of Misdea, a young soldier of about twenty-one, unintelligent but not vicious. Although subject to epileptic fits, he had served for some years in the army when suddenly, for some trivial cause, he attacked and killed eight of his superior officers and comrades. His horrible work accomplished, he fell into a deep slumber, which lasted twelve hours and on waking appeared to have no recollection of what had happened. Misdea, while representing the most ferocious type of animal, manifested, in addition, all the phenomena of epilepsy, which appeared to be hereditary in all the members of his family. It flashed across my mind that many criminal characteristics not attributable to atavism, such as facial asymmetry, cerebral sclerosis, impulsiveness, instantaneousness, the periodicity of criminal acts, the desire of evil for evil's sake, were morbid characteristics common to epilepsy, mingled with others due to atavism.
>
> Thus were traced the first clinical outlines of my work which had hitherto been entirely anthropological. The clinical outlines confirmed the anthropological contours, and *vice versa;* for the greatest criminals showed themselves to be epileptics, and, on the other hand, epileptics manifested the same anomalies as criminals. Finally it was shown that epilepsy frequently reproduced atavistic characteristics, including even those common to lower animals. (Lombroso, 1911/1972, pp. xxv–xxvi)

In summary, Lombroso looks at the criminal rather than the crime, implying the importance of examining the individual rather than his or her social conditions; determines that the relevant characteristics for crime causation are physical, inborn (thus, "the criminal man"), and atavistic; and declares the essence of this "born criminal" to be "epilepsy." According to Wolfgang, "Epilepsy becomes the 'uniting bond,' the morbid condition 'that unites and bases the moral imbecile and the born criminal in the same natural family'" (1961, p. 371).

And what were the implications of Lombrosian formulations for people with epilepsy? Stephen Jay Gould, discussing the 60-year period extending from Lombroso's initial writings on this topic through the beginning of World War II, notes:

> The added burden imposed by Lombroso's theory upon thousands of epileptics cannot be calculated; they became a major target of eugenical schemes in part because Lombroso had explicated their illness as a mark of moral degeneracy. (1981, p. 134)

Finally, it is also crucial to emphasize the enormous impact that Lombroso had on criminology in general. Savitz writes: "One must admit that modern criminology stems directly from the activities and dedication of a single man, Cesare Lombroso" (1972, p. vi). Jeffery adds: "Whereas the Classical School focused attention on the *crime,* the Positive School [founded by Lombroso and others] shifted the emphasis to the *criminal!*" (emphasis in the original) (1959, p. 18).

EPILEPSY AND SOCIETY

We have spent some time describing the factors and processes that brought Lombroso to the notion of the "criminal man" and the role of epilepsy in his conception. We believe that his formulation has no intrinsic correctness and in fact that there is a coherent world view that would serve to explain "Lombroso-like" examples better. We present three such examples and discuss reasonable "non-Lombrosian" explanations.

It probably makes most sense for us to begin where Lombroso did—with Misdea, "a young soldier of about twenty-one" who "for some trivial cause ... attacked and killed eight of his superior officers and comrades" and who "manifested ... all the phenomena of epilepsy" (Lombroso, 1911/1972, pp. xxv–xxvi). As we saw this was the pivotal incident for Lombroso's schema. Yet, in describing this incident for what would likely be the last time, he provides few details and his daughter's summary of his work contains little more information. We learn from her that Misdea was "the son of degenerate parents" and "killed his superior officer and eight or ten soldiers who tried to overpower him" (Lombroso-Ferrero, 1911/1972, p. 92), and that he was once "roused to fury by dismissal from his post [and] broke four razors into small pieces with his teeth" (p. 65). This is all we are told here, but it would be helpful to know what evidence of epilepsy existed, the conditions of Misdea's army life, his relations with his fellow soldiers, and even how he killed these people. We ask these questions because a recent prominent parallel suggests a nonepilepsy interpretation.

One way to search for the cause of a foot soldier killing a commanding officer is to look within that soldier's brain for misfiring neurons, that is, to look for epilepsy. There are other possible explanations. During the Vietnam War, there were hundreds of cases of drafted U.S. soldiers attempting to kill their commanding officers. The practice was so common it was given a name—"fragging." And the numbers were astounding. According to sources in the Department of Defense, there were 551 officially documented cases "in which [U.S.] soldiers threw fragmentation grenades in attempts to kill or maim their superior officers or other enemies" in the U.S. Army between July 1968 and July 1972. The sources noted that 86 deaths occurred during this interval (Caldwell, 1972). To our knowledge, no one thought that these fraggings were caused by epilepsy. It is more likely that they were perceived as a way, even if extreme, for soldiers fighting a highly controversial war to express their anger at inept or reckless officers, and other very complex social dynamics. One wonders if the story of Misdea might not have a similar explanation.

Let us now consider a second example. In the mid-1950s, black people in the United States organized themselves to work in opposition to the racial discrimination that had long dominated their lives. Using many methods of peaceful struggle such as demonstrations, sit-ins, and law suits, they tried to convince the United States to end the injustices that black people had been subjected to for the past 350 years (Sitkoff, 1981). During this period, major black leaders such as Malcolm X, Martin Luther King, Jr., and Fred Hampton were assassinated, the Black Panther Party was attacked by police forces across the United States, and a "counterintelligence" program, named COINTELPRO, was initiated by the Federal Bureau of Investigation (Blackstock, 1976) to destroy black organizing efforts and their leaders, including Martin Luther King, Jr. (Garrow, 1981). In response to enduring social inequalities, black people rebelled in many urban areas—New York, Los Angeles, Chicago, Newark, Detroit, and other places as well. According to a Ford Foundation report, there were "1893 individual racial disorders from 1964 to 1969" (Thomas, 1981, p. 28). Buildings were burned, stores were looted, and large neighborhoods were totally destroyed. Damage ran into the hundreds of millions of dollars (Kerner et al., 1968).

While some analysts attempted to understand the social causes of these rebellions (Boesel & Rossi, 1971; Kerner et al., 1968), three physicians who specialized in the study of the brain looked elsewhere. In a long letter to the *Journal of the American Medical Association,* Mark, Sweet, and Ervin (1967) wrote that although unemployment, poor housing, and inadequate education were indeed problems,

> these causes may have blinded us to the subtle role of other possible factors, including brain dysfunction in the rioters . . . besides the need to study the social fabric that creates the riot atmosphere, we need intensive research and clinical studies of the *individuals* committing the violence. The goal of such studies would be to pinpoint, diagnose, and treat those people with low violence thresholds before they contribute to further tragedies [emphasis in the original]. (p. 895)

This call for "treatment" is noteworthy since these authors were leading advocates of psychosurgery as a cure for patients with a history of violence (Mark & Ervin, 1970), an approach that has been criticized by many (Chavkin, 1978; Chorover, 1974, 1980).

We have discussed this as one of our examples because it presents a sharp choice between a biological and a social explanation of violence. It involves the central social phenomenon of racism in the United States, three well-known Harvard University physicians, and an influential medical journal. The analysis of Mark, Sweet, and Ervin urges us to look for causes of urban rebellions in discharging neurons rather than relevant social ills. The cure would presumably require a similar perspective. Interestingly, this theme has not disappeared from scientific research. Recently it has been suggested that a controlled experiment be done to study whether "episodic violence" might be treated with anticonvulsant medication (Pincus, 1980).

The third and final example is a murder case that was closely chronicled in the news media.

On Thanksgiving Day, 1976, New York City police officer Robert Torsney pulled his pistol and shot a bullet at "point-blank" range into the head of 15-year-old Randolph Evans, who had stopped to ask him a question (Siegel, 1976). Torsney, who is white, claimed that Evans, who was black, pulled a gun, but all witnesses said this was not true; no gun was ever found (Dunning, 1977b).

Soon afterward, Torsney claimed epilepsy as a defense, saying that he killed Evans during an episode of "automatism of Penfield," and also claimed insanity ("Accused policeman," 1977). He was acquitted on these grounds (Dunning, 1977a) and eventually confined at Creedmore Psychiatric Hospital.

In November of 1978, two years after the death of Evans, Torsney was released because he "could function in society and was not a danger to himself or others" (Kifner, 1978, p. B5). In this same article, Dr. Deborah Kaiser, who was in charge of Torsney's examination, is quoted as follows: "Since we have received him he has shown no evidence of psychosis or any kind of cerebral dysfunction, nor a hysterical disassociative reaction, which was the original diagnosis" (p. B5).

Reina Berner, the Executive Director of the Epilepsy Institute of New York, wrote about this case:

> Significantly, no newspaper stated that testimony from neurologists who specialize in epilepsy was heard. Was this because the defense knew that no complicated behavior such as pulling out a gun, aiming and shooting, can occur during a seizure? . . . It is truly amazing how old myths and stigmas are perpetuated at every level of our society. . . . And to the 4 million people who have epilepsy, no, you can't kill a person during seizure. (1978, p. A5)

There were frequent demonstrations by black people in New York City over the killing of Randolph Evans. These demonstrations maintained that the murder of Evans was an example of still another black person being murdered without reason by the New York City Police Department. The demonstrators thus presented a coherent non-Lombrosian explanation for why the murdered youth never reached his 16th birthday.

We would like to emphasize that these three examples of epilepsy serving as explanation for violence are not exceptions, nor are they the most outlandish. One recent article reports that epilepsy has been used as a defense in murder or homicide trials at least 20 times since 1977 (Pollak, 1984). Another article, on serial killers (people who kill several people), appeared recently in *Life* magazine and maintained that "quite a few [serial killers] showed signs of psychomotor epilepsy, a form of the disease that is rare in the general population *but frequent among violent criminals*" (our emphasis) (Darrach & Norris, 1984, p. 68). Finally, a letter to the prestigious *New England Journal of Medicine* suggested "capital punishment for a person [imprisoned for a violent crime] whose EEG did not become normal within a given period (such as five years)" (Freeman, 1970, p. 603).

CONCLUSION

About Epilepsy

We placed this chapter at the end of the book because we believe the issues raised by looking into the relationship between epilepsy and violence are the same issues that run all through the epilepsy/psychopathology debate. What policy is suggested by the approaches we have discussed?

On October 26, 1982, C. Everett Koop, Surgeon General of the United States, addressed the annual meeting of the American Academy of Pediatrics. He was concerned about the "surge in youth violence" and "urged the pediatricians to bend their efforts to spotting family problems and other conditions that often lead to violence in the young" (Webster, 1982, p. 13). He added, "Some of the conditions to watch for . . . were *psychomotor seizures,* mothers under psychiatric care, violence between parents, youngsters without friends, and attempted suicide" (our emphasis) (Webster, 1982, p. 13). Quite likely, this reference to epilepsy was inspired by a long interview by the *New York Times* that had appeared just 1 month earlier (Collins, 1982). Lewis and Pincus were both interviewed and asked for their opinions of the causes of adolescent violence. Using their research, which we have described, they maintained that psychomotor seizures were a predictor of violence in children. The belief that epilepsy and violence are linked thus persists. Furthermore, it is now espoused by the highest ranking U.S. government health expert.

We have tried to show in this chapter that there is no remotely persuasive evidence linking epilepsy to violence/aggression and that the theory that suggested such a link was initiated by Lombroso and founded on intuition—"flashes of insight" and no data. On the basis of such myth and prejudice many people with epilepsy have been stigmatized and discriminated against.

To researchers in this area we emphasize that neither seizure type (TLE) nor any other epilepsy-specific variable has ever been shown to be *consistently* related to violence. It is thus time to turn our attention to societal factors. To medicolegal workers we emphasize that never has it been demonstrated that any crime was committed due to a seizure and never has it been demonstrated that people with epilepsy commit more crimes than other people who are similarly situated in life. There is thus no basis for defense efforts that suggest that epilepsy is the cause of crime. The data we present in this chapter may be properly seen as a challenge. To deny the conclusions supported by the data is to perpetuate myth and stigma against people with epilepsy and to obscure the role of important social factors.

Beyond Epilepsy

The second part of our conclusion takes us beyond the data and even beyond the debate over the alleged epilepsy-violence link. However, we think this excursion is relevant. Trying to understand how a specific scientific debate—in this case, over the relationship between epilepsy and violence—fits into larger scientific and social themes (biological determinism or "sociobiology") is a valuable endeavor because it can shed light on both the specific debate and the larger themes.

In 1975, E. O. Wilson, a Harvard professor of entomology, published a 700-page book entitled *Sociobiology: The New Synthesis*. In this book he wrote, "Sociobiology is the systematic study of the biological basis of all forms of social behavior, including sexual and parental, in all kinds of organisms including man" (p. 547). This is not the only definition of sociobiology but it is probably representative, coming, as it does, from the world's leading and best known sociobiologist. The two central themes of sociobiology are that aspects of biology determine human behavior and that these aspects are genetically transmitted.

Today's epilepsy-determined violence argument is thus not a "full" sociobiological model since it is generally not claimed that such behavior is inherited. Nonetheless, the epilepsy/violence model synergistically feeds into and draws from sociobiology. It was, after all, early Lombrosian criminology (often called "criminal anthropology") that set the stage for current theories like "biosocial criminology" (Jeffery, 1978; Mednick & Christiansen, 1977) and the XYY genotype controversy in particular (Chorover, 1980). As Lewontin, Rose, and Kamin (1984) point out:

> While no one now would give serious consideration to Lombroso's idea that one can tell a murderer by the shape of his or her head, it is now said that one can do so by the shape of his or her chromosomes. There is an unbroken line of science from the criminal anthropology of 1876 to the criminal cytogenetics of 1975, yet the evidence and argument of determinist claims remain as weak now as they were a hundred years ago. (p. 25)

Sociobiology offers a very troublesome conceptualization of the world. In declaring biology the basis of all behavior, sociobiology says, in effect, that our general condition is natural and, by implication, subject only to biological, and not social, influence. Thus, if we are competitive it is natural; if we make war or rape or are racist or sexist, it is natural—it is all "human nature." (See Lewontin et al. [1984] and Rose [1980] for expositions of this issue.)

If sociobiologists were engaged in exciting new research, reaction to their work might be more tempered. But this has not been the case. Gould (1977) has noted that the data produced by sociobiologists are not demonstrably linked to the larger claims being made, which suggests other dynamics. He writes:

> Science, we are told, progresses by accumulating new information and using it to improve or replace old theories. But the new biological determinism rests upon no recent fund of information and can cite in its behalf not a single unambiguous fact. Its renewed support must have some other basis, most likely social or political in nature. (Gould, 1977, p. 238)

No matter how sincere, socially conscious, and scientifically honest sociobiologists are, their research must lead in one direction—to an inevitability of the status quo. The theory of Mark et al. (1967) may have gone a "bit too far" beyond the data. Freedman, who writes that "racial antagonisms are more or less built into the species" (in Beckwith, 1981–1982, p. 314), and David Barash, a leading sociobiologist who maintains that "sociobiology explains why women have almost universally found themselves relegated to the nursery while men derive their greatest satisfaction from their jobs" (in Beckwith, 1981–1982, p. 313), may also have gone a "bit too far." The problem is, however, that sociobiology has nowhere else to go. Put simply, it is an ideology of limits that says things cannot change.

Long ago, in response to early arguments of biological determinism, J. S. Mill wrote:

> Of all the vulgar modes of escaping from the consideration of the effect of social and moral influences upon the human mind, the most vulgar is that of attributing the diversities of conduct and character to inherent natural differences. (Pastore, 1949, p. 7)

This, for us, is the essence of the matter.

In this chapter, we have tried to suggest that the theory of epilepsy (biologically) determined crime is a regressive one that does not fit the facts, stigmatizes people with epilepsy, and promotes models of generalized biologically determined behavior. Biological determinism, which obtained substantial early support from epilepsy/violence research, now has run into a prominent barrier from that same field of investigation. We hope that further research into the relationship between epilepsy and violence—and between epilepsy and psychopathology in general—will guard against easy but incorrect and dangerous theories that are overdependent on biological explanations.

REFERENCES

Accused policeman pleads insanity. (1977, November 10). *The New York Times*, p. B16.

Arangio, A. (1975). The stigma of epilepsy. *American Rehabilitation* 2, 273.

Arangio, A. (1980), The social worker and epilepsy: A description of assessment and treatment variables. In B. P. Hermann (Ed.), *A multidisciplinary handbook of epilepsy*. Springfield, IL: Thomas.

Beckwith, J. (1981–1982). The political uses of sociobiology in the United States and Europe. *Philosophical Forum* 13, 311–21.

Berner, R. (1978, January 7). Torsney verdict: A medical view. *Amsterdam News*, p. A5.

Blackstock, N. (1976). *COINTELPRO: The FBI's secret war on political freedom*. New York: Vintage Books.

Boesel, D., & P. H. Rossi. (Eds.). (1971). *Cities under siege*. New York: Basic Books.

Cairns, V. M. (1974). Epilepsy, personality and behavior. In P. Harris & C. Mawdsley (Eds.), *Epilepsy: Proceedings of the Hans Berger Centenary Exposition*. Edinburgh: Churchill-Livingstone.

Caldwell, E. (1972, September 22). Grenade death court-martial unexpectedly recessed on coast. *The New York Times*, p. 14.

Chase, A. (1977). *The legacy of Malthus*. New York: Knopf.

Chavkin, S. (1978). *The mind stealers*. Westport, CT: Lawrence Hill.

Chorover, S. (1974, May). The pacification of the brain. *Psychology Today*, 59, 60; 63, 64; 66; 69.

Chorover, S. (1980). *From genesis to genocide*. Cambridge, MA: MIT Press.

Collins, G. (1982, September 27). The violent child: Some patterns emerge. *The New York Times*, p. B10.

Darrach, B., & J. Norris. (1984, August). An American tragedy. *Life*, pp. 58–72.

Delgado-Escueta, A. V., F. E. Bascal, & D. M. Treiman. (1982). Complex partial seizures on closed-circuit television and EEG: A study of 691 attacks in 79 patients. *Annals of Neurology* 11, 292–300.

Delgado-Escueta, A. V., U. Kunze, G. Waddell, J. Boxley, & A. Nadel. (1977). Lapse of consciousness and automatisms in temporal lobe epilepsy: A videotape analysis. *Neurology* 27, 144–55.

Delgado-Escueta, A. V., R. Mattson, L. King, E. S. Goldensohn, H. Speigel, J. Madsen, P. Crandall, F. Dreifuss, & R. J. Porter. (1981). The nature of aggression during epileptic seizures. *New England Journal of Medicine* 305, 711–16.

Dunning, J. (1977a, December 1). Officer Torsney acquitted as jury rules him insane in killing of boy. *The New York Times*, pp. A1; B18.

Dunning, J. (1977b, November 29). Torsney's insanity defense linked to fact slaying victim had no gun. *The New York Times*, p. 30.

Eichelman, B. (1983). The limbic system and aggression in humans. *Neuroscience and Biobehavioral Reviews* 7, 391–94.

Freeman, W. E. (1970). Another arbiter role for the EEG. *New England Journal of Medicine* 283, 603.

Garrow, D. J. (1981). *The FBI and Martin Luther King, Jr.* New York: Norton.

Goldstein, M. (1974). Brain research and violent behavior. *Archives of Neurology* 30, 1–35.

Gould, S. J. (1977). *Ever since Darwin*. New York: Norton.

Gould, S. J. (1981). *The mismeasure of man.* New York: Norton.

Guerrant, J., W. W. Anderson, A. Fischer, M. R. Weinstein, J. M. Jarros, & A. Deskins. (1962). *Personality in epilepsy.* Springfield, IL: Thomas.

Gunn, J. (1977). *Epileptics in prison.* New York: Academic Press.

Gunn, J., & G. Fenton. (1971). Epilepsy, automatism, and crime. *Lancet,* June 5, 1173–76.

Hauser, W. A., & L. T. Kurland. (1975). The epidemiology of epilepsy in Rochester, Minnesota, 1935 through 1967. *Epilepsia* 16, 1–66.

Hauser, W. A., K. Tabaddor, P. R. Factor, & C. Finer (1984). Seizures and head injury in an urban community. *Neurology* 34, 746–51.

Hermann, B. P., & S. Whitman. (1984). Behavioral and personality correlates of epilepsy: A review, methodological critique and conceptual model. *Psychological Bulletin* 95, 451–96.

Jeffery, C. R. (1959). The historical development of criminology. *Journal of Criminal Law, Criminology and Police Science* 50, 3–19.

Jeffery, C. R. (1978). *Crime prevention through environmental design.* Beverly Hills, CA: Sage.

Kerner, O., J. V. Lindsay, F. R. Harris, E. W. Brooke, J. C. Corman, W. M. McCulloch, I. W. Abel, C. B. Thornton, R. Wilkins, K. G. Peden, & H. Jenkins. (1968). *Report of the National Advisory Commission on Civil Disorders.* New York: Bantam Books.

Kifner, J. (1978, November 15). Officer in mental care after youth's slaying is certified for release. *The New York Times,* pp. A1; B5.

Lewis, D. O. (1976). Delinquency, psychomotor epileptic symptoms, and paranoid ideation: A triad. *American Journal of Psychiatry* 133, 1395–98.

Lewis, D. O., J. H. Pincus, S. S. Shanok, & G. H. Glaser. (1982). Psychomotor epilepsy and violence in a group of incarcerated adolescent boys. *American Journal of Psychiatry* 139, 882–87.

Lewis, D. O., S. S. Shanok, J. H. Pincus, & G. H. Glaser. (1979). Violent juvenile delinquents. *Journal of the American Academy of Child Psychiatry* 18, 307–19.

Lewontin, R. C., S. Rose, & L. J. Kamin. (1984). *Not in our genes.* New York: Pantheon.

Lindesmith, A. R., & Y. Levin. (1937). The Lombrosian myth in criminology. *American Journal of Sociology* 42, 897–99.

Lombroso, C. (1972). Introduction. In G. Lombroso-Ferrero, *Criminal man according to the classification of Cesare Lombroso.* Montclair, NJ: Patterson Smith. (Original work published 1911)

Lombroso-Ferrero, G. (1972). *Criminal man according to the classification of Cesare Lombroso.* Montclair, NJ: Patterson Smith. (Original work published 1911)

Mark, V. H., & F. R. Ervin. (1970). *Violence and the brain.* New York: Harper & Row.

Mark, V. H., W. H. Sweet, & F. R. Ervin. (1967). Role of brain disease in riots and urban violence. *Journal of the American Medical Association* 201, 894–95.

Mednick, S., & K. O. Christiansen. (1977). *Biosocial bases of criminal behavior.* New York: Gardner Press.

Mungas, D. (1983). An empirical analysis of specific syndromes of violent behavior. *Journal of Nervous and Mental Disease* 171, 243–71.

Nelson, S. D. (1974). Nature/nurture revisited I: A review of the biological bases of conflict. *Journal of Conflict Resolution* 18, 285–335.

Pastore, N. (1949). *The nature–nurture controversy.* New York: King's Crown Press.

Pincus, J. H. (1980). Can violence be a manifestation of epilepsy? *Neurology* 30, 304–7.

Pincus, J. H. (1981). Violence and epilepsy. *New England Journal of Medicine* 305, 696–98.

Pollak, R. (1984, May). The epilepsy defense. *Atlantic Monthly*, pp. 20–28.

Ramani, V., & R. J. Gumnit. (1981). Intensive monitoring of epileptic patients with a history of episodic aggression. *Archives of Neurology* 38, 570–71.

Rodin, E. A. (1973). Psychomotor epilepsy and aggressive behavior. *Archives of General Psychiatry* 28, 210–13.

Rodin, E. A. (1982). Aggression and epilepsy. In T. L. Riley & A. Roy (Eds.), *Pseudoseizures*. Baltimore: Williams & Wilkins.

Rose, S. (1980). "It's only human nature": The sociobiologist's fairyland. In A. Montagu (Ed.), *Sociobiology examined*. New York: Oxford University Press.

Rosenberg, C. E. (1976). *No other gods: On science and American social thought*. Baltimore: Johns Hopkins University Press.

Saint-Hilaire, J. M., M. Gilbert, G. Bouvier, & A. Barbeau. (1980). Epilepsy and aggression: Two cases with depth electrode studies. In P. Robb (Ed.), *Epilepsy updated: Causes and treatment*. Miami: Symposia Specialists.

Savitz, L. D. (1972). Introduction. In G. Lombroso-Ferrero, *Criminal man according to the classification of Cesare Lombroso*. Montclair, NJ: Patterson Smith.

Schneider, J., & P. Conrad. (1983). *Having epilepsy*. Philadelphia: Temple University Press.

Shamansky, S. L., & G. H. Glaser. (1979). Socioeconomic characteristics of childhood seizure disorders in the New Haven area: An epidemiological study. *Epilepsia* 20, 457–74.

Siegel, M. H. (1976, November 27). Boy, 15, shot to death point-blank; officer arrested in east New York. *The New York Times*, pp. 1–2; 16.

Sitkoff, H. (1981). *The struggle for black equality, 1954–1980*. New York: Hill & Wang.

Sourcebook of Criminal Justice Statistics—1981. (1982). U. S. Department of Justice, Bureau of Justice Statistics. Washington, DC: U.S. Government Printing Office.

Standage, K. F., & G. W. Fenton. (1975). Psychiatric symptom profiles of patients with epilepsy: A controlled investigation. *Psychological Medicine* 5, 152–60.

Stevens, J. R., & B. P. Hermann. (1981). Temporal lobe epilepsy, psychopathology, and violence: The state of the evidence. *Neurology* 31, 1127–32.

Temkin, O. (1971). *The falling sickness* (2nd ed.). Baltimore: Johns Hopkins University Press.

Thomas, J. (1981, May 17). Study finds Miami riot was unlike those of 60's. *The New York Times*, p. 28.

Treiman, D. M., & A. V. Delgado-Escueta. (1983). Violence and epilepsy: A critical review. In T. A. Pedley and B. S. Meldrum (Eds.), *Recent advances in epilepsy*. London: Churchill-Livingstone.

Webster, B. (1982, October 27). Koop cites surge in youth violence. *The New York Times*, p. 13.

Whitman, S., T. Coleman, B. Berg, L. N. King, & B. Desai. (1980). Epidemiological insights into the socioeconomic correlates of epilepsy. In B. Hermann (Ed.), *A multidisciplinary handbook of epilepsy*. Springfield, IL: Thomas.

Whitman, S., T. Coleman, C. Patmon, B. T. Desai, R. L. Cohen, & L. N. King.

(1984). Epilepsy in prison: Elevated prevalence and no relationship to violence. *Neurology* 34, 775–82.

Wilson, E. O. (1975). *Sociobiology: The new synthesis.* Cambridge, MA: Harvard University Press.

Wolfgang, M. E. (1961). Cesare Lombroso: 1835–1909. *Journal of Criminal Law, Criminology and Police Science* 52, 361–91.

Index

Page numbers followed by *t* indicate tables.